T0074153

Dawn E. Holmes and Lakhmi C. Jain (Eds.)

Data Mining: Foundations and Intelligent Paradigms

Intelligent Systems Reference Library, Volume 24

Editors-in-Chief

Prof. Janusz Kacprzyk
Systems Research Institute
Polish Academy of Sciences
ul. Newelska 6
01-447 Warsaw
Poland
E-mail: kacprzyk@ibspan.waw.pl

Prof. Lakhmi C. Jain
University of South Australia
Adelaide
Mawson Lakes Campus
South Australia 5095
Australia
E-mail: Lakhmi.jain@unisa.edu.au

Further volumes of this series can be found on our homepage: springer.com

Vol. 1. Christine L. Mumford and Lakhmi C. Jain (Eds.)
Computational Intelligence: Collaboration, Fusion and Emergence, 2009
ISBN 978-3-642-01798-8

Vol. 2. Yuehui Chen and Ajith Abraham
Tree-Structure Based Hybrid Computational Intelligence, 2009
ISBN 978-3-642-04738-1

Vol. 3. Anthony Finn and Steve Scheding
Developments and Challenges for Autonomous Unmanned Vehicles, 2010
ISBN 978-3-642-10703-0

Vol. 4. Lakhmi C. Jain and Chee Peng Lim (Eds.)
Handbook on Decision Making: Techniques and Applications, 2010
ISBN 978-3-642-13638-2

Vol. 5. George A. Anastassiou
Intelligent Mathematics: Computational Analysis, 2010
ISBN 978-3-642-17097-3

Vol. 6. Ludmila Dymowa
Soft Computing in Economics and Finance, 2011
ISBN 978-3-642-17718-7

Vol. 7. Gerasimos G. Rigatos
Modelling and Control for Intelligent Industrial Systems, 2011
ISBN 978-3-642-17874-0

Vol. 8. Edward H.Y. Lim, James N.K. Liu, and Raymond S.T. Lee
Knowledge Seeker – Ontology Modelling for Information Search and Management, 2011
ISBN 978-3-642-17915-0

Vol. 9. Menahem Friedman and Abraham Kandel
Calculus Light, 2011
ISBN 978-3-642-17847-4

Vol. 10. Andreas Tolk and Lakhmi C. Jain
Intelligence-Based Systems Engineering, 2011
ISBN 978-3-642-17930-3

Vol. 11. Samuli Niiranen and Andre Ribeiro (Eds.)
Information Processing and Biological Systems, 2011
ISBN 978-3-642-19620-1

Vol. 12. Florin Gorunescu
Data Mining, 2011
ISBN 978-3-642-19720-8

Vol. 13. Witold Pedrycz and Shyi-Ming Chen (Eds.)
Granular Computing and Intelligent Systems, 2011
ISBN 978-3-642-19819-9

Vol. 14. George A. Anastassiou and Oktay Duman
Towards Intelligent Modeling: Statistical Approximation Theory, 2011
ISBN 978-3-642-19825-0

Vol. 15. Antonino Freno and Edmondo Trentin
Hybrid Random Fields, 2011
ISBN 978-3-642-20307-7

Vol. 16. Alexiei Dingli
Knowledge Annotation: Making Implicit Knowledge Explicit, 2011
ISBN 978-3-642-20322-0

Vol. 17. Crina Grosan and Ajith Abraham
Intelligent Systems, 2011
ISBN 978-3-642-21003-7

Vol. 18. Achim Zielesny
From Curve Fitting to Machine Learning, 2011
ISBN 978-3-642-21279-6

Vol. 19. George A. Anastassiou
Intelligent Systems: Approximation by Artificial Neural Networks, 2011
ISBN 978-3-642-21430-1

Vol. 20. Lech Polkowski
Approximate Reasoning by Parts, 2011
ISBN 978-3-642-22278-8

Vol. 21. Igor Chikalov
Average Time Complexity of Decision Trees, 2011
ISBN 978-3-642-22660-1

Vol. 22. Przemysław Różewski, Emma Kusztina, Ryszard Tadeusiewicz, and Oleg Zaikin
Intelligent Open Learning Systems, 2011
ISBN 978-3-642-22666-3

Vol. 23. Dawn E. Holmes and Lakhmi C. Jain (Eds.)
Data Mining: Foundations and Intelligent Paradigms, 2012
ISBN 978-3-642-23165-0

Vol. 24. Dawn E. Holmes and Lakhmi C. Jain (Eds.)
Data Mining: Foundations and Intelligent Paradigms, 2012
ISBN 978-3-642-23240-4

Dawn E. Holmes and Lakhmi C. Jain (Eds.)

Data Mining: Foundations and Intelligent Paradigms

Volume 2: Statistical, Bayesian, Time Series and other Theoretical Aspects

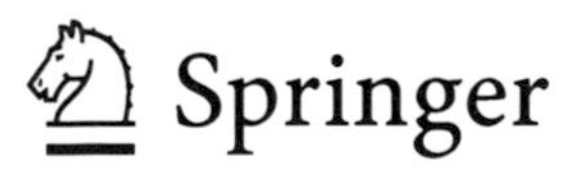

Prof. Dawn E. Holmes
Department of Statistics and Applied Probability
University of California
Santa Barbara,
CA 93106
USA
E-mail: holmes@pstat.ucsb.edu

Prof. Lakhmi C. Jain
Professor of Knowledge-Based Engineering
University of South Australia
Adelaide
Mawson Lakes, SA 5095
Australia
E-mail: Lakhmi.jain@unisa.edu.au

ISBN 978-3-642-23240-4 e-ISBN 978-3-642-23241-1

DOI 10.1007/978-3-642-23242-8

Intelligent Systems Reference Library ISSN 1868-4394

Library of Congress Control Number: 2011936705

Typeset & Cover Design: Scientific Publishing Services Pvt. Ltd., Chennai, India.

Printed on acid-free paper

9 8 7 6 5 4 3 2 1

springer.com

Preface

There are many invaluable books available on data mining theory and applications. However, in compiling a volume titled "DATA MINING: Foundations and Intelligent Paradigms: Volume 2: Core Topics including Statistical, Time-Series and Bayesian Analysis" we wish to introduce some of the latest developments to a broad audience of both specialists and non-specialists in this field.

The term 'data mining' was introduced in the 1990's to describe an emerging field based on classical statistics, artificial intelligence and machine learning. Important core areas of data mining such as support vector machines, a kernel based learning method, have been very productive in recent years as attested by the rapidly increasing number of papers published each year. Time series analysis and prediction have been enhanced by methods in neural networks, particularly in the area of financial forecasting. Bayesian analysis is of primary importance in data mining research, with ongoing work in prior probability distribution estimation.

In compiling this volume we have sought to present innovative research from prestigious contributors in these particular areas of data mining. Each chapter is self-contained and is described briefly in Chapter 1.

This book will prove valuable to theoreticians as well as application scientists/ engineers in the area of Data Mining. Postgraduate students will also find this a useful sourcebook since it shows the direction of current research.

We have been fortunate in attracting top class researchers as contributors and wish to offer our thanks for their support in this project. We also acknowledge the expertise and time of the reviewers. Finally, we also wish to thank Springer for their support.

Dr. Dawn E. Holmes
University of California
Santa Barbara, USA

Dr. Lakhmi C. Jain
University of South Australia
Adelaide, Australia

Contents

Editors

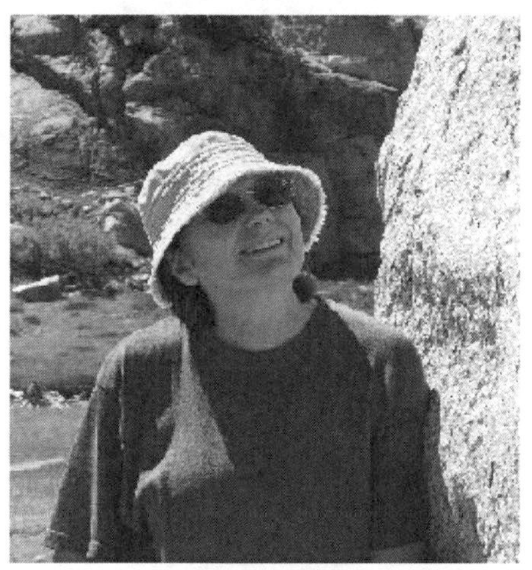

Dr. Dawn E. Holmes serves as Senior Lecturer in the Department of Statistics and Applied Probability and Senior Associate Dean in the Division of Undergraduate Education at UCSB. Her main research area, Bayesian Networks with Maximum Entropy, has resulted in numerous journal articles and conference presentations. Her other research interests include Machine Learning, Data Mining, Foundations of Bayesianism and Intuitionistic Mathematics. Dr. Holmes has co-edited, with Professor Lakhmi C. Jain, volumes 'Innovations in Bayesian Networks' and 'Innovations in Machine Learning'. Dr. Holmes teaches a broad range of courses, including SAS programming, Bayesian Networks and Data Mining. She was awarded the Distinguished Teaching Award by Academic Senate, UCSB in 2008.

As well as being Associate Editor of the International Journal of Knowledge-Based and Intelligent Information Systems, Dr. Holmes reviews extensively and is on the editorial board of several journals, including the Journal of Neurocomputing. She serves as Program Scientific Committee Member for numerous conferences; including the International Conference on Artificial Intelligence and the International Conference on Machine Learning. In 2009 Dr. Holmes accepted an invitation to join Center for Research in Financial Mathematics and Statistics (CRFMS), UCSB. She was made a Senior Member of the IEEE in 2011.

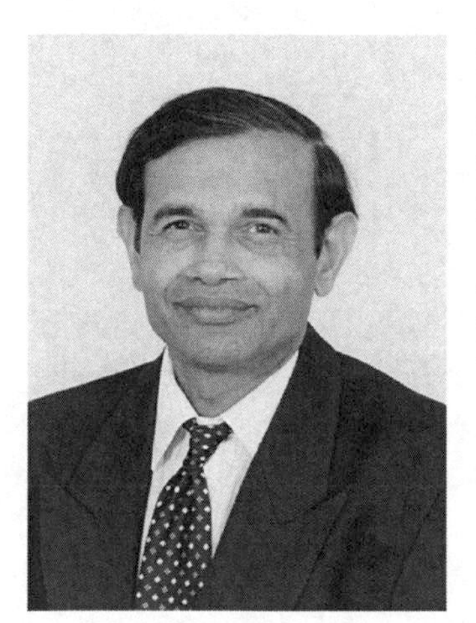

Professor Lakhmi C. Jain is a Director/Founder of the Knowledge-Based Intelligent Engineering Systems (KES) Centre, located in the University of South Australia. He is a fellow of the Institution of Engineers Australia.

His interests focus on the artificial intelligence paradigms and their applications in complex systems, art-science fusion, e-education, e-healthcare, unmanned air vehicles and intelligent agents.

Chapter 1
Advanced Modelling Paradigms in Data Mining

Dawn E. Holmes[1], Jeffrey Tweedale[2], and Lakhmi C. Jain[2]

[1] Department of Statistics and Applied Probability
University of California Santa Barbara
Santa Barbara
CA 93106-3110
USA

[2] School of Electrical and Information Engineering
University of South Australia
Adelaide
Mawson Lakes Campus
South Australia SA 5095
Australia

1 Introduction

As discussed in the previous volume, the term *Data Mining* grew from the relentless growth of techniques used to interrogation masses of data. As a myriad of databases emanated from disparate industries, enterprise management insisted their information officers develop methodology to exploit the knowledge held in their repositories. Industry has invested heavily to gain knowledge they can exploit to gain a market advantage. This includes extracting hidden data, trends or pattern from what was traditionally considered noise. For instance most corporations track sales, stock, pay role and other operational information. Acquiring and maintaing these repositories relies on mainstream techniques, technology and methodologies. In this book we discuss a number of founding techniques and expand into intelligent paradigms.

2 Foundations

Management relies heavily of information systems to gain market advantage. For this reason they invest heavily in Information Technology (IT) systems that enable them to acquire, retain and manipulate industry related facts. Payroll and accounting systems were traditionally based on statistical manipulation, however have evolved to include machine learning and artificial intelligence [1]. A non-exhaustive list of existing techniques would include:

- Artificial Intelligence (AI) Class introduction;
- Bayesian Networks;
- Biosurveillance;
- Cross-Validation;
- Decision Trees;

D.E. Holmes, L.C. Jain (Eds.): Data Mining: Found. & Intell. Paradigms, ISRL 24, pp. 1–7.
springerlink.com

- Eight Regression Algorithms;
- Elementary probability;
- Game Tree Search Algorithms;
- Gaussian Bayes Classifiers and Mixture Models;
- Genetic Algorithms;
- K-means and Hierarchical Clustering;
- Markov Decision Processes and Hidden Markov Models;
- Maximum Likelihood Estimation;
- Neural Networks;
- Predicting Real-valued Outputs;
- Probability Density Functions;
- Probably Approximately Correct Learning;
- Reinforcement Learning;
- Robot Motion Planning.
- Search - Hill Climbing, Simulated Annealing and A-star Heuristic Search;
- Spatial Surveillance;
- Support Vector Machines;
- Time Series Methods;
- Time-series-based anomaly detection;
- Visual Constraint Satisfaction Algorithms; and
- Zero and non-zero-Sum Game Theory.

2.1 Statistical Modelling

Using statistics we are able to gain useful information from raw data. Based on a founding knowledge of probability theory, statistical data analysis provides historical measures from empirical data. Based on this premise, there has been an evolutionary approach in *Statistical Modelling* techniques [2]. A recent example is Exceptional Model Mining (EMM). This is a framework that allows for more complicated target concepts. Rather than finding subgroups based on the distribution of a single target attribute, EMM finds subgroups where a model fitted to that subgroup is somehow exceptional. These models enable experts to discover historical results, but work has also been done on prediction using analytical techniques.

2.2 Predictions Analysis

In order to gain a market advantage, industry continues to seek, forecast or predict future trends [3]. Many algorithms have been developed to enable us to perform prediction and forecasting. Many of these focus on improving performance by altering the means of interacting with data. For example, Time Series Predictions is widely applied across various domains. There is a growing trend for industry to automate this process. Many now produce annual lists that indexes or rates their competitors based on a series of business parameters. Focuses on a series of observations that are statistically analyzed to generate a prediction based on a predefined number of previous values. A recent example in this book uses the average sum of nth-order difference of series terms with limited range margins. The algorithm performances are evaluated using measurement data-sets of monthly average Sunspot Number, Earthquakes and Pseudo-Periodical Synthetic Time Series. An alternative algorithm using time-discrete target-environment regulatory systems (TE-systems) under ellipsoidal uncertainty is also examined. More sophisticated data analysis tools have also emanated in this area.

2.3 Data Analysis

Not long ago, accountants manually manipulated data to extract patterns or trends. Researchers have continued to evolve methodology to automate this process in many domains. Data analysis is the process of applying one or more models to data in the effort to discover knowledge or even predict patterns. This process has proven useful, regardless of the repository source or size. There are many commercial data mining methods, algorithms and applications, with several that have had major impact. Examples include: *SAS*[1], *SPSS*[2] and *Statistica*[3]. The analysis methodology is mature enough to produce visualised representations that make results easier to interpret by management. The emerging field of Visual Analytics combines several fields. Highly complexity data mining tasks often require employing a multi-level top-down approach. The uppermost level conducts a qualitative analysis of complex situations in an attempt to discover patterns. This chapter focuses on the concept of using Monotone Boolean Function Visual Analytics (MBFVA) and provides an application framework named DIS3GNO. The visualization shows the border between a number of classes and displays any location of the case of interest relative to the border between the patterns. Detection of abnormal case buried *inside the abnormals area, is visually* highlighted when the results show a significant separation from the border typically depicting *normal* and *abnormal* classes. Based on the anomaly, an analyst can extort this manifestation by following any *relationship chains* determined prior to the interrogation.

2.4 Chains of Relationships

Often we choose to follow several relationships within a set of data. For instance a *dietitian* may wish to report on good nutrition from food labels. Using the same data they may need to identify products or suppliers suitable for specific groups of the population. Typically data mining considers a single relation that relates two different attributes [4]. In real life it is often the case that we have multiple attributes related through chains of relations. The final chapter of this book discusses various algorithms and identify the conditions when *apriori* techniques can be used. This chapter experimentally demonstrates the effectiveness and efficiency of an algorithm using a three-level chain relation. This discussion focuses on four common problems, namely frequency [5], authority [6], the program committee [7] and classification problems [8]. Chains of relationships must be identified before investigating the use of any intelligent paradigm techniques.

---

[1] See `http://www.sas.com/`

[2] See `http://www.spss.com/`

[3] See `http://www.statsoft.com/`

3 Intelligent Paradigms

A number of these techniques include decision-trees, rule-based techniques, Bayesian, rough sets, dependency networks, reinforcement learning, Support Vector Machines (SVM), Neural Networkss (NNs), genetic algorithms, evolutionary algorithms and swarm intelligence. Many of these topics are covered in this book. An example of intelligence is to use AI search algorithms to create automated macros or templates [9]. Again Genetic Algorithm (GA) can be employed to induce rules using rough sets or numerical data. A simple search on data mining will reveal numerous paradigms, many of which are intelligent. The scale of search escalates with the volume of data, hence the reason to model data. As data becomes ubiquitous, there is increasing pressure to provide an on-line presence to enable access to public information repositories and warehouses. Industry is also increasingly providing access to certain types of information using kiosks or paid web services. Data warehousing commonly uses the following steps to model information:

- data extraction,
- data cleansing,
- modeling data,
- applying data mining algorithm,
- pattern discovery, and
- data visualization.

Any number of paradigms are used to mine data and visualize queries. For instance, the popular *six-sigma* approach (define, measure, analyse, improve and control) is used to eliminate defects, waste and quality issues. An alternative is the SEMMA (sample, explore, modify, model and assess). Other intelligent techniques are also commonly employed. Although we don't provide a definitive list of such techniques, this book focuses on many of the most recent paradigms being developed, such as Bayesian analysis, SVMs and learning techniques.

3.1 Bayesian Analysis

Bayesian methods have been used to discover patterns and represent uncertainty in many domains. It has proven valuable in modeling certainty and uncertainty in data mining. It can be used to explicitly indicate a statistical dependence or independence of isolated parameters in any repository. Biomedical and healthcare data presents a wide range of uncertainties [10]. Bayesian analysis techniques can deal with missing data by explicitly isolating statistical dependent or independent relationships. This enables the integration of both biomedical and clinical background knowledge. These requirements have given rise to an influx of new methods into the field of data analysis in healthcare, in particular from the fields of machine learning and probabilistic graphical models.

3.2 Support Vector Machines

In data mining there is always a need to model information using classification or regression. An SVM represents a suitable robust tool for use in noisy, complex domains

[11]. Their major feature is the use of generalization theory or non-linear kernel functions. SVMs provide flexible machine learning techniques that can fit complex nonlinear mappings. They transform the input variables into a high dimensional feature space and then finds the best hyperplane that models the data in the feature space. SVMs are gaining the attention of the data mining (community and are particularly useful when simpler data models fail to provide satisfactory predictive models.

3.3 Learning

Decision trees use a combination of statistics and machine learning as a predictive tool to map observations about a specific item based on a given value. Decision trees are generally generated using two methods; classification and regression. Regardless of the methodology, decision trees provide many advantages. They are:

- able to handle both numerical and categorical data,
- generally use a white box model,
- perform well with large data in a short time
- possible to validate a model using statistical tests,
- requires little data preparation,
- robust, and
- simple to understand and interpret.

A well known methodology of learning decision trees is the use of data streams. Some aspects of decision tree learning still need solving. For example, numerical attribute discretization. The best-known discretization approaches are unsupervised equal-width and equal-frequency binning. Other learning methods include:

- Association Rules,
- Bayesian Networks,
- Classification Rules,
- Clustering,
- Extending Linear Models,
- Instance-Based Learning,
- Multi-Instance Learning,
- Numeric Prediction with Local Linear Models,
- Semisupervised Learning, and
- 'Weka' Implementations.

There is a significant amount of research on these topics. This book provide a collection of recent and topical techniques. A description of these topics is outlined next.

4 Chapters Included in the Book

This book includes eleven chapters. Each chapter is self-contained and is briefly described below. Chapter 1 provides an introduction to data mining and presents a brief abstract of each chapter included in the book. Chapter 2 is on data mining with Multi-Layer Perceptronss (MLPs) and SVMs. The author demonstrates the applications of MLPs and SVMs to the real world classification and regression data mining applications.

Chapter 3 is on regulatory networks under ellipsoidal uncertainty. The authors have introduced and analyzed time-discrete target-environment regulatory systems under ellipsoidal uncertainty. Chapter 4 is on visual environment for designing and running data mining workflows in the knowledge grid.

Chapter 5 is on formal framework for the study of algorithmic properties of objective interestingness measures. Chapter 6 is on Non-negative Matrix Factorization (NMF). The author presents a survey of NMF in terms of the model formulation and its variations and extensions, algorithms and applications, as well as its relations with *k* means and probabilistic latent semantic indexing.

Chapter 7 is on visual data mining and discovery with binarized vectors. The authors present the concept of monotone Boolean function visual analytics for top level pattern discovery. Chapter 8 is on a new approach and its applications for time series analysis and prediction. The approach focuses on a series of observations with the aim of using mathematical and artificial intelligence techniques for analyzing, processing and predicting on the next most probable value based on a number of previous values. The approach is validated for its superiority.

Chapter 9 is on Exceptional Model Mining (EMM). It allows for more complicated target concepts. The authors have discussed regression as well as classical models and defined quality measures that determine how exceptional a given model on a subgroup is. Chapter 10 is on online ChiMerge algorithm. The authors have shown that a sampling theoretical attribute discretization algorithm ChiMerge can be implemented efficiently in online setting. A comparative evaluation of the algorithm is presented. Chapter 11 is on mining chains of relations. The authors formulated a generic problem of finding selector sets such that the projected dataset satisfies a specific property. The effectiveness of the technique is demonstrated experimentally.

5 Conclusion

This chapter presents a collection of selected contribution of leading subject matter experts in the field of data mining. This book is intended for students, professionals and academics from all disciplines to enable them the opportunity to engage in the state of art developments in:

- Data Mining with Multilayer Perceptrons and Support Vector Machines;
- Regulatory Networks under Ellipsoidal Uncertainty - Data Analysis and Prediction;
- A Visual Environment for Designing and Running Data Mining Workflows in the Knowledge Grid;
- Formal framework for the Study of Algorithmic Properties of Objective Interestingness Measures;
- Nonnegative Matrix Factorization: Models, Algorithms and Applications;
- Visual Data Mining and Discovery with Binarized Vectors;
- A New Approach and Its Applications for Time Series Analysis and Prediction based on Moving Average of nth-order Difference;
- Exceptional Model Mining;

- Online ChiMerge Algorithm; and
- Mining Chains of Relations.

Readers are invited to contact individual authors to engage with further discussion or dialog on each topic.

References

1. Abraham, A., Hassanien, A.E., Carvalho, A., Snášel, V. (eds.): Foundations of Computational Intelligence. SCI, vol. 6. Springer, New York (2009)
2. Hill, T., Lewicki, P.: Statistics: Methods and Applications. StatSoft, Tulsa (2007)
3. Nimmagadda, S., Dreher, H.: Ontology based data warehouse modeling and mining of earthquake data: prediction analysis along eurasian-australian continental plates. In: 5th IEEE International Conference on Industrial Informatics, Vienna, Austria, June 23-27, vol. 2, pp. 597–602. IEEE Press, Piscataway (2007)
4. Agrawal, R., Imielinski, T., Swami, A.N.: Mining association rules between sets of items in large databases. In: Buneman, P., Jajodia, S. (eds.) International Conference on Management of Data, Washington, D.C, May 26-28. ACM SIGMOD, pp. 207–216. ACM Press, New York (1993)
5. Nwana, H.S., Ndumu, D.T., Lee, L.: Zues: An advanced tool-kit for engineering distributed multi-agent systems. Applied AI 13:1(2), 129–1185 (1998)
6. Afrati, F., Das, G., Gionis, A., Mannila, H., Mielikäinen, T., Tsaparas, P.: Mining chains of relations. In: ICDM, pp. 553–556. IEEE Press, Los Alamitos (2005)
7. Jaschke, R., Hotho, A., Schmitz, C., Ganter, B., Gerd, S.: Trias–an algorithm for mining iceberg tri-lattices. In: Sixth International Conference on Data Mining, pp. 907–911. IEEE Computer Society, Washington, DC, USA (2006)
8. Anthony, M., Biggs, N.: An introduction to computational learning theory. Cambridge University Press, Cambridge (1997)
9. Lin, T., Xie, Y., Wasilewska, A., Liau, C.J. (eds.): Data Mining: Foundations and Practice. Studies in Computational Intelligence, vol. 118. Springer, New York (2008)
10. Lucas, P.: Bayesian analysis, pattern analysis, and data mining in health care. In: Curr. Opin. Crit. Care, pp. 399–403 (2004)
11. Burbidge, R., Buxton, B.: An introduction to support vector machines for data mining, pp. 3–15. Operational Research Society, University of Nottingham (2001)

Chapter 2
Data Mining with Multilayer Perceptrons and Support Vector Machines

Paulo Cortez

Centro Algoritmi, Departamento de Sistemas de Informação,
Universidade do Minho, 4800-058 Guimarães, Portugal
pcortez@dsi.uminho.pt

Abstract. Multilayer perceptrons (MLPs) and support vector machines (SVMs) are flexible machine learning techniques that can fit complex nonlinear mappings. MLPs are the most popular neural network type, consisting on a feedforward network of processing neurons that are grouped into layers and connected by weighted links. On the other hand, SVM transforms the input variables into a high dimensional feature space and then finds the best hyperplane that models the data in the feature space. Both MLP and SVM are gaining an increase attention within the data mining (DM) field and are particularly useful when more simpler DM models fail to provide satisfactory predictive models. This tutorial chapter describes basic MLP and SVM concepts, under the CRISP-DM methodology, and shows how such learning tools can be applied to real-world classification and regression DM applications.

1 Introduction

The advances in information technology has led to an huge growth of business and scientific databases. Powerful information systems are available in virtually all organizations and each year more procedures are being automatized, increasing data accumulation over operations and activities. All this data (often with high complexity), may hold valuable information, such as trends and patterns, that can be used to improve decision making and optimize success. The goal of data mining (DM) is to use (semi-)automated tools to analyze raw data and extract useful knowledge for the domain user or decision-maker [16][35]. To achieve such goal, several steps are required. For instance, the CRISP-DM methodology [6] divides a DM project into 6 phases (e.g. data preparation, modeling and evaluation).

In this chapter, we will address two important DM goals that work under the supervised learning paradigm, where the intention is to model an unknown function that maps several input variables with one output target [16]:

classification – labeling a data item into one of several predefined classes (e.g. classify the type of credit client, "good" or "bad", given the status of her/his bank account, credit purpose and amount, etc.); and

D.E. Holmes, L.C. Jain (Eds.): Data Mining: Found. & Intell. Paradigms, ISRL 24, pp. 9–25.
springerlink.com

regression – estimate a real-value (the *dependent variable*) from several (*independent*) attributes (e.g. predict the price of a house based on its number of rooms, age and other characteristics).

Typically, a data-driven approach is used, where the model is fitted with a training set of examples (i.e. past data). After training, the DM model is used to predict the responses related to new items. For the classification example, the training set could be made of thousands of past records from a banking system. Once the DM model is built, it can be fed with the details of a new credit request (e.g. amount), in order to estimate the credit worthiness (i.e. "good" or "bad").

Given the interest in DM, several learning techniques are available, each one with its own purposes and advantages. For instance, the linear/multiple regression (MR) has been widely used in regression applications, since it is simple and easy to interpret due to the additive linear combination of its independent variables. Multilayer perceptrons (MLPs) and support vector machines (SVMs) are more flexible models (i.e. no *a priori* restriction is imposed) that can cope with noise and complex nonlinear mappings. Both models are being increasingly used within the DM field and are particularly suited when more simpler learning techniques (e.g. MR) do not provide sufficiently accurate predictions [20][35]. While other DM models are easier to interpret (e.g. MR), it is still possible to extract knowledge from MLPs and SVMs, given in terms of input variable relevance [13] or by extracting a set of rules [31]. Examples of three successful DM applications performed by the author of this chapter (and collaborators) are: assessing organ failure in intensive care units (three-class classification using MLP) [32]; spam email filtering (binary classification using SVM) [12]; and wine quality prediction (regression/ordinal classification using SVM, some of the details are further described in Sect. 4.1) [11].

This chapter is focused on the use of MLPs and SVMs for supervised DM tasks. First, supervised learning, including MLP and SVM, is introduced (Sect. 2). Next, basic concepts of DM and use of MLP/SVM under the CRISP-DM methodology are presented (Sect. 3). Then, two real-world datasets from the UCI repository (i.e. white wine quality assessment and car price prediction) [1] are used to show the MLP and SVM capabilities (Sect. 4). Finally, conclusions are drawn in Sect. 5.

2 Supervised Learning

DM learning techniques mainly differ on two aspects: model representation and search algorithm used to adjust the model parameters [25]. A supervised model is adjusted to a dataset, i.e. training data, made up of $k \in \{1,...,N\}$ examples. An example maps an input vector $\mathbf{x}_k = (x_{k,1},\ldots,x_{k,I})$ to a given output target y_k. Each input (x_i) or output variable (y) can be categorical or continuous. A classification task assumes a categorical output with $G \in \{G_1,\ldots,G_{N_G}\}$ groups, while regression a continuous one (i.e. $y \in \Re$). Discrete data can be further classified into:

binary – with N_G =2 possible values (e.g. $G \in$ {yes, no});
ordered – with N_G >2 ordered values (e.g. $G \in$ {low, medium, high});
nominal – non-ordered with N_G >2 classes (e.g. $G \in$ {red, blue, yellow}).

Due to its historical importance, this section starts by presenting two classical methods: multiple and logistic regression. Then, the MLP is introduced, followed by the SVM.

2.1 Classical Regression

The linear/multiple regression (MR) is the classical approach for regression [20]:

$$\hat{y}_k = w_0 + \sum_{i=1}^{I} w_i x_{k,i} \tag{1}$$

where $\hat{y}_k$ denotes the predicted value for example k and $\{w_0, \ldots, w_I\}$ the parameters to be adjusted (e.g. by using a least squares algorithm). This model can also be used in binary classification, for instance using the encoding $y \in \{G_1 = 0, G_2 = 1\}$ and assigning the rule: G_2 if $\hat{y}_k > 0.5$ else G_1.

For binary classification, the logistic regression (LR) is a popular choice (e.g. in Medicine) that operates a smooth nonlinear logistic transformation over the MR model and allows the estimation of class probabilities [36]:

$$p(G_c|\mathbf{x}_k) = \frac{1}{1 + exp(w_0 + \sum_{i=1}^{I} w_i x_{k,i})} \tag{2}$$

where $p(G_c|\mathbf{x})$ denotes the probability of event $G_c \in G$ given the example $\mathbf{x}_k$. There is also the multinomial logistic regression variant, which extends the LR model to multi-class tasks.

Both MR and LR are easy to interpret, due to the additive linear combination of its independent variables (i.e. $\mathbf{x}$). Yet, these models are quite rigid and can only model adequately linear or logistic relationships in the data. While there are other variants (e.g. polynomial regression), the classical statistical approach requires a priori knowledge or trial-and-error experiments to set/select the type of model used (e.g. order of the polynomial regression). In contrast, there are learning techniques, such as MLP and SVM, that use a more flexible representation and are universal approximators, i.e. capable in theory to learn any type of mapping, provided there is an implicit relationship between the inputs and the desired output target [21]. MLP and SVM require more computation and are more difficult to interpret when compared with the MR and LR models. Yet, they tend to give more accurate predictions and this is an important factor in several real-world applications. Moreover, it is possible to extract knowledge from MLP and SVM, as described in Sec. 3.

2.2 Multilayer Perceptron

Since the advent of the backpropagation algorithm in 1986, the multilayer perceptron (MLP) has become the most popular NN architecture [21] (Fig. 1). The MLP is activated by feeding the input layer with the input vector and then propagating the activations in a feedforward fashion, via the weighted connections, through the entire network. For a given input $\mathbf{x}_k$ the state of the i-th neuron (s_i) is computed by:

$$s_i = f(w_{i,0} + \sum_{j \in P_i} w_{i,j} \times s_j) \tag{3}$$

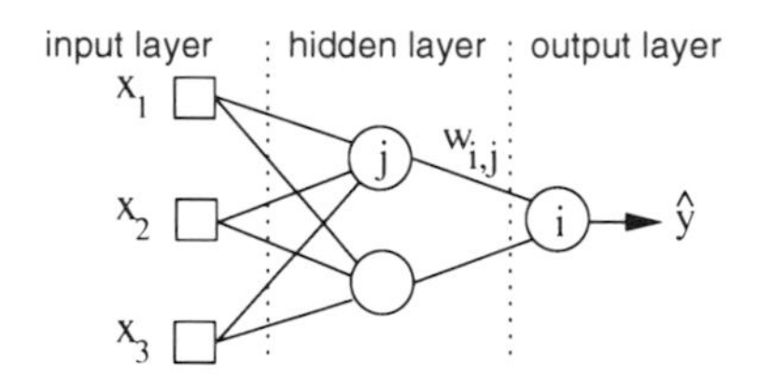

Fig. 1. Example of a multilayer perceptron with 3 input, 2 hidden and 1 output nodes

where P_i represents the set of nodes reaching node i; f the activation function; $w_{i,j}$ the weight of the connection between nodes j and i; and $s_1 = x_{k,1}, \ldots, s_I = x_{k,I}$. The $w_{i,0}$ connections are called bias and are often included to increase the MLP learning flexibility.

While several hidden layers can be used for complex tasks (e.g. two-spirals), the most common approach is to use one hidden layer of H hidden nodes with the the logistic ($f(x) = \frac{1}{1+exp(-x)}$) activation function. For binary classification, one output node with logistic function is often used, in a configuration that allows to interpret the output as a probability and also equivalent to the LR model when H=0. For multi-class tasks (with $N_G > 2$ output classes), usually there are N_G output linear nodes ($f(x) = x$) and the softmax function is used to transform these outputs into class probabilities [30]:

$$p(G_c|\mathbf{x}_k) = \frac{exp(\hat{y}_{k,c})}{\sum_{j=1}^{N_G} exp(\hat{y}_{k,j})} \tag{4}$$

where $\hat{y}_{k,c}$ is the MLP output for class G_c. For regression, typically one linear output neuron is used, since outputs may lie out of the logistic range ($[0,1]$). When $H = 0$, this network is equivalent to MR.

MLPs learn through an iterative algorithm that starts from random initial weights (e.g. within $[-0.7, +0.7]$). Next, a training algorithm adjusts the weights to the desired target values. Several training algorithms have been developed for MLPs. The standard backpropagation is quite used, but there are variants that often lead to a faster convergence (e.g. QuickProp, RProp) [24]. Other fast alternatives are the Levenberg-Marquardt and BFGS algorithms [30][36]. During the training, several cost functions can be used. Often, minimization of the squared error is used for regression, while the likelihood is maximized for classification [20]. The training is usually stopped when the error slope approaches zero, when the validation error arises (if early stopping is used) or after a maximum number of epochs. Since the NN cost function is nonconvex (with multiple minima), N_R runs can be applied to each MLP configuration, being selected the MLP with the lowest error. Another option is to use an ensemble of all MLPs and output the average of the individual predictions [10].

Under this settings, performance is heavily dependent on tuning one hyperparameter [20]: weight decay ($\lambda \in [0,1]$) or number of hidden nodes ($H \in \{0,1,\ldots\}$). The former option includes fixing H to a high value and then search for the best λ, which is a penalty value that shrinks the size of the weights, i.e. a higher λ produces a simpler

MLP. The latter strategy ($\lambda = 0$) searches for the best H value. The simplest MLP will have $H = 0$, while more complex models will use a high H value.

2.3 Support Vector Machines

Support vector machine (SVM) is a powerful learning tool that is based in a statistical learning theory and was developed in the 1990s, due to the work of Vapnik and its collaborators (e.g. [9]). SVMs present theoretical advantages over MLPs, such as the absence of local minima in the learning phase. In effect, the SVM was recently considered one of the most influential DM algorithms, in particular due to its high performance on classification tasks [40]. The basic idea is transform the input $\mathbf{x}$ into a high m-dimensional feature space ($m > I$) by using a nonlinear mapping. Then, the SVM finds the best linear separating hyperplane, related to a set of support vector points, in the feature space (Fig. 2). The transformation depends on a nonlinear mapping (ϕ) that does not need to be explicitly known but that depends of a kernel function $K(x,x') = \sum_{i=1}^{m} \phi_i(x)\phi_i(x')$. The gaussian kernel is popular option and presents less hyperparameters and numerical difficulties than other kernels (e.g. polynomial or sigmoid):

$$K(x,x') = exp(-\gamma||x-x'||^2),\ \gamma > 0 \tag{5}$$

For binary classification, the output target is encoded in the range $y \in \{G_1 = -1, G_2 = 1\}$ and the classification function is:

$$f(\mathbf{x}_k) = \sum_{j=1}^{m} y_j \alpha_j K(\mathbf{x}_j, \mathbf{x}_k) + b \tag{6}$$

where b and α_j are coefficients of the model and m is the number of support vectors. The discriminant rule is given by G_2 if $f(\mathbf{x}_k) > 0$ else G_1. The probabilistic SVM output is given by [39]:

$$p(G_2|\mathbf{x}_k) = 1/(1 + exp(Af(\mathbf{x}_k) + B)) \tag{7}$$

where A and B are determined by solving a regularized maximum likelihood problem. When $N_G > 2$, the one-against-one approach is often used, which trains $N_G(N_G - 1)/2$ binary classifiers and the output is given by a pairwise coupling [39]. For regression, the ε-insensitive cost function is commonly used [33], which sets a tube around the residuals, being the tiny errors within this tube discarded (Fig. 2). Then, SVM finds the best linear separating hyperplane:

$$\hat{y}_k = w_0 + \sum_{i=1}^{m} w_i \phi_i(\mathrm{x}_k) \tag{8}$$

For all these SVM variants, the sequential minimal optimization (SMO) is the most commonly used training algorithm.

Under these settings, classification performance is affected by two hyperparameters: γ, the parameter of the kernel, and $C > 0$, a penalty parameter of the error term. For regression, there is the additional hyperparameter $\varepsilon > 0$. The gaussian parameter has a strong impact in performance, with too low (γ=0) or too large ($\gamma \approx \infty$) leading to poor generalizations [37]. During model selection, exponentially growing search sequences are often used to set these parameters [5], such as $\gamma \in \{2^{-15}, 2^{-13}, \ldots, 2^{3}\}$, $C \in \{2^{-5}, 2^{-3}, \ldots, 2^{15}\}$ and $\varepsilon \in \{2^{-8}, 2^{-7}, \ldots, 2^{-1}\}$.

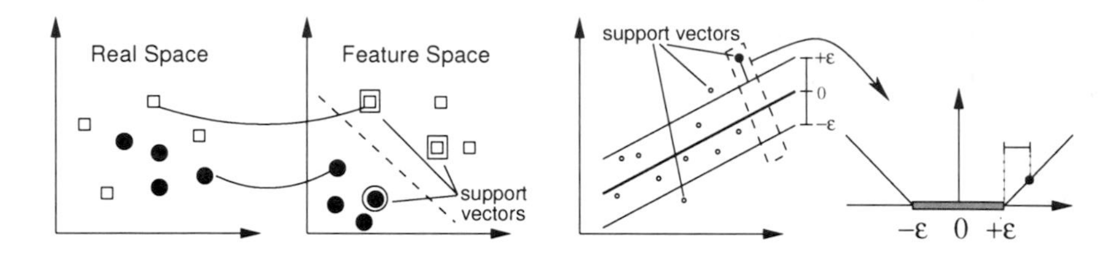

Fig. 2. Example of a SVM classification (left) and regression using the ε-insensitive tube (right)

3 Data Mining

DM is an iterative process that consists in several steps. The CRISP-DM [6], a tool-neutral methodology supported by the industry (e.g. SPSS, DaimlerChryslyer), partitions a DM project into 6 phases (Fig. 3): 1) business understanding; 2) data understanding; 3) data preparation; 4) modeling; 5) evaluation; and 6) deployment. The next subsections address these steps, with an emphasis on the use of MLPs and SVMs to solve classification and regression goals.

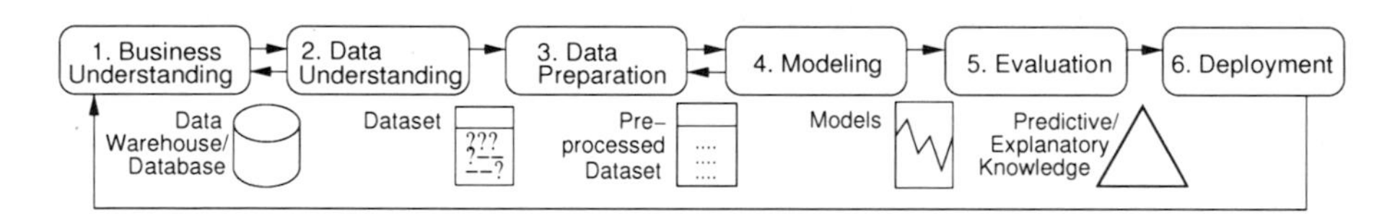

Fig. 3. The CRISP-DM methodology (adapted from [6])

3.1 Business Understanding

The first phase involves tasks such as learning the business domain, goals and success criteria, setting DM goals, project plan and inventory of resources, including personnel and software tools. Currently, there are dozens of software solutions that offer MLP/SVM capabilities for DM tasks [26]. Examples of commercial tools that implement both MLP and SVM are IBM SPSS Modeler (former Clementine), GhostMiner and Matlab. There are also open source tools, such as RapidMiner, WEKA and R. Most of these solutions follow the guidelines described in this chapter (e.g. data preparation).

3.2 Data Understanding

The second phase comprehends data collection, description, exploration and quality verification. Data collection may involve data loading and integration from multiple sources. The remaining phase tasks allow the identification of the data main characteristics (e.g. use of histograms) and data quality problems.

3.3 Data Preparation

It is assumed that a dataset, with past examples of the learning goal, is available. Preprocessing involves tasks such as data selection, cleaning, transformation [28]. Using examples and attributes that are more related with the learning goal will improve the DM project success. Data selection can be guided by domain knowledge or statistics (e.g. for outlier removal) and includes selection of attributes (columns) and also examples (rows). Since MLP and SVM work only with numeric values, data cleaning and transformation are key prerequisites.

Missing data is quite common, due to several reasons, such as procedural factors or refusal of response. To solve this issue, there are several solutions, such as [4]:

- use complete data only;
- for categorical data, treat missing values as an additional "unknown" class;
- perform data imputation (e.g. substitute by mean, median or values found in other data sources);
- model-based imputation, where a DM model (e.g. k-nearest neighbor) is used to first model the variable relationship to the remaining attributes in the dataset and then the model predictions are used as substitute values.

The first strategy is suited when there is few missing data. Imputation methods allow the use of all cases, but may introduce "wrong" values. For instance, mean substitution is simple and popular method based on the assumption that it is a reasonable estimate, yet it may distort the variable distribution values. Model-based imputation is a more sophisticated method that estimates the missing value from the remaining dataset (e.g. most similar case).

Before fitting a MLP or SVM, categorical values need to be transformed. Binary attributes can be easily encoded into 2 values (e.g. {-1,1} or {0,1}). Ordered variables can be encoded in a scale that preserves the order (e.g. low→-1, medium→0, high→1). For nominal attributes, the One-of-N_G remapping is the most adopted solution, where one binary variable is assigned to each class (e.g. red→(1,0,0); blue→(0,1,0); yellow→(0,0,1)), allowing the definition of in between items (e.g. orange→(0.5,0,0.5)). Other m-of-N_G remappings may lead to more useful transformations but require domain knowledge (e.g. encode a U.S. state under 2 geographic coordinates) [28].

Another common MLP/SVM transformation is to rescale the data, for instance by standardizing each x_a attribute according to:

$$x'_a = \frac{x_a - \overline{x_a}}{s_{x_a}} \tag{9}$$

where $\overline{x_a}$ and s_{x_a} are the mean and sample standard deviation of x_a (measured over the training data). This transformation has the advantage of rescaling all inputs to the same range, thus assigning them an equal importance. Also, it reduces numerical difficulties related to MLP and SVM learning algorithms [30].

3.4 Modeling

This stage involves selecting the learning models, estimation method, design strategy, building and assessing the models.

3.4.1 Estimation Method

Powerful learners, such as MLP and SVM, can overfit the data by memorizing all examples. Thus, the generalization capability needs to be assessed on unseen data. To achieve this, the holdout validation is commonly used. This method randomly partitions the data into training and test subsets. The former subset is used to fit the model (typically with $2/3$ of the data), while the latter (with the remaining $1/3$) is used to compute the estimate. A more robust estimation procedure is the K-fold cross-validation [14], where the data is divided into K partitions of equal size. One subset is tested each time and the remaining data are used for fitting the model. The process is repeated sequentially until all subsets have been tested. Therefore, under this scheme, all data are used for training and testing. However, this method requires around K times more computation, since K models are fitted. In practice, the 10-fold estimation is a common option when there are a few thousands or hundreds of samples. If very few samples are available (e.g. $N < 100$), the N-fold validation, also known as leave-one-out, is used. In contrast, if the number of samples is too large (e.g. $N > 5000$) then the simpler holdout method is a more reasonable option.

The estimation method is stochastic, due to the random train/test partition. Thus, several R runs should be applied. A large R value increases the robustness of the estimation but also the computational effort. R should be set according to the data size and computational effort available (common R values are 5, 10, 20 or 30). When $R > 1$, results should be reported using mean or median values and statistical tests (e.g. t-test) should be used to check for statistical differences [17].

3.4.2 Design Strategy

As describe in Sect. 2, both MLP and SVM have several configuration details that need to be set (e.g. number of hidden layers, kernel function or learning algorithm). Furthermore, for a given setup there are hyperparameters that need to be set (e.g. number of hidden nodes or kernel parameter). The design of the best model that can be solved by using heuristic rules, a simple grid search or more advanced optimization algorithms, such as evolutionary computation [29]. For example, the WEKA environment uses the default rule for setting $H = I/2$ in MLP classification tasks [38]. Such heuristic rules require few computation but may lead to models that are far from the optimum. The grid search a popular approach, usually set by defining an internal estimation method (e.g. holdout or K-fold) over the training data, i.e., the training data is further divided into training and validation sets. A grid of parameters (e.g. $H \in \{2,4,6,8\}$ for MLP) is set for the search and the model that produces the best generalization estimate is selected.

The design strategy may also include variable selection, which is quite valuable when the number of inputs is large ($I \gg$). Variable selection [19] is useful to discard irrelevant inputs, leading to simpler models that are easier to interpret and that usually give better performances. Such selection can be based on heuristic or domain related rules (e.g. use of variables that are more easy to collect). Another common approach is the use of variable selection algorithms (e.g. backward and forward selection or evolutionary computation). Also, variable and model selection should be performed simultaneously.

Table 1. The 2×2 confusion matrix

↓ **actual** \ **predicted** →	**negative**	**positive**
negative	TN	FP
positive	FN	TP

TN - true negative, FP - false positive, FN - false negative, TP - true positive.

3.4.3 Model Assessment

This section describes the most common classification and regression metrics (e.g. confusion matrix and MAE). The confusion matrix [23] is commonly used for classification analysis, a matrix of size $N_G \times N_G$ (Table 1). The matrix is created by matching the predicted ($\hat{y}$) with the desired (y) values. From the matrix, several metrics can be computed, such as: the accuracy (ACC) or correct classification rate; the true positive rate (TPR) or recall/sensitivity; and the true negative rate (TNR) or specificity. These metrics can be computed using the equations:

$$\begin{aligned} TPR &= \frac{TP}{FN+TP} \times 100\,(\%) \\ TNR &= \frac{TN}{TN+FP} \times 100\,(\%) \\ ACC &= \frac{TN+TP}{TN+FP+FN+TP} \times 100\,(\%) \end{aligned} \quad (10)$$

A classifier should present high values of ACC, TPR and TNR. When there are different FP and FN costs and/or balanced (i.e. towards a given class) output targets, the ACC metric is not sufficient and both TPR and TNR such be used, as there is often a trade-off between the two. The receiver operating characteristic (ROC) curve shows the performance of a two class classifier across the range of possible threshold (D) values, plotting FPR$=1-$TNR (x-axis) versus TPR (y-axis) [15]. When the output is modeled as a probability, then $D \in [0.0, 1.0]$ and the output class G_c is positive if $p(G_c|\mathbf{x}) > D$. The global accuracy is given by the area under the curve (AUC$=\int_0^1 ROC dD$). A random classifier will have an AUC of 0.5, while the ideal value should be close to 1.0. The ROC analysis has the advantage of being insensitive to the output class distribution. Moreover, it provides a wide range of FPR/TPR points to the domain user, which can later, based on her/his knowledge, select the most advantageous setup.

For multi-class tasks, the $N_G \times N_G$ confusion matrix can be converted into a 2×2 one by selecting a given class (G_c) as the positive concept and $\neg G_c$ as the negative one. Also, a global AUC can also be defined by weighting the AUC for each class according its prevalence in the data [27].

The error of a regression model is given by $e_k = y_k - \hat{y}_k$. The overall performance is computed by a global metric, such as mean absolute error (MAE), relative absolute error (RAE), root mean squared error (RMSE), root relative squared error (RRSE), which can be computed as [38]:

$$\begin{array}{l} MAE = 1/N \times \sum_{i=1}^{N} |y_i - \hat{y}_i| \\ RAE = MAD / \sum_{i=1}^{N} |y_i - \overline{y}_i| \times 100\,(\%) \\ RMSE = \sqrt{\sum_{i=1}^{N} (y_i - \hat{y}_i)^2 / N} \\ RRSE = \sqrt{\frac{\sum_{i=1}^{N} (y_i - \hat{y}_i)^2}{\sum_{i=1}^{N} (y_i - \overline{y}_i)^2}} \times 100\,(\%) \end{array} \quad (11)$$

where N denotes the number of examples (or cases) considered. A good regressor should present a low error. The RAE, RRSE and MAPE metrics are scale independent, where 100% denotes an error similar to the naive average predictor ($\overline{y}$).

3.5 Evaluation

The previous phase leads to a model with some given accuracy. In this phase, the aim is to assess if the such model meets the business goals and if it is interesting. The former issue involves analyzing the model in terms of business criteria for success. For instance, when considering the bank credit example (Sect. 1), the best model could present a ROC curve with an AUC=0.9 (high discrimination power). Still, such ROC curve presents several FPR vs TPR points. A business analysis should select the best ROC point based on the expected profit and cost. The latter issue (i.e. model interestingness) involves checking if the model makes sense to the domain experts and if it unveils useful or challenging information. When using MLPs or SVMs, this can be achieved by measuring input importance or by extracting rules from fitted models.

Input variable importance can be estimated from any supervised model (after training) by adopting a sensitivity analysis procedure. The basic idea is to measure how much the predictions are affected when the inputs are varied through their range of values. For example, a computationally efficient sensitivity analysis version was proposed in [22] and works as follows. Let $\hat{y}_{a,j}$ denote the output obtained by holding all input variables at their average values except x_a, which varies through its entire range ($x_{a,j}$, with $j \in \{1,\ldots,L\}$ levels). If a given input variable ($x_a \in \{x_1,\ldots,x_I\}$) is relevant then it should produce a high variance (V_a). For classification tasks, V_a can be computed over output probabilities. If $N_G > 2$ (multi-class), V_a can be set as the sum of the variances for each output class probability ($p(G_c)|\mathbf{x}_{a,j}$) [10]. The input relative importance (R_a) is given by $R_a = V_a / \sum_{i=1}^{I} V_i \times 100\,(\%)$. For a more detailed individual input influence analysis, the variable effect characteristic (VEC) curve [13] can be used, which plots the $x_{a,j}$ values (x-axis) versus the $y_{a,j}$ predictions (y-axis).

The extraction of knowledge from MLPs and SVMs is still an active research area [31][2]. The two main approaches are based on decompositional and pedagogical techniques. The former extracts first rules from a lower level, such as a rule for each individual neuron of a MLP. Then, the subsets of rules are aggregated to form the global knowledge. The latter approach extracts the direct relationships (e.g. by applying a decision tree) between the inputs and outputs of the model. By using a black-box point of view, less computation effort is required and a simpler set of rules may be achieved.

3.6 Deployment

The aim is to use the data mining results in the business or domain area. This includes monitoring and maintenance, in order to deal with issues such as: user feedback, checking if there have been changes in the environment (i.e. concept drift or shift) and if the DM model needs to be updated or redesigned. Regarding the use of the model, MLP and SVMs should be integrated into a friendly business intelligence or decision support system. This can be achieved by using the DM tool to export the best model into a standard format, such as the predictive model markup language (PMML) [18], and then loading this model into a standalone program (e.g. written in C or Java).

4 Experiments

The UCI machine learning is a public repository that includes a wide range of real-world problems that are commonly used to test classification and regression algorithms [1]. The next subsections address two UCI tasks: white wine quality (classification) and automobile (regression). Rather than presenting state of the art results, the intention is to show tutorial examples of the MLP and SVM capabilities. All experiments were conducted under the rminer library [10], which facilitates the use of MLP and SVM algorithms in the R open source tool. The rminer library and code examples are available at: http://www3.dsi.uminho.pt/pcortez/rminer.html.

4.1 Classification Example

The **wine quality** data [11] includes 4898 white *vinho verde* samples from the north-west region of Portugal. The goal is to predict human expert taste preferences based on 11 analytical tests (continuous values, such as pH or alcohol levels) that are easy to collect during the wine certification step. The output variable is categorical and ordered, ranging from 3 (low quality) to 9 (high quality).

In this example, a binary classification was adopted, where the goal is to predict very good wine (i.e. $G_2 = 1$ if quality> 6) based on the 11 input variables. Also, three DM models were tested (LR, MLP and SVM), where each model output probabilities ($p(G_2|\mathrm{x}_k)$). Before fitting the models, the data was first standardized to a zero mean and one standard deviation (using only training data). The MLP was set with logistic activation functions, one hidden layer with H hidden nodes, one output node. The initial weights were randomly set within the range [-0.7,0.7]. Both LR and MLP were trained with 100 epochs of the BFGS algorithm for a likelihood maximization. The final MLP output is given by the average of an ensemble of $N_R = 5$ MLPs. The best MLP setup was optimized using a grid search with $H \in \{0,1,2,\ldots,9\}$ (in a total of 10 searches) using an internal (i.e. using only training data) 3-fold validation. The best H corresponds to the MLP setup that provides the highest AUC value under a ROC analysis. After selecting H, the final MLP ensemble was retrained with all training data. The SVM probabilistic output model uses a gaussian kernel and is fit using the SMO algorithm. To reduce the search space, the simple heuristic rule $C = 3$ [7] was adopted and the gaussian hyperparameter was set using a grid search ($\gamma \in \{2^3, 2^1, \ldots, 2^{-15}\}$ [37]) that works similarly to the MLP search (e.g. use of 3-fold internal validation).

Each selected model was evaluated using $R = 10$ runs of an external 3-fold cross-validation (since the dataset is quite large). The results are summarized in Table 2. The first row presents the average hyperparameter values, the second row shows the computational effort, in terms of time elapsed, and the last row contains the average test set

AUC value (with the respective 95% confidence intervals under a t-student distribution). In this example, the LR requires much less computation when compared with MLP and SVM. The high H and γ values suggest that this task is highly nonlinear. In effect, both MLP and SVM outperform the simpler LR model in terms of discriminatory power (i.e. AUC values). When comparing SVM against MLP, the average AUC is slightly higher, although the difference is not statistically significant under a t-test (p-value=0.2).

A more detailed analysis is given by the ROC test set curves (Fig. 4). In the figure, baseline gray curve denotes the performance of a random classifier, while the whiskers show the 95% t-student confidence intervals for the 10 runs. Both SVM and MLP curves are clearly above the LR performance. Selecting the best model depends on the TNR/TPR gains and FN/FP costs. The DM model could be used to assist and speed up the wine expert evaluations (e.g. the expert could repeat is evaluation only if it differs from the DM prediction) [11]. Hence, it should be the expert to select the best ROC point (i.e. TNR vs TPR tradeoff). For a better TNR the best choice is SVM (when FPR< 0.25), else the best option is to use the MLP. As an example of explanatory knowledge, the left of Fig. 4 plots the relevance of the 11 inputs (ordered by importance) as measured by a sensitivity analysis procedure ($L = 6$) described in Sec.3.5. The plot shows that the most important input is alcohol, followed by the volatile acidity, pH and sulphates.

Table 2. The white wine quality results (best values in **bold**)

	LR	MLP	SVM
Parameter	–	$\overline{H}$=8.4	$\overline{\gamma} = 2^{0.27}$
Time (s)	**14**	1699	2520
AUC	78.9%±0.1	85.9%±0.2	**86.3%**±0.6

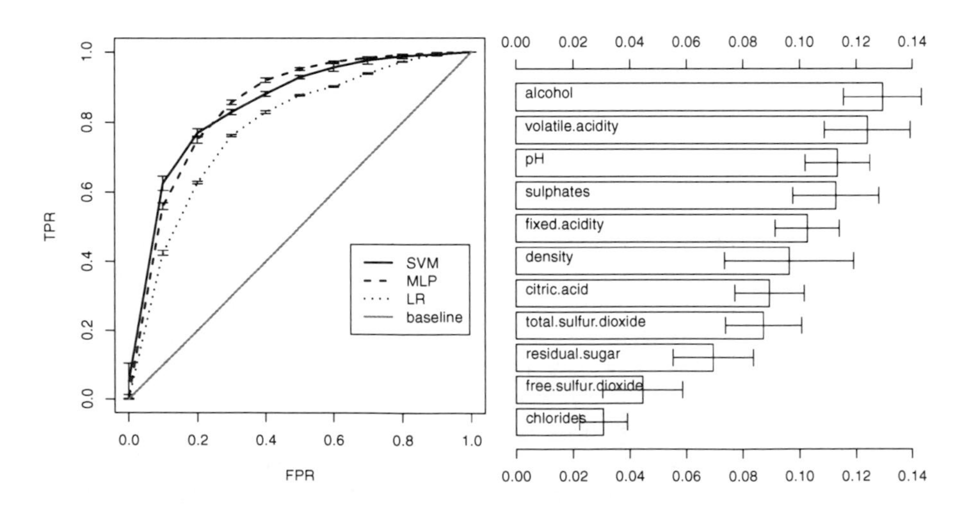

Fig. 4. ROC curves for the white wine quality task (left) and SVM input importances (right)

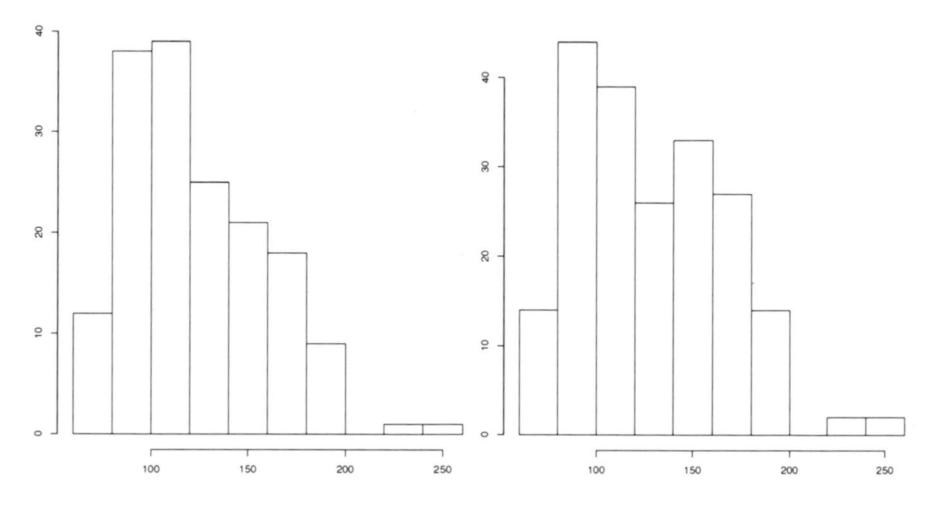

Fig. 5. Histogram for the normalized losses with missing data (left) and after model-based imputation (right)

4.2 Regression Example

The **automobile** dataset goal is to predict car prices using 25 continuous and categorical attributes. To simplify the example, only 9 inputs were used: normalized losses (continuous), fuel type (categorical, $N_G = 2$), aspiration ($N_G = 2$), number of doors ($N_G = 2$), body style ($N_G = 5$), drive wheels ($N_G = 3$), curb weight (cont.), horsepower (cont.) and peak rpm (cont.). The data includes 205 instances, although there are several missing values. To deal with missing data, two strategies were adopted. First, the two examples with missing values in the output variable were deleted. Second, the remaining missing values (37 in normalized losses; 2 in number of doors, horsepower and peak rpm) were replaced using a model-based (i.e. 1-nearest neighbor) imputation (as described in Sect. 3.3). Fig. 5 plots two histograms for the normalized losses input (with 37 missing values), before and after the model-based imputation. In general, it can be seen that this imputation method maintains the original distribution values.

Before fitting the models, the categorical attributes were remapped using a One-of-N_G transformation, leading to a total of 1+2+2+2+5+3+1+1+1=18 inputs. Also, the numeric values were standardized to a zero mean and one standard deviation. Three models were tested during the modeling phase: MR, MLP and SVM. Each model was set similarly to the wine quality example, except for the following differences: MR and MLP were fit using the BGFS algorithm under a least squares minimization; MLP has a linear output node and the ensemble uses $N_R = 7$ MLPs; the ε-insensitive cost function was used for SVM, with the heuristic rule $\varepsilon = 3\sigma_y\sqrt{\log(N)/N}$, where σ_y denotes the standard deviation of the predictions of given by a 3-nearest neighbor [7]; and the RMSE metric was used to select the best model during the grid search (for MLP and SVM).

Since the number of samples is rather small (i.e. 203), the models were evaluated using $R = 10$ runs of a 10-fold validation and the obtained results are shown in Table 3.

Again, the MR algorithm requires less computation when compared with SVM and MLP. Yet, MR presents the worst predictive results. The best predictive model is SVM (RRSE=47.4%, 52.6 pp better than the average naive predictor), followed by MLP (the differences are statistically significant under paired t-tests). The quality of the SVM predictions is shown in the left of Fig. 6, which plots the observed vs predicted values. In the scatter plot, the diagonal line denotes the ideal method. Most of the SVM predictions follow this line, although the model tends to give higher errors for highly costly cars (top right of the plot). Only using domain knowledge it is possible to judge the quality of this predictive performance (although it should be stressed that better results can be achieved for this dataset, as in this example only 9 inputs were used). Assuming it is interesting, in the deployment phase the SVM model could be integrated into a decision support system (e.g used by car auction sites). Regarding the extraction of knowledge, the sensitivity analysis procedure revealed the curb weight as the most relevant factor. For demonstration purposes, the VEC curve (left of Fig. 6) shows that this factor produces a positive effect in the price (in an expected outcome), particularly within the range [2500,3500].

Table 3. The automobile results (best values in **bold**)

	LR	MLP	SVM
Parameter	–	$\overline{H}$=4.3	$\overline{\gamma} = 2^{-3.1}$
Time (s)	**15**	918	230
RMSE	3760±49	3234±174	**2822**±128
RRSE	47.4%±0.6	40.8%±2.2	**35.6%**±1.6

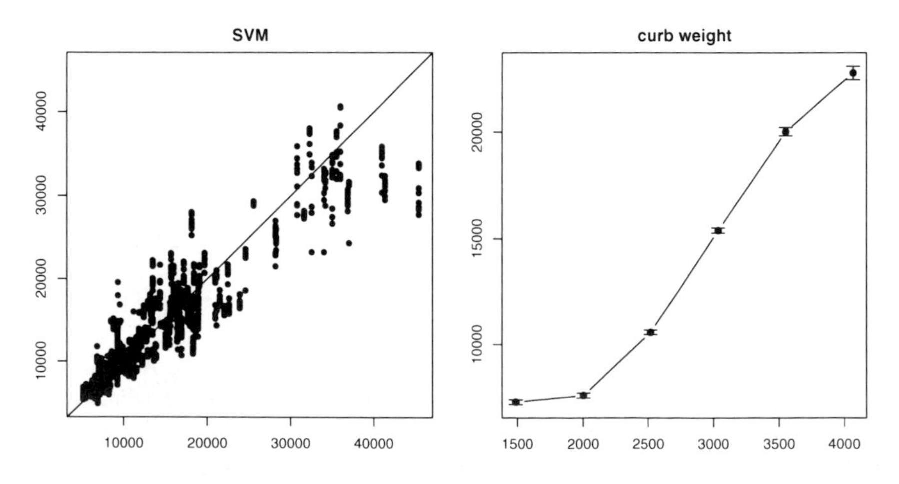

Fig. 6. Scatter plot for the best automobile predictive model (left, x-axis denotes target values and y-axis the predictions) and VEC curve for the curb weight influence (right, x-axis denotes the 6 curb weight levels and y-axis the SVM average response variation)

5 Conclusions and Further Reading

In the last few decades, powerful learning techniques, such as multilayer perceptrons (MLPs) and more recently support vector machines (SVMs) are emerging. Both techniques are flexible models (i.e. no a priori restriction is required) that can cope with complex nonlinear mappings. Hence, the use of MLPs and SVMs in data mining (DM) classification and regression tasks is increasing. In this tutorial chapter, basic MLP and SVM concepts were first introduced. Then, the CRISP-DM methodology, which includes 6 phases, was used to describe how such models can be used in a real DM project. Next, two real-world applications were used to demonstrate the MLP and SVM capabilities: wine quality assessment (binary classification) and car price estimation (regression). In both cases, MLP and SVM have outperformed more simpler methods (e.g. logistic and multiple regression). Also, it was shown how knowledge can be extracted from MLP/SVM models, in terms of input relevance.

For more solid mathematical explanation on MLPs and SVMs, the recommended books are [3], [20] and [21]. Additional details about the CRISP-DM methodology can be found in [6] and [8]. Reference [35] shows examples of MLP/SVM DM applications and their integration into business intelligence and decision support systems. The kdnuggets web portal aggregates information about DM in general and includes an extensive list of commercial and free DM tools [26]. There are also web sites with lists of tools (and other useful details) that specifically target MLPs [30] and SVMs [34].

References

1. Asuncion, A., Newman, D.: UCI Machine Learning Repository, Univ. of California Irvine (2007), http://www.ics.uci.edu/~mlearn/MLRepository.html
2. Barakat, N., Diederich, J.: Learning-based rule-extraction from support vector machines. In: 14th International Conference on Computer Theory and Applications ICCTA, Citeseer, vol. 2004 (2004)
3. Bishop, C.M., et al.: Pattern recognition and machine learning. Springer, New York (2006)
4. Brown, M., Kros, J.: Data mining and the impact of missing data. Industrial Management & Data Systems 103(8), 611–621 (2003)
5. Chang, C., Hsu, C., Lin, C.: A Practical Guide to Support Vector Classification. Technical report, National Taiwan University (2003)
6. Chapman, P., Clinton, J., Kerber, R., Khabaza, T., Reinartz, T., Shearer, C., Wirth, R.: CRISP-DM 1.0: Step-by-step data mining guide. CRISP-DM consortium (2000)
7. Cherkassy, V., Ma, Y.: Practical Selection of SVM Parameters and Noise Estimation for SVM Regression. Neural Networks 17(1), 113–126 (2004)
8. CRISP-DM consortium. CRISP-DM Web Site (2010), http://www.crisp-dm.org/
9. Cortes, C., Vapnik, V.: Support Vector Networks. Machine Learning 20(3), 273–297 (1995)
10. Cortez, P.: Data Mining with Neural Networks and Support Vector Machines Using the R/rminer Tool. In: Perner, P. (ed.) ICDM 2010. LNCS(LNAI), vol. 6171, pp. 572–583. Springer, Heidelberg (2010)
11. Cortez, P., Cerdeira, A., Almeida, F., Matos, T., Reis, J.: Modeling wine preferences by data mining from physicochemical properties. Decision Support Systems 47(4), 547–553 (2009)
12. Cortez, P., Correia, A., Sousa, P., Rocha, M., Rio, M.: Spam Email Filtering Using Network-Level Properties. In: Perner, P. (ed.) ICDM 2010. LNCS(LNAI), vol. 6171, pp. 476–489. Springer, Heidelberg (2010)

13. Cortez, P., Teixeira, J., Cerdeira, A., Almeida, F., Matos, T., Reis, J.: Using data mining for wine quality assessment. In: Gama, J., Costa, V.S., Jorge, A.M., Brazdil, P.B. (eds.) DS 2009. LNCS, vol. 5808, pp. 66–79. Springer, Heidelberg (2009)
14. Dietterich, T.: Approximate Statistical Tests for Comparing Supervised Classification Learning Algorithms. Neural Computation 10(7), 1895–1923 (1998)
15. Fawcett, T.: An introduction to ROC analysis. Pattern Recognition Letters 27, 861–874 (2006)
16. Fayyad, U., Piatetsky-Shapiro, G., Smyth, P.: Advances in Knowledge Discovery and Data Mining. MIT Press, Cambridge (1996)
17. Flexer, A.: Statistical Evaluation of Neural Networks Experiments: Minimum Requirements and Current Practice. In: Proceedings of the 13th European Meeting on Cybernetics and Systems Research, Vienna, Austria, vol. 2, pp. 1005–1008 (1996)
18. Grossman, R., Hornick, M., Meyer, G.: Data Mining Standards Initiatives. Communications of ACM 45(8), 59–61 (2002)
19. Guyon, I., Elisseeff, A.: An introduction to variable and feature selection. Journal of Machine Learning Research 3, 1157–1182 (2003)
20. Hastie, T., Tibshirani, R., Friedman, J.: The Elements of Statistical Learning: Data Mining, Inference, and Prediction, 2nd edn. Springer, Heidelberg (2008)
21. Haykin, S.S.: Neural networks and learning machines. Prentice-Hall, Englewood Cliffs (2009)
22. Kewley, R., Embrechts, M., Breneman, C.: Data Strip Mining for the Virtual Design of Pharmaceuticals with Neural Networks. IEEE Trans. Neural Networks 11(3), 668–679 (2000)
23. Kohavi, R., Provost, F.: Glossary of Terms. Machine Learning 30(2/3), 271–274 (1998)
24. Mendes, R., Cortez, P., Rocha, M., Neves, J.: Particle Swarms for Feedforward Neural Network Training. In: Proceedings of The 2002 International Joint Conference on Neural Networks (IJCNN 2002), May 2002, pp. 1895–1899. IEEE Computer Society Press, Honolulu, Havai, USA (2002)
25. Mitchell, T.: Machine Learning. McGraw-Hill, New York (1997)
26. Piatetsky-Shapiro, G.: Software Suites for Data Mining, Analytics, and Knowledge Discovery (2010), http://www.kdnuggets.com/software/suites.html
27. Provost, F., Domingos, P.: Tree Induction for Probability-Based Ranking. Machine Learning 52(3), 199–215 (2003)
28. Pyle, D.: Data Preparation for Data Mining. Morgan Kaufmann, San Francisco (1999)
29. Rocha, M., Cortez, P., Neves, J.: Evolution of Neural Networks for Classification and Regression. Neurocomputing 70, 2809–2816 (2007)
30. Sarle, W.: Neural Network Frequently Asked Questions (2002), ftp://ftp.sas.com/pub/neural/FAQ.html
31. Setiono, R.: Techniques for Extracting Classification and Regression Rules from Artificial Neural Networks. In: Fogel, D., Robinson, C. (eds.) Computational Intelligence: The Experts Speak, pp. 99–114. IEEE, Piscataway (2003)
32. Silva, Á., Cortez, P., Santos, M.F., Gomes, L., Neves, J.: Rating organ failure via adverse events using data mining in the intensive care unit. Artificial Intelligence in Medicine 43(3), 179–193 (2008)
33. Smola, A., Schölkopf, B.: A tutorial on support vector regression. Statistics and Computing 14, 199–222 (2004)
34. Smola, A., Schölkopf, B.: Kernel-Machines.Org (2010), http://www.kernel-machines.org/

35. Turban, E., Sharda, R., Delen, D.: Decision Support and Business Intelligence Systems, 9th edn. Prentice Hall, Englewood Cliffs (2010)
36. Venables, W., Ripley, B.: Modern Applied Statistics with S, 4th edn. Springer, Heidelberg (2003)
37. Wang, W., Xu, Z., Lu, W., Zhang, X.: Determination of the spread parameter in the Gaussian kernel for classification and regression. Neurocomputing 55(3), 643–663 (2003)
38. Witten, I.H., Frank, E.: Data Mining: Practical Machine Learning Tools and Techniques with Java Implementations. Morgan Kaufmann, San Francisco (2005)
39. Wu, T.F., Lin, C.J., Weng, R.C.: Probability estimates for multi-class classification by pairwise coupling. The Journal of Machine Learning Research 5, 975–1005 (2004)
40. Wu, X., Kumar, V., Quinlan, J., Gosh, J., Yang, Q., Motoda, H., MacLachlan, G., Ng, A., Liu, B., Yu, P., Zhou, Z., Steinbach, M., Hand, D., Steinberg, D.: Top 10 algorithms in data mining. Knowledge and Information Systems 14(1), 1–37 (2008)

Chapter 3
Regulatory Networks under Ellipsoidal Uncertainty – Data Analysis and Prediction by Optimization Theory and Dynamical Systems

Erik Kropat[1], Gerhard-Wilhelm Weber[2], and Chandra Sekhar Pedamallu[3]

[1] Universität der Bundeswehr München, Institute for Theoretical Computer Science, Mathematics and Operations Research
Werner-Heisenberg-Weg 39, 85577 Neubiberg, Germany
erik.kropat@unibw.de

[2] Middle East Technical University, Institute of Applied Mathematics, 06531 Ankara, Turkey
Faculty of Economics, Business and Law, University of Siegen, Germany;
Center for Research on Optimization and Control, University of Aveiro, Portugal;
Faculty of Science, Universiti Teknologi Malaysia, Skudai, Malaysia
gweber@metu.edu.tr

[3] Bioinformatics Group, New England Biolabs Inc,
240 County Road, Ipswich, MA 01938, USA
pcs.murali@gmail.com

Abstract. We introduce and analyze time-discrete target-environment regulatory systems (TE-systems) under ellipsoidal uncertainty. The uncertain states of clusters of target and environmental items of the regulatory system are represented in terms of ellipsoids and the interactions between the various clusters are defined by affine-linear coupling rules. The parameters of the coupling rules and the time-dependent states of clusters define the regulatory network. Explicit representations of the uncertain multivariate states of the system are determined with ellipsoidal calculus. In addition, we introduce various regression models that allow us to determine the unknown system parameters from uncertain (ellipsoidal) measurement data by applying semidefinite programming and interior point methods. Finally, we turn to rarefications of the regulatory network. We present a corresponding mixed integer regression problem and achieve a further relaxation by means of continuous optimization. We analyze the structure of the optimization problems obtained, especially, in view of their solvability, we discuss the structural frontiers and research challenges, and we conclude with an outlook.

Keywords: regulatory systems, continuous optimization, mixed integer programming, mathematical modeling, uncertainty, networks, operations research, parameter estimation, dynamical systems, gene-environment networks, eco-finance networks.

1 Introduction

Regulatory networks are often characterized by the presence of a large number of variables and parameters resulting in a complexity which is beyond man's everyday

D.E. Holmes, L.C. Jain (Eds.): Data Mining: Found. & Intell. Paradigms, ISRL 24, pp. 27–56.
springerlink.com

perception. The development of high throughput technologies led to a generation of massive quantities of data and this technological progress has been accompanied by the development of new mathematical methods for the analysis of highly interconnected systems that allows to gain deeper insights in the dynamic behaviour and the topological aspects of complex regulatory systems in biology, finance and engineering sciences.

In this paper, we address the special class of so-called *TE-regulatory systems* (Target-Environment regulatory systems). These systems are composed of two distinct groups of data, exhibiting a completely different behaviour, although they are strongly related. The first group consists of the *targets*; these are the most important variables of the system and they depend on an additional group of so-called *environmental items*. This specific type of regulatory systems occurs in many applications. For example, in modeling and prediction of gene-expression and environmental patterns, so-called *gene-environment networks* are investigated in order to determine the complex interactions between genes and other components of cells and tissues. Here, the target variables are the expression values of the genes while the environmental items are given by toxins, transcription factors, radiation, etc. [1, 19, 24, 25, 26, 27, 28, 29, 35, 38, 55, 57, 66, 67, 68, 75, 76, 82, 83, 88, 89, 90, 91, 94, 95].

In Operational Research, *eco-finance networks* were introduced in [43] and applied to an extension of the Technology-Emissions-Means Model (in short: TEM-model), which allows a simulation of the cooperative economic behaviour of countries or enterprises with the aim of a reduction of greenhouse gas emissions. Here, the target variables are the emissions that the actors wish to reduce and the required financial means act as additional environmental items [36, 39, 40, 41, 47, 59, 60, 61, 62].

As it is clearly understood today, environmental factors constitute an essential group of regulating components and by including these additional variables the models performance can be significantly improved. The advantage of such an refinement has been demonstrated for example in [48], where it is shown that prediction and classification performances of supervised learning methods for the most complex genome-wide human disease classification can be greatly improved by considering environmental aspects. Many other examples from biology and life sciences refer to TE-regulatory systems where environmental effects are strongly involved. Among them are, e.g., *metabolic networks* [17, 58, 88], *immunological networks* [32], *social-* and *ecological networks* [30]. We refer to [27, 36, 66, 67, 68, 94, 95] for applications, practical examples and numerical calculations.

TE-models are usually based on measurements which are always effected by random noise and uncertainty. In order to include errors and uncertainty in TE-regulatory systems various regression models based on interval arithmetics but also on spline regression and stochastic differential equations have been developed. In particular, *generalized additive models* and models based on *multivariate adaptive regression splines* (MARS) have been introduced and the related *Tikhonov regularization problem* was treated by methods from *conic quadratic programming* [69, 70, 71, 72, 73, 74, 92, 93]. In general, for data corrupted by random noise the probability function is usually assumed to be Gaussian. This assumption has computational advantages but this approach is not sufficient as in case of real world data one has to include non-Gaussian or non-white noise. To overcome these difficulties, set theoretic approaches can be used where bounds on the uncertain variable are imposed. Here, we focus on *ellipsoids* which have proved to be suitable for data corrupted by noise. Ellipsoids are very flexible with respect to correlations of the data, while intervals and parallelpipes usually come from a perspective where stochastic dependencies among any two of the errors made in the measurements of the expression values of targets and environmental levels are not taken into account explicitly [8]. Moreover, these sets are usually smaller than the ellipsoids and their orthogonal projections into the 2-dimensional Cartesian planes, respectively [8]. Indeed, those confidence ellipsoids are obtained with respect to stochastic dependencies of the error variables. Those dependencies are the case in reality, e.g., in microarray experiments and in environmental studies as well. In reverse, any ellipsoid can be inscribed into a sufficiently large parallelpipe which, in addition, could be suitably located and directed in space around its eigenaxes.

There is a rich list of roles and performances delivered which are associated and assigned to ellipsoids. They include: *(i)* encompassing of objects, *(ii)* inner or outer approximation of shapes and bodies, of discrete or continuous kinds of sets, *(iii)* support for classification of objects and discrimination of different objects, *(iv)* defining critical points or contours which mark tails of higher dimensional and connected versions of tails that describe neighbourhoods of infinity, usually with small values of small probabilities assigned, *(v)* set-valued generalizations of numbers, and generalizations of balls with a reduced wealth of symmetries but still highly symmetrical, *(vi)* geometrical representation of linear mappings which execute certain expansions and contractions (herewith, deformation; e.g., applied to a ball) and rotations, with respect to axes in an orthogonal system of coordinates, *(vi)* geometrical representation of some symmetry breakings, compared with balls, *(vii)* geometrical representation of dependencies, especially, of variances and correlations, *(viii)* easy measurability and support for an approximate measuring of other sets and subsets.

Clustering and *classification* provides an insight in the structure of the data and allows to identify groups of data items jointly acting on other clusters of target and environmental items. The uncertain states of these clusters are represented by ellipsoids and ellipsoidal calculus is applied to model the dynamics of the TE-regulatory system. *Affine-linear transformations* define the coupling rules which describe the multiple interactions between the clusters and lead to a propagation of ellipsoidal states. The unknown parameters of the time-discrete TE-model are also arranged in clusters and have to be adapted according to uncertain (ellipsoidal) measurement data. Various *regression models* will be introduced which compare measurements and predictions. For parameter estimation we have to measure the size of certain ellipsoids which will be expressed by nonnegative criteria functions associated with the configuration matrix of the ellipsoid. The trace, the trace of square, the determinant or the volume are examples of such measures and they lead to different regression models for parameter estimation of the TE-model. In particular, *semidefinite programming* as well as *conic programming* and *interior point methods* can be applied to solve the various regression models.

Complex regulatory systems usually consist of a large number of interconnected components and the TE-regulatory network is highly structured with multiple interactions between many different clusters. For practical reasons, it may be necessary to reduce the number of branches of the TE-regulatory network. In this situation, bounds on the indegrees of the nodes (clusters) can reduce the complexity of the model. Binary constraints can be used to decide whether or not there is a connection between pairs of clusters. Adding these additional constraints to the objective function of the regression problem, we obtain a *mixed integer optimization problem* which corresponds to our network rarefication. However, binary constraints are very strict and in some situations they can even destroy the connectivity of the regulatory network. In order to avoid these difficulties, the binary constraints can be replaced by more flexible continuous constraints leading to a further *relaxation* in terms of *continuous optimization*.

The paper is organized as follows: In Section 2, we state some basic facts about ellipsoids and introduce basic operations of ellipsoidal calculus. In Section 3, we introduce the time-discrete TE-model under ellipsoidal uncertainty. Explicit representations of the predictions of this model are given in Section 3.2. In Section 4, we turn to an estimation of parameters of the TE-model and introduce various regression models. We discuss their solvability by semidefinite programming and interior point methods. Reduction of complexity will be addressed in Section 5, where an associated mixed integer approximation problem and a further relaxation based on continuous optimization are introduced.

2 Ellipsoidal Calculus

The states of target and environmental variables of our TE-model will be represented in terms of ellipsoids. In this section, we introduce the basic operations needed to deal with ellipsoidal uncertainty such as *sums*, *intersections (fusions)* and *affine-linear transformations* of ellipsoids. The family of ellipsoids in $\mathbb{R}^p$ is closed with respect to affine-linear transformations but neither the sum nor the intersection is generally ellipsoidal, so both must be approximated by ellipsoidal sets.

2.1 Ellipsoidal Descriptions

An *ellipsoid* in $\mathbb{R}^p$ will be parameterized in terms of its center $c \in \mathbb{R}^p$ and a symmetric non-negative definite *configuration matrix* $\Sigma \in \mathbb{R}^{p \times p}$ as

$$\mathcal{E}(c, \Sigma) = \{\Sigma^{1/2}u + c \,|\, \|u\| \leq 1\},$$

where $\Sigma^{1/2}$ is any matrix square root satisfying $\Sigma^{1/2}(\Sigma^{1/2})^T = \Sigma$. When Σ is of full rank, the non-degenerate ellipsoid $\mathcal{E}(c, \Sigma)$ may be expressed as

$$\mathcal{E}(c, \Sigma) = \{x \in \mathbb{R}^p \,|\, (x - c)^T \Sigma^{-1} (x - c) \leq 1\}.$$

The eigenvectors of Σ point in the directions of principal semiaxes of $\mathcal{E}$. The lengths of the semiaxes of the ellipsoid $\mathcal{E}(c, \Sigma)$ are given by $\sqrt{\lambda_i}$, where λ_i are the eigenvalues of Σ for $i = 1, \ldots, p$. The volume of the ellipsoid $\mathcal{E}(c, \Sigma)$ is given by $\operatorname{vol} \mathcal{E}(c, \Sigma) = V_p \sqrt{\det(\Sigma)}$, where V_p is the volume of the unit ball in $\mathbb{R}^p$, i.e.,

$$V_p = \begin{cases} \dfrac{\pi^{p/2}}{(p/2)!} & , \text{ for even } p \\[2ex] \dfrac{2^p \pi^{(p-1)/2}((p-1)/2)!}{p!} & , \text{ for odd } p. \end{cases}$$

2.2 Affine Transformations

The family of ellipsoids is closed with respect to *affine transformations*. Given an ellipsoid $\mathcal{E}(c, \Sigma) \subset \mathbb{R}^p$, matrix $A \in \mathbb{R}^{m \times p}$ and vector $b \in \mathbb{R}^m$ we get $A\mathcal{E}(c, \Sigma) + b = \mathcal{E}(Ac + b, A\Sigma A^T)$. Thus, ellipsoids are preserved under affine transformation. If the rows of A are linearly independent (which implies $m \leq p$), and $b = 0$, the affine transformation is called *projection* [45].

2.3 Sums of Two Ellipsoids

Given two non-degenerate ellipsoids $\mathcal{E}_1 = \mathcal{E}(c_1, \Sigma_1)$ and $\mathcal{E}_2 = \mathcal{E}(c_2, \Sigma_2)$, their *geometric (Minkowksi) sum* $\mathcal{E}_1 + \mathcal{E}_1 = \{z_1 + z_2 \,|\, z_1 \in \mathcal{E}_1,\ z_2 \in \mathcal{E}_2\}$ is not generally an ellipsoid. However, it can be tightly approximated by parameterized families of external ellipsoids. The range of values of $\mathcal{E}_1 + \mathcal{E}_1$ is contained in the ellipsoid

$$\mathcal{E}_1 \oplus \mathcal{E}_1 := \mathcal{E}(c_1 + c_2, \Sigma(s))$$

for all $s > 0$, where

$$\Sigma(s) = (1 + s^{-1})\Sigma_1 + (1 + s)\Sigma_2.$$

For a *minimal* and *unique* external ellipsoidal approximation an additional condition has to be fulfilled. The value of s is commonly chosen to minimize either the trace or the determinant of $\Sigma(s)$. If we select

$$s = \frac{(\mathrm{Tr}\,\Sigma_1)^{1/2}}{(\mathrm{Tr}\,\Sigma_2)^{1/2}},$$

then this value defines the ellipsoid containing the sum that has minimal trace, or, sum of squares of semiaxes. We note that the minimum trace calculation can also be used in case of degenerate ellipsoids [22, 44, 45].

2.4 Sums of K Ellipsoids

Given K bounded ellipsoids of $\mathbb{R}^p$, $\mathcal{E}_k = \mathcal{E}(c_k, \Sigma_k)$, $k = 1, \ldots, K$. We adapt the notion of the minimal trace ellipsoid from [21] and introduce the outer ellipsoidal approximation $\mathcal{E}(\sigma, P) = \oplus_{k=1}^{K} \mathcal{E}_k$ containing the sum $\mathcal{S} = \sum_{k=1}^{K} \mathcal{E}_k$ of ellipsoids which is defined by

$$\sigma = \sum_{k=1}^{K} c_k$$

and

$$P = \left(\sum_{k=1}^{K} \sqrt{\mathrm{Tr}\,\Sigma_k}\right)\left(\sum_{k=1}^{K} \frac{\Sigma_k}{\sqrt{\mathrm{Tr}\,\Sigma_k}}\right).$$

2.5 Intersection of Ellipsoids

As the intersection of two ellipsoids is generally not an ellipsoid we replace this set by the outer ellipsoidal approximation of minimal volume. We adapt the notion of *fusion* of ellipsoids from [64]. Given two non-degenerate ellipsoids $\mathcal{E}(c_1, \Sigma_1)$ and $\mathcal{E}(c_2, \Sigma_2)$ in $\mathbb{R}^p$ with $\mathcal{E}(c_1, \Sigma_1) \cap \mathcal{E}(c_2, \Sigma_2) \neq \emptyset$ we define an ellipsoid

$$\begin{aligned}\mathcal{E}_\lambda(c_0, \Sigma_0) := \{x \in \mathbb{R}^p \mid \lambda(x - c_1)^T \Sigma_1^{-1}(x - c_1) \\ + (1 - \lambda)(x - c_2)^T \Sigma_2^{-1}(x - c_2) \leq 1\},\end{aligned}$$

where $\lambda \in [0, 1]$.

The ellipsoid $\mathcal{E}_\lambda(c_0, \Sigma_0)$ coincides with $\mathcal{E}(c_1, \Sigma_1)$ and $\mathcal{E}(c_2, \Sigma_2)$ for $\lambda = 1$ and $\lambda = 0$, respectively. In order to determine a tight external ellipsoidal approximation $\mathcal{E}_\lambda(c_0, \Sigma_0)$ of the intersection of $\mathcal{E}(c_1, \Sigma_1)$ and $\mathcal{E}(c_2, \Sigma_2)$, we introduce

$$\mathcal{X} := \lambda \Sigma_1^{-1} + (1 - \lambda)\Sigma_2^{-1}$$

and

$$\tau := 1 - \lambda(1 - \lambda)(c_2 - c_1)^T \Sigma_2^{-1} \mathcal{X}^{-1} \Sigma_1^{-1}(c_2 - c_1).$$

The ellipsoid $\mathcal{E}_\lambda(c_0, \Sigma_0)$ is given by the center

$$c_0 = \mathcal{X}^{-1}(\lambda \Sigma_1^{-1} c_1 + (1 - \lambda)\Sigma_2^{-1} c_2)$$

and configuration matrix

$$\Sigma_0 = \tau \mathcal{X}^{-1}.$$

The *fusion* of $\mathcal{E}(c_1, \Sigma_1)$ and $\mathcal{E}(c_2, \Sigma_2)$, whose intersection is a nonempty bounded region, is defined as the ellipsoid $\mathcal{E}_\lambda(c_0, \Sigma_0)$ for the value $\lambda \in [0, 1]$ that minimizes its volume [64]. The fusion of $\mathcal{E}(c_1, \Sigma_1)$ and $\mathcal{E}(c_2, \Sigma_2)$ is $\mathcal{E}(c_1, \Sigma_1)$, if $\mathcal{E}(c_1, \Sigma_1) \subset \mathcal{E}(c_2, \Sigma_2)$; or $\mathcal{E}(c_2, \Sigma_2)$, if $\mathcal{E}(c_2, \Sigma_2) \subset \mathcal{E}(c_1, \Sigma_1)$; otherwise, it is $\mathcal{E}_\lambda(c_0, \Sigma_0)$ defined as above where λ is the only root in $(0, 1)$ of the following polynomial of degree $2p - 1$:

$$\begin{aligned}&\tau(\det \mathcal{X}) \operatorname{Tr}(\operatorname{co}(\mathcal{X})(\Sigma_1^{-1} - \Sigma_2^{-1})) - p(\det \mathcal{X})^2 \\ &\times (2c_0^T \Sigma_1^{-1} c_1 - 2c_0^T \Sigma_2^{-1} c_2 + c_0^T (\Sigma_2^{-1} - \Sigma_1^{-1}) c_0 - c_1^T \Sigma_1^{-1} c_1 + c_2^T \Sigma_2^{-1} c_2) = 0.\end{aligned}$$

Here, $\operatorname{co}(\mathcal{X})$ denotes the matrix of cofactors of $\mathcal{X}$. Since $\mathcal{X}^{-1} = \operatorname{co}(\mathcal{X})/\det \mathcal{X}$, we represent this polynomial as

$$\begin{aligned}&\tau(\det \mathcal{X})^2 \operatorname{Tr}(\mathcal{X}^{-1}(\Sigma_1^{-1} - \Sigma_2^{-1})) - p(\det \mathcal{X})^2 \\ &\times (2c_0^T \Sigma_1^{-1} c_1 - 2c_0^T \Sigma_2^{-1} c_2 + c_0^T (\Sigma_2^{-1} - \Sigma_1^{-1}) c_0 - c_1^T \Sigma_1^{-1} c_1 + c_2^T \Sigma_2^{-1} c_2) = 0.\end{aligned}$$

We note that it is also possible to define an inner ellipsoidal approximation. The method of finding the internal ellipsoidal approximation of the intersection of two ellipsoids is described in [77].

3 Target-Environment Regulatory Systems under Ellipsoidal Uncertainty

In this section, we introduce a time-discrete model for TE-regulatory systems under ellipsoidal uncertainty. This approach is based on clustering of the sets of targets and environmental items what refers to combinations of variables commonly exerting influence on other groups of system variables. The uncertain states of these clusters are represented in terms of ellipsoids which provide a more detailed description of uncertainty that reflects the correlation of data items. The dynamic behaviour of the clusters and their interactions are determined by clusters of unknown parameters which directly depend on the structure of the system variables. This approach further extends the time-discrete models developed for an analysis of gene-environment networks and eco-finance networks where errors and uncertainty are represented by intervals [43, 84, 85, 87].

3.1 The Time-Discrete Model

In our time-discrete TE-regulatory system, we consider n target variables and m environmental factors. Motivated by the applications presented in the introduction we assume that functionally related groups of targets and environmental items are identified in a preprocessing step of clustering and data analysis. In particular, the set of targets can be divided in R disjoint or overlapping clusters $C_r \subset \{1, \ldots, n\}$, $r = 1, \ldots, R$. Similarly, the set of all environmental items can be divided in S (disjoint or overlapping) clusters $D_s \subset \{1, \ldots, m\}$, $s = 1, \ldots, S$. In case of disjoint clusters the relations $C_{r_1} \cap C_{r_2} = \emptyset$ for all $r_1 \neq r_2$ and $D_{s_1} \cap D_{s_2} = \emptyset$ for all $s_1 \neq s_2$ are fulfilled. The papers [2, 11, 12, 56, 78] introduce into clustering theory as a central element of unsupervised learning and data mining, and they discuss the questions of how to determine the number of clusters and of the stability of the clustering. For clustering techniques based on *nonsmooth optimization* we refer to [9, 10].

Since each cluster corresponds to a functionally related group of data items, the uncertain states of these clusters are represented in terms of ellipsoids

$$\mathcal{E}(\mu_r, \Sigma_r) \subset \mathbb{R}^{|C_r|}, \quad \mathcal{E}(\rho_s, \Pi_s) \subset \mathbb{R}^{|D_s|}.$$

We note that ellipsoids can be identified with intervals if clusters are singletons. In addition, flat ellipsoids $\mathcal{E}(\mu_r, \Sigma_r)$ and $\mathcal{E}(\rho_s, \Pi_s)$ would refer to data sets where at least one of the variables is exactly known, but, if necessary in the approximating sense, we can avoid this by an artificial extension in the corresponding coordinate directions of length $\varepsilon > 0$. In other words, one can impose lower bounds on the semiaxes lengths. Similarly, one can control the extension by imposing sufficiently large upper bounds and, thus, avoid needle-shaped or degenerate ellipsoids.

The dynamic behaviour of the time-discrete TE-regulatory system is governed by affine-linear coupling rules which describe the interactions between the various clusters. These affine-linear relations have to reflect the mutual dependence of pairs of clusters but also overlaps of clusters have to be taken into account.

The *regulatory system of the target items* is defined by

(1) the interactions between the clusters of target items
(represented by an $n \times n$-*interaction matrix* A^{TT} and an n-*intercept vector* V^{TT}),

(2) the effects of the clusters of environmental items on the target clusters
(represented by an $n \times m$ *interaction-matrix* A^{TE} and an n-*intercept vector* V^{TE}).

The entries of the interaction matrices A^{TT}, A^{TE} and the intercept vectors V^{TT}, V^{TE} comprise the unknown parameters of the regulatory system. Clusters of parameters, given by specific sub-matrices and sub-vectors of A^{TT}, A^{TE} and V^{TT}, V^{TE}, define the affine-linear coupling rules. In order to describe the interactions between the clusters of target items we assign a sub-matrix $\Gamma_{jr}^{TT} \in \mathbb{R}^{|C_j| \times |C_r|}$ of A^{TT} to each pair C_j and C_r (the elements of C_j and C_r determine the indices of rows and columns). This sub-matrix can in turn be considered as a *connectivity matrix* between the clusters C_j and C_r that represents the (uncertain) degree of connectivity between the elements of the two clusters of targets. Later we will add an additional shift (intercept) by the sub-vector $\Phi_j^{TT} \in \mathbb{R}^{|C_j|}$ of V^{TT}. We note that the sub-matrices Γ_{jr}^{TT} and sub-vectors Φ_j^{TT} will be partly composed of the same elements in case of overlapping clusters.

In an analogous manner we can describe the effects of the clusters of environmental items on the target clusters. For each pair of target clusters C_j and environmental clusters D_s we define a sub-matrix $\Gamma_{js}^{TE} \in \mathbb{R}^{|C_j| \times |D_s|}$ (the elements of C_j and D_s determine the indices of rows and columns) and a sub-vector $\Phi_j^{TE} \in \mathbb{R}^{|C_j|}$ of V^{TE}. The sub-matrix Γ_{js}^{TE} acts as a *connectivity matrix* between the clusters C_j and D_s and Φ_j^{TE} acts as a shift.

Beside the regulatory system of target variables, there can be an additional *environmental regulatory system* which is defined by

(3) the interactions between the clusters of environmental items
(represented by an $m \times m$ interaction-matrix A^{EE} and an m-intercept vector V^{EE}),

(4) the effects of the target clusters on the environmental clusters
(represented by an $m \times n$ interaction-matrix A^{ET} and an m-intercept vector V^{ET}).

The degree of connectivity between pairs of environmental clusters D_i and D_s or a pair of environmental and target clusters, D_i and C_r, is given by the sub-matrices $\Gamma_{is}^{EE} \in \mathbb{R}^{|D_i| \times |D_s|}$ of A^{EE} and $\Gamma_{ir}^{ET} \in \mathbb{R}^{|D_i| \times |C_r|}$ of A^{ET} as well as the sub-vectors $\Phi_i^{EE} \in \mathbb{R}^{|D_i|}$ of V^{EE} and $\Phi_i^{ET} \in \mathbb{R}^{|D_i|}$ of V^{ET}.

Now we introduce our time-discrete model that allows us to calculate predictions $X_r^{(k)}$ and $E_s^{(k)}$ of the ellipsoidal states targets and environmental variables.

TE-Model

For $k = 0, 1, 2, \ldots$

For $j = 1, 2, \ldots, R$:

(1) **Interactions between the clusters of targets**

(A) Effect of cluster C_r on cluster C_j

$$G_{jr}^{(k)} = \Gamma_{jr}^{TT} \cdot X_r^{(k)} + \Phi_j^{TT}, \ r = 1, 2, \ldots, R$$

(B) Sum of the effects of all clusters of targets on cluster C_j

$$G_j^{(k)} = \bigoplus_{r=1}^{R} G_{jr}^{(k)}$$

(2) **Effects of the environmental clusters on the clusters of targets**

(A) Effect of environmental cluster D_s on target cluster C_j

$$H_{js}^{(k)} = \Gamma_{js}^{TE} \cdot E_s^{(k)} + \Phi_j^{TE}, \ s = 1, 2, \ldots, S$$

(B) Sum of the effects of all environmental clusters on cluster C_j

$$H_j^{(k)} = \bigoplus_{s=1}^{S} H_{js}^{(k)}$$

(3) **Sum of effects on the target clusters**

$$\boldsymbol{X}_j^{(k+1)} = \boldsymbol{G}_j^{(k)} \oplus \boldsymbol{H}_j^{(k)}$$

For $i = 1, 2, \ldots, S$:

(1) **Interactions between the clusters of environmental items**

(A) Effect of cluster D_s on cluster D_i

$$M_{is}^{(k)} = \Gamma_{is}^{EE} \cdot E_s^{(k)} + \Phi_i^{EE}, \ s = 1, 2, \ldots, S$$

(B) Sum of the effects of all environmental clusters on cluster D_i

$$M_i^{(k)} = \bigoplus_{s=1}^{S} M_{is}^{(k)}$$

(2) **Effects of the target clusters on the clusters of environmental items**

(A) Effect of target cluster C_r on environmental cluster D_i

$$N_{ir}^{(k)} = \Gamma_{ir}^{ET} \cdot X_r^{(k)} + \Phi_i^{ET}, \ r = 1, 2, \ldots, R$$

(B) Sum of the effects of all target clusters on environmental cluster D_i

$$N_i^{(k)} = \bigoplus_{r=1}^{R} N_{ir}^{(k)}$$

(3) **Sum of effects on clusters of environmental items**

$$\boldsymbol{E}_i^{(k+1)} = \boldsymbol{M}_i^{(k)} \oplus \boldsymbol{N}_i^{(k)}$$

Since $\Gamma_{jr}^{TT} \cdot X_r^{(k)} + \Phi_j^{TT}$, $\Gamma_{js}^{TE} \cdot E_s^{(k)} + \Phi_j^{TE}$, $\Gamma_{is}^{EE} \cdot E_s^{(k)} + \Phi_i^{EE}$ and $\Gamma_{ir}^{ET} \cdot X_r^{(k)} + \Phi_i^{ET}$ are affine-linear transformations, the sets $G_{jr}^{(k)}$, $H_{js}^{(k)}$, $M_{is}^{(k)}$ and $N_{ir}^{(k)}$ are ellipsoids. In addition, $G_j^{(k)}$, $H_j^{(k)}$, $M_i^{(k)}$ and $N_i^{(k)}$ are defined as sums of ellipsoids and, therefore, constitute ellipsoids themselves. Therefore, the above algorithm allows us to calculate predictions

$$\left(X_1^{(k+1)}, \ldots, X_R^{(k+1)}, E_1^{(k+1)}, \ldots, E_S^{(k+1)}\right)$$

of the ellipsoidal states of targets and environmental items. In the next subsection, we investigate the structure of the ellipsoids and determine the corresponding centers and configuration matrices.

$$A^{TT} = \left[\begin{array}{cc|cc|cc} a_{11}^{TT} & a_{12}^{TT} & a_{13}^{TT} & a_{14}^{TT} & a_{15}^{TT} & a_{16}^{TT} \\ a_{21}^{TT} & a_{22}^{TT} & a_{23}^{TT} & a_{24}^{TT} & a_{25}^{TT} & a_{26}^{TT} \\ \hline a_{31}^{TT} & a_{32}^{TT} & a_{33}^{TT} & a_{34}^{TT} & a_{35}^{TT} & a_{36}^{TT} \\ a_{41}^{TT} & a_{42}^{TT} & a_{43}^{TT} & a_{44}^{TT} & a_{45}^{TT} & a_{46}^{TT} \\ \hline a_{51}^{TT} & a_{52}^{TT} & a_{53}^{TT} & a_{54}^{TT} & a_{55}^{TT} & a_{56}^{TT} \\ a_{61}^{TT} & a_{62}^{TT} & a_{63}^{TT} & a_{64}^{TT} & a_{65}^{TT} & a_{66}^{TT} \end{array}\right], \qquad \Phi^{TT} = \left[\begin{array}{c} \Phi_1^{TT} \\ \Phi_2^{TT} \\ \hline \Phi_3^{TT} \\ \Phi_4^{TT} \\ \hline \Phi_5^{TT} \\ \Phi_6^{TT} \end{array}\right]$$

$$G_{23}^{(k)} = \Gamma_{23}^{TT} \cdot X_3^{(k)} + \Phi_2^{TT} = \begin{pmatrix} a_{33}^{TT} & a_{34}^{TT} \\ a_{43}^{TT} & a_{44}^{TT} \end{pmatrix} \cdot X_3^{(k)} + \begin{pmatrix} \Phi_3^{TT} \\ \Phi_4^{TT} \end{pmatrix}$$

Fig. 1. Interaction matrices and intercept vectors. In a TE-regulatory network with six targets and three target clusters $C_1 = \{1,2\}$, $C_2 = \{3,4\}$, $C_3 = \{5,6\}$, the interaction between target clusters C_2 and C_3 is determined by the affine-linear transformation $\Gamma_{23}^{TT} \cdot X_3^{(k)} + \Phi_2^{TT}$ given by the corresponding parts $\Gamma_{23}^{TT} = \begin{pmatrix} a_{33}^{TT} & a_{34}^{TT} \\ a_{43}^{TT} & a_{44}^{TT} \end{pmatrix}$ of the interaction matrix A^{TT} and $\Phi_2^{TT} = \begin{pmatrix} \Phi_{33}^{TT} \\ \Phi_{34}^{TT} \end{pmatrix}$ of the intercept vector Φ^{TT}.

REMARK. In the above model, the state of each cluster depends on the state of this cluster at the previous time-step. We can avoid this by introducing the following cluster interaction formulas:

$$\begin{aligned} G_{jr}^{(k)} &= (1-\delta_{jr}) \cdot \left(\Gamma_{jr}^{TT} \cdot X_r^{(k)} + \Phi_j^{TT}\right), \ r = 1,2,\ldots,R \\ H_{js}^{(k)} &= (1-\delta_{js}) \cdot \left(\Gamma_{js}^{TE} \cdot E_s^{(k)} + \Phi_j^{TE}\right), \ s = 1,2,\ldots,S \\ M_{is}^{(k)} &= (1-\delta_{is}) \cdot \left(\Gamma_{is}^{EE} \cdot E_s^{(k)} + \Phi_i^{EE}\right), \ s = 1,2,\ldots,S \\ N_{ir}^{(k)} &= (1-\delta_{ir}) \cdot \left(\Gamma_{ir}^{ET} \cdot X_r^{(k)} + \Phi_i^{ET}\right), \ r = 1,2,\ldots,R, \end{aligned}$$

where $\delta_{\alpha\beta}$ denotes the Kronecker-Delta.

REMARK. The relations and interconnections between the various clusters of target and environmental items of the regulatory system can be represented in terms of a highly interconnected *TE-regulatory network* (Target-Environment regulatory network). The nodes of this network are given by the clusters and the branches are weighted by the matrices and vectors that determine the affine linear coupling rules of the TE-model. Additional weights can be assigned to the nodes of the network. This can be, e.g., the ellipsoids (or some measures of the size of the ellipsoids) associated with the clusters. Although the weights of the branches are static, the evolution of ellipsoids leads to a time-dependent *TE-regulatory network*. Hereby, discrete mathematics and its network algorithms in both versions, statically and dynamically, becomes applicable on subjects such as connectedness, components, clusters, cycles, shortest paths or further subnetworks. Beside these discrete-combinatorial aspects, combinatorial relations between graphs and (nonlinear) optimization problems as well as topological properties of regulatory networks can be analyzed [42]. When we regard the matrices of interactions as a map, then we can "navigate" between the different entries [82, 83]. This can be considered as a focus and control about the dynamics of, e.g., medical, environmental or financial items and their change rates. This kind of navigation is represented by discrete homotopies within the matrices and by continuous homotopies between the underlying ellipsoids. This very much depends on the structures of overlapping or (projective) intersections of these ellipsoidal sets, which are of a polynomial definition [13, 15, 31]. Via such intersections and, covering the paths of navigation, unions of ellipsoids, we in fact arrive at real semialgebraic sets. Then, these classes represent the uncertainty which we study in this paper and take the place of σ-algebras that we would employ from an alternative stochastic viewpoint. We note that the study of our paths of navigation can be analyzed by homotopy theory [31]. The paper [63] gives example how conic, especially, semidefinite programming comes into play via introducing semialgebraic sets, and we remark that the normal forms (sums of squares of polynomials) relate with regression theory where also conic quadratic programming serves for [13, 15, 31]. In forthcoming papers, we shall work out these various new aspects.

3.2 Algorithm

With the TE-Model we can calculate predictions of the ellipsoidal states $X_r^{(k)}$ and $E_s^{(k)}$ of targets and environmental items in terms of subsets of $\mathbb{R}^{|C_r|}$ and $\mathbb{R}^{|D_s|}$, respectively. Now, we introduce an algorithm that can be used to determine centers and configuration matrices of the predictions obtained from the TE-model.

At time step $k \in \mathbb{N}_0$ these predictions are given by the ellipsoids

$$X_r^{(k)} = \mathcal{E}\big(\mu_r^{(k)}, \Sigma_r^{(k)}\big) \quad \text{and} \quad E_s^{(k)} = \mathcal{E}\big(\rho_s^{(k)}, \Pi_s^{(k)}\big).$$

Applying the ellipsoidal calculus from Section 2, we obtain the following algorithm:

TE-Model: Centers and Configuration Matrices

For $k = 0, 1, 2, \ldots$

For $j = 1, 2, \ldots, R$:

(1) **Interactions between the clusters of targets**

(A) Effect of cluster C_r on cluster C_j

$$g_{jr}^{(k)} = \Gamma_{jr}^{TT} \mu_r^{(k)} + \Phi_j^{TT} \quad , \; r = 1, 2, \ldots, R$$
$$\mathcal{G}_{jr}^{(k)} = \Gamma_{jr}^{TT} \Sigma_r^{(k)} (\Gamma_{jr}^{TT})^T \; , \; r = 1, 2, \ldots, R$$
$$G_{jr}^{(k)} = \mathcal{E}\big(g_{jr}^{(k)}, \mathcal{G}_{jr}^{(k)}\big) \quad , \; r = 1, 2, \ldots, R$$

(B) Sum of the effects of all clusters of targets on cluster C_j

$$g_j^{(k)} = \sum_{r=1}^{R} g_{jr}^{(k)}$$
$$\mathcal{G}_j^{(k)} = \Big(\sum_{r=1}^{R} \sqrt{\operatorname{Tr} \mathcal{G}_{jr}^{(k)}} \Big) \cdot \Big(\sum_{r=1}^{R} \frac{\mathcal{G}_{jr}^{(k)}}{\sqrt{\operatorname{Tr} \mathcal{G}_{jr}^{(k)}}} \Big)$$
$$G_j^{(k)} = \mathcal{E}\big(g_j^{(k)}, \mathcal{G}_j^{(k)}\big)$$

(2) **Effects of the environmental clusters on the clusters of targets**

(A) Effect of environmental cluster D_s on target cluster C_j

$$h_{js}^{(k)} = \Gamma_{js}^{TE} \rho_s^{(k)} + \Phi_j^{TE} \quad , \; s = 1, 2, \ldots, S$$
$$\mathcal{H}_{js}^{(k)} = \Gamma_{js}^{TE} \Pi_s^{(k)} (\Gamma_{js}^{TE})^T, \; s = 1, 2, \ldots, S$$
$$H_{js}^{(k)} = \mathcal{E}\big(h_{js}^{(k)}, \mathcal{H}_{js}^{(k)}\big) \quad , \; s = 1, 2, \ldots, S$$

(B) Sum of the effects of all environmental clusters on cluster C_j

$$h_j^{(k)} = \sum_{s=1}^{S} h_{js}^{(k)}$$
$$\mathcal{H}_j^{(k)} = \Big(\sum_{s=1}^{S} \sqrt{\operatorname{Tr} \mathcal{H}_{js}^{(k)}} \Big) \cdot \Big(\sum_{s=1}^{S} \frac{\mathcal{H}_{js}^{(k)}}{\sqrt{\operatorname{Tr} \mathcal{H}_{js}^{(k)}}} \Big)$$
$$H_j^{(k)} = \mathcal{E}\big(h_j^{(k)}, \mathcal{H}_j^{(k)}\big)$$

(3) **Sum of effects on the target clusters**

$$\mu_j^{(k+1)} = g_j^{(k)} + h_j^{(k)}$$
$$\Sigma_j^{(k+1)} = \Big(\sqrt{\operatorname{Tr} \mathcal{G}_j^{(k)}} + \sqrt{\operatorname{Tr} \mathcal{H}_j^{(k)}} \Big) \cdot \Big(\frac{\mathcal{G}_j^{(k)}}{\sqrt{\operatorname{Tr} \mathcal{G}_j^{(k)}}} + \frac{\mathcal{H}_j^{(k)}}{\sqrt{\operatorname{Tr} \mathcal{H}_j^{(k)}}} \Big)$$
$$X_j^{(k+1)} = \mathcal{E}\big(\mu_j^{(k+1)}, \Sigma_j^{(k+1)}\big)$$

TE-Model: Centers and Configuration Matrices (continued)

For $i = 1, 2, \ldots, S$:

(1) **Interactions between the clusters of environmental items**

(A) Effect of cluster D_s on cluster D_i

$$\begin{aligned} m_{is}^{(k)} &= \Gamma_{is}^{EE} \rho_s^{(k)} + \Phi_i^{EE} \quad , \; s = 1, 2, \ldots, S \\ \mathcal{M}_{is}^{(k)} &= \Gamma_{is}^{EE} \Pi_s^{(k)} (\Gamma_{is}^{EE})^T, \; s = 1, 2, \ldots, S \\ M_{is}^{(k)} &= \mathcal{E}\big(m_{is}^{(k)}, \mathcal{M}_{is}^{(k)}\big) \quad , \; s = 1, 2, \ldots, S \end{aligned}$$

(B) Sum of the effects of all environmental clusters on cluster D_i

$$\begin{aligned} m_i^{(k)} &= \sum_{s=1}^{S} m_{is}^{(k)} \\ \mathcal{M}_i^{(k)} &= \Big(\sum_{s=1}^{S} \sqrt{\operatorname{Tr} \mathcal{M}_{is}^{(k)}} \Big) \cdot \Big(\sum_{s=1}^{S} \frac{\mathcal{M}_{is}^{(k)}}{\sqrt{\operatorname{Tr} \mathcal{M}_{is}^{(k)}}} \Big) \\ M_i^{(k)} &= \mathcal{E}\big(m_i^{(k)}, \mathcal{M}_i^{(k)}\big) \end{aligned}$$

(2) **Effects of the target clusters on the clusters of environmental items**

(A) Effect of target cluster C_r on environmental cluster D_i

$$\begin{aligned} n_{ir}^{(k)} &= \Gamma_{ir}^{ET} \mu_r^{(k)} + \Phi_i^{ET} \quad , \; r = 1, 2, \ldots, R \\ \mathcal{N}_{ir}^{(k)} &= \Gamma_{ir}^{ET} \Sigma_r^{(k)} (\Gamma_{ir}^{ET})^T \quad , \; r = 1, 2, \ldots, R \\ N_{ir}^{(k)} &= \mathcal{E}\big(n_{ir}^{(k)}, \mathcal{N}_{ir}^{(k)}\big) \quad , \; r = 1, 2, \ldots, R \end{aligned}$$

(B) Sum of the effects of all target clusters on environmental cluster D_i

$$\begin{aligned} n_i^{(k)} &= \sum_{r=1}^{R} n_{ir}^{(k)} \\ \mathcal{N}_i^{(k)} &= \Big(\sum_{r=1}^{R} \sqrt{\operatorname{Tr} \mathcal{N}_{ir}^{(k)}} \Big) \cdot \Big(\sum_{r=1}^{R} \frac{\mathcal{N}_{ir}^{(k)}}{\sqrt{\operatorname{Tr} \mathcal{N}_{ir}^{(k)}}} \Big) \\ N_i^{(k)} &= \mathcal{E}\big(n_i^{(k)}, \mathcal{N}_i^{(k)}\big) \end{aligned}$$

(3) **Sum of effects on clusters of environmental items**

$$\begin{aligned} \rho_i^{(k+1)} &= m_i^{(k)} + n_i^{(k)} \\ \Pi_i^{(k+1)} &= \Big(\sqrt{\operatorname{Tr} \mathcal{M}_i^{(k)}} + \sqrt{\operatorname{Tr} \mathcal{N}_i^{(k)}} \Big) \cdot \Big(\frac{\mathcal{M}_i^{(k)}}{\sqrt{\operatorname{Tr} \mathcal{M}_i^{(k)}}} + \frac{\mathcal{N}_i^{(k)}}{\sqrt{\operatorname{Tr} \mathcal{N}_i^{(k)}}} \Big) \\ \boldsymbol{E_i^{(k+1)}} &= \boldsymbol{\mathcal{E}\big(\rho_i^{(k+1)}, \Pi_i^{(k+1)}\big)} \end{aligned}$$

4 The Regression Problem

We now turn to an estimation of parameters of the time-discrete TE-model with ellipsoidal states. As mentioned before, the states of predictions of targets and environmental items depend on the unknown entries of the interaction matrices A^{TT}, A^{TE}, A^{EE}, A^{ET} and vectors V_j^{TT}, V_j^{TE}, V_i^{EE} and V_i^{ET}. For an estimation of parameters we compare the predictions

$$\widehat{X}_r^{(\kappa)} = \mathcal{E}\big(\widehat{\mu}_r^{(\kappa)}, \widehat{\Sigma}_r^{(\kappa)}\big), \quad \widehat{E}_s^{(\kappa)} = \mathcal{E}\big(\widehat{\rho}_s^{(\kappa)}, \widehat{\Pi}_s^{(\kappa)}\big)$$

calculated with the algorithm from Subsection 3.2 with the data

$$\overline{X}_r^{(\kappa)} = \mathcal{E}\big(\overline{\mu}_r^{(\kappa)}, \overline{\Sigma}_r^{(\kappa)}\big), \quad \overline{E}_s^{(\kappa)} = \mathcal{E}\big(\overline{\rho}_s^{(\kappa)}, \overline{\Pi}_s^{(\kappa)}\big),$$

obtained from measurements of target and environmental items at sampling times $t_0 < t_1 < \ldots < t_T$. The initial values of the algorithm may be given by $\widehat{X}_r^{(0)} := \overline{X}_r^{(0)}$ and $\widehat{E}_s^{(0)} := \overline{E}_s^{(0)}$ (here, $r = 1, \ldots, R$, $s = 1, \ldots, S$, $\kappa = 0, 1, \ldots, T$).

As the predictions and measurement values (both ellipsoids) should overlap as much as possible, we introduce the ellipsoids

$$\Delta X_r^{(\kappa)} := \widehat{X}_r^{(\kappa)} \cap \overline{X}_r^{(\kappa)} \quad \text{and} \quad \Delta E_s^{(\kappa)} := \widehat{E}_s^{(\kappa)} \cap \overline{E}_s^{(\kappa)}.$$

In addition, the centers of the ellipsoids are adjusted, so that their distance

$$\Delta\mu_r^{(\kappa)} := \widehat{\mu}_r^{(\kappa)} - \overline{\mu}_r^{(\kappa)} \quad \text{and} \quad \Delta\rho_s^{(\kappa)} := \widehat{\rho}_s^{(\kappa)} - \overline{\rho}_s^{(\kappa)}$$

becomes minimized (cf. Figure 2). This leads us to the following regression problem:

$$(R) \quad \text{Maximize} \quad \sum_{\kappa=1}^{T} \Big\{ \sum_{r=1}^{R} \Big(\| \Delta X_r^{(\kappa)} \|_* - \| \Delta\mu_r^{(\kappa)} \|_2^2 \Big) + \sum_{s=1}^{S} \Big(\| \Delta E_s^{(\kappa)} \|_* - \| \Delta\rho_s^{(\kappa)} \|_2^2 \Big) \Big\}.$$

Here, $\| \cdot \|_*$ denotes a measure that reflects the geometrical size of the intersections (fusions) and we assume that $\|\Delta X_r^{(\kappa)}\|_* = 0$, if $\Delta X_r^{(\kappa)} = \emptyset$ and $\|\Delta E_s^{(\kappa)}\|_* = 0$, if $\Delta E_s^{(\kappa)} = \emptyset$. There exist various measures that are related to the shape of the intersections, e.g., the *volume* (which corresponds to the ellipsoid matrix determinant), the *sum of squares of semiaxes* (which corresponds to the trace of the configuration matrix), the *length of the largest semiaxes* (which corresponds to the eigenvalues of the configuration matrix). All these examples lead to specific formulations of the regression problem (R) and they depend on the configuration matrices of the fusions $\Delta X_r^{(\kappa)}$ and $\Delta E_s^{(\kappa)}$ as well as the distances $\Delta\mu_r^{(\kappa)}$ and $\Delta\rho_s^{(\kappa)}$.

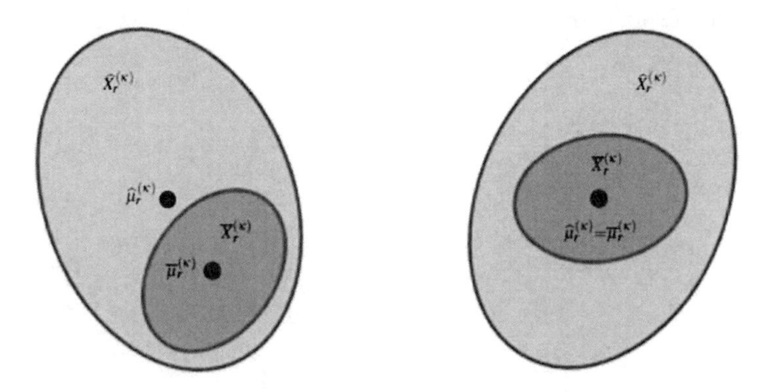

Fig. 2. Overlap of ellipsoids: The intersections of the two ellipsoids $\widehat{X}_r^{(\kappa)}$ and $\overline{X}_r^{(\kappa)}$ have the same geometrical size with the same measure of fusions on the left and the right side. On the right side, the centers $\widehat{\mu}_r^{(\kappa)}$ and $\overline{\mu}_r^{(\kappa)}$ are adjusted in order to minimize the difference between the centers of ellipsoids.

For a deeper analysis of the above stated regression problem (R), explicit representations of the fusions $\Delta X_r^{(\kappa)}$ and $\Delta\Sigma_r^{(\kappa)}$ are required. The fusion $\Delta X_r^{(\kappa)} = \widehat{X}_r^{(\kappa)} \cap \overline{X}_{C_r}^{(\kappa)}$ is an ellipsoid $\mathcal{E}\big(\Delta\mu_r^{(\kappa)}, \Delta\Sigma_r^{(\kappa)}\big)$ with center

$$\Delta\mu_r^{(\kappa)} = \big[\mathcal{X}_r^{(\kappa)}\big]^{-1}\big(\lambda\big[\widehat{\Sigma}_r^{(\kappa)}\big]^{-1}\widehat{\mu}_r^{(\kappa)} + (1-\lambda)\big[\overline{\Sigma}_r^{(\kappa)}\big]^{-1}\overline{\mu}_r^{(\kappa)}\big)$$

and configuration matrix

$$\Delta\Sigma_r^{(\kappa)} = \xi_r^{(\kappa)}\,\big[\mathcal{X}_r^{(\kappa)}\big]^{-1},$$

where

$$\mathcal{X}_r^{(\kappa)} := \lambda\big[\widehat{\Sigma}_r^{(\kappa)}\big]^{-1} + (1-\lambda)\big[\overline{\Sigma}_r^{(\kappa)}\big]^{-1}$$

and

$$\xi_r^{(\kappa)} := 1 - \lambda(1-\lambda)\big(\overline{\mu}_r^{(\kappa)} - \widehat{\mu}_r^{(\kappa)}\big)^T\big[\overline{\Sigma}_r^{(\kappa)}\big]^{-1}\big[\mathcal{X}_r^{(\kappa)}\big]^{-1}\big[\widehat{\Sigma}_r^{(\kappa)}\big]^{-1}\big(\overline{\mu}_r^{(\kappa)} - \widehat{\mu}_r^{(\kappa)}\big).$$

The parameter λ is the only root in $(0,1)$ of the following polynomial of degree $2|C_r| - 1$:

$$\begin{aligned}
&\xi_r^{(\kappa)}\big(\det\mathcal{X}_r^{(\kappa)}\big)^2\,\mathrm{Tr}\Big(\big[\mathcal{X}_r^{(\kappa)}\big]^{-1}\Big(\big[\widehat{\Sigma}_r^{(\kappa)}\big]^{-1} - \big[\overline{\Sigma}_r^{(\kappa)}\big]^{-1}\Big)\Big) - |C_r|\big(\det\mathcal{X}_r^{(\kappa)}\big)^2\\
&\times\Big(2\big[\Delta\mu_r^{(\kappa)}\big]^T\big[\widehat{\Sigma}_r^{(\kappa)}\big]^{-1}\widehat{\mu}_r^{(\kappa)} - 2\big[\Delta\mu_r^{(\kappa)}\big]^T\big[\overline{\Sigma}_r^{(\kappa)}\big]^{-1}\overline{\mu}_r^{(\kappa)}\\
&+\big[\Delta\mu_r^{(\kappa)}\big]^T\Big(\big[\overline{\Sigma}_r^{(\kappa)}\big]^{-1} - \big[\widehat{\Sigma}_r^{(\kappa)}\big]^{-1}\Big)\Delta\mu_r^{(\kappa)} - \big[\widehat{\mu}_r^{(\kappa)}\big]^T\big[\widehat{\Sigma}_r^{(\kappa)}\big]^{-1}\widehat{\mu}_r^{(\kappa)}\\
&+\big[\overline{\mu}_r^{(\kappa)}\big]^T\big[\overline{\Sigma}_r^{(\kappa)}\big]^{-1}\overline{\mu}_r^{(\kappa)}\Big) = 0.
\end{aligned}$$

Similarly, the fusion $\Delta E_s^{(\kappa)} = \widehat{E}_s^{(\kappa)} \cap \overline{E}_s^{(\kappa)}$ is an ellipsoid $\mathcal{E}\big(\Delta\rho_s^{(\kappa)}, \Delta\Pi_s^{(\kappa)}\big)$ with center

$$\Delta\rho_s^{(\kappa)} = \big[\mathcal{Y}_s^{(\kappa)}\big]^{-1}\big(\lambda\big[\widehat{\Pi}_s^{(\kappa)}\big]^{-1}\widehat{\rho}_s^{(\kappa)} + (1-\lambda)\big[\overline{\Pi}_s^{(\kappa)}\big]^{-1}\overline{\rho}_s^{(\kappa)}\big)$$

and configuration matrix

$$\Delta\Pi_s^{(\kappa)} = \eta_s^{(\kappa)}\,\big[\mathcal{Y}_s^{(\kappa)}\big]^{-1},$$

where

$$\mathcal{Y}_s^{(\kappa)} := \lambda\big[\widehat{\Pi}_s^{(\kappa)}\big]^{-1} + (1-\lambda)\big[\overline{\Pi}_s^{(\kappa)}\big]^{-1}$$

and

$$\eta_s^{(\kappa)} := 1 - \lambda(1-\lambda)\big(\overline{\rho}_s^{(\kappa)} - \widehat{\rho}_s^{(\kappa)}\big)^T\big[\overline{\Pi}_s^{(\kappa)}\big]^{-1}\big[\mathcal{Y}_s^{(\kappa)}\big]^{-1}\big[\widehat{\Pi}_s^{(\kappa)}\big]^{-1}\big(\overline{\rho}_s^{(\kappa)} - \widehat{\rho}_s^{(\kappa)}\big).$$

The parameter λ is the only root in $(0,1)$ of the following polynomial of degree $2|D_s|-1$:

$$\begin{aligned}
&\eta_s^{(\kappa)}\big(\det\mathcal{Y}_s^{(\kappa)}\big)^2\,\mathrm{Tr}\Big(\big[\mathcal{Y}_s^{(\kappa)}\big]^{-1}\Big(\big[\widehat{\Pi}_s^{(\kappa)}\big]^{-1} - \big[\overline{\Pi}_s^{(\kappa)}\big]^{-1}\Big)\Big) - |D_s|\big(\det\mathcal{Y}_s^{(\kappa)}\big)^2\\
&\times\Big(2\big[\Delta\rho_s^{(\kappa)}\big]^T\big[\widehat{\Pi}_s^{(\kappa)}\big]^{-1}\widehat{\rho}_s^{(\kappa)} - 2\big[\Delta\rho_s^{(\kappa)}\big]^T\big[\overline{\Pi}_s^{(\kappa)}\big]^{-1}\overline{\rho}_s^{(\kappa)}\\
&+\big[\Delta\rho_s^{(\kappa)}\big]^T\Big(\big[\overline{\Pi}_s^{(\kappa)}\big]^{-1} - \big[\widehat{\Pi}_s^{(\kappa)}\big]^{-1}\Big)\Delta\rho_s^{(\kappa)} - \big[\widehat{\rho}_s^{(\kappa)}\big]^T\big[\widehat{\Pi}_s^{(\kappa)}\big]^{-1}\widehat{\rho}_s^{(\kappa)}\\
&+\big[\overline{\rho}_s^{(\kappa)}\big]^T\big[\overline{\Pi}_s^{(\kappa)}\big]^{-1}\overline{\rho}_s^{(\kappa)}\Big) = 0.
\end{aligned}$$

As a measure for the size of a p-dimensional ellipsoid $\mathcal{E}(0,Q)$ (here, the size of the fusion) we use nonnegative-valued criteria functions $\psi(\mathcal{E}(0,Q))$ defined on the set of all nondegenerate ellipsoids and which are monotonous by increasing with respect to inclusion, i.e., $\psi(\mathcal{E}_1) \leq \psi(\mathcal{E}_2)$ if $\mathcal{E}_1 \subseteq \mathcal{E}_2$. Such measures are, e.g.,

(a) *the trace of* Q,

$$\psi_T(\mathcal{E}(0,Q)) := \mathrm{Tr}\,Q = \lambda_1 + \ldots + \lambda_p,$$

where λ_i are the eigenvalues of Q (i.e., $\mathrm{Tr}\,Q$ is equal to the sum of the squares of the semiaxes),

(b) *the trace of square of* Q,

$$\psi_{TS}(\mathcal{E}(0,Q)) := \mathrm{Tr}\,Q^2,$$

(c) *the determinant of* Q,

$$\psi_{Det}(\mathcal{E}(0,Q)) := \det Q = \lambda_1 \cdot \ldots \cdot \lambda_p,$$

which is equal to the product of eigenvalues and proportional to the volume

$$\mathrm{vol}\,\mathcal{E}(0,Q) = \pi^{\frac{p}{2}}\,(\det Q)^{\frac{1}{2}}\big(\Gamma\big(\tfrac{p}{2}+1\big)\big)^{-1}$$

of the ellipsoid, where Γ stands for the Gamma-function,

(d) *the diameter*,

$$\psi_{Dia}(\mathcal{E}(0,Q)) := \operatorname{diam}(\mathcal{E}(0,Q)) := d,$$

where

$$\max\{\lambda_i \in \mathbb{R} \mid i = 1,\ldots,p\} = \left(\frac{d}{2}\right)^2,$$

so that $d/2$ is the radius of the smallest p-dimensional ball that includes $\mathcal{E}(0,Q)$.

For further details on criteria functions we refer to [44], p. 101. The measures stated above lead to different representations of the regression problem (R) and we study them now in more detail.

4.1 The Trace Criterion

The first regression problem is based on the traces of the configuration matrices of the ellipsoids $\Delta X_r^{(\kappa)}$ and $\Delta E_s^{(\kappa)}$:

$$(R_{Tr}) \qquad \text{Maximize} \quad \sum_{\kappa=1}^{T} \left\{ \sum_{r=1}^{R} \left(\operatorname{Tr}\left(\Delta\Sigma_r^{(\kappa)}\right) - \|\Delta\mu_r^{(\kappa)}\|_2^2 \right) + \sum_{s=1}^{S} \left(\operatorname{Tr}\left(\Delta\Pi_s^{(\kappa)}\right) - \|\Delta\rho_s^{(\kappa)}\|_2^2 \right) \right\}.$$

As the trace of the configuration matrix is equal to the sum of the squares of the semi-axes, the regression problem takes the form

$$(R'_{Tr}) \qquad \text{Maximize} \quad \sum_{\kappa=1}^{T} \left\{ \sum_{r=1}^{R} \left(\sum_{j=1}^{|C_r|} \lambda_{r,j}^{(\kappa)} - \|\Delta\mu_r^{(\kappa)}\|_2^2 \right) + \sum_{s=1}^{S} \left(\sum_{i=1}^{|D_s|} \Lambda_{s,i}^{(\kappa)} - \|\Delta\rho_s^{(\kappa)}\|_2^2 \right) \right\},$$

where $\lambda_{r,j}^{(\kappa)}$ and $\Lambda_{s,i}^{(\kappa)}$ are the eigenvalues of $\Delta\Sigma_r^{(\kappa)}$ and $\Delta\Pi_s^{(\kappa)}$, respectively.

4.2 The Trace of the Square Criterion

Another variant of our regression problem can be obtained with the traces of the squares of the configuration matrices of the ellipsoids $\Delta X_r^{(\kappa)}$ and $\Delta E_s^{(\kappa)}$:

$$(R_{TS}) \qquad \text{Maximize} \quad \sum_{\kappa=1}^{T} \left\{ \sum_{r=1}^{R} \left(\operatorname{Tr}\left(\Delta\Sigma_r^{(\kappa)}\right)^2 - \|\Delta\mu_r^{(\kappa)}\|_2^2 \right) + \sum_{s=1}^{S} \left(\operatorname{Tr}\left(\Delta\Pi_s^{(\kappa)}\right)^2 - \|\Delta\rho_s^{(\kappa)}\|_2^2 \right) \right\}.$$

4.3 The Determinant Criterion

Referring to the determinants of the configuration matrices of the ellipsoids $\Delta X_r^{(\kappa)}$ and $\Delta E_s^{(\kappa)}$, we obtain the following model:

$$(R_{Det}) \qquad \text{Maximize} \quad \sum_{\kappa=1}^{T} \Big\{ \sum_{r=1}^{R} \Big(\det \big(\Delta \Sigma_r^{(\kappa)} \big) - \| \Delta \mu_r^{(\kappa)} \|_2^2 \Big) + \sum_{s=1}^{S} \Big(\det \big(\Delta \Pi_s^{(\kappa)} \big) - \| \Delta \rho_s^{(\kappa)} \|_2^2 \Big) \Big\}.$$

Equivalent formulations of (R_{Det}) can be given in terms of the eigenvalues of the configuration matrices

$$(R'_{Det}) \qquad \text{Maximize} \quad \sum_{\kappa=1}^{T} \Big\{ \sum_{r=1}^{R} \Big(\prod_{j=1}^{|C_r|} \lambda_{r,j}^{(\kappa)} - \| \Delta \mu_r^{(\kappa)} \|_2^2 \Big) + \sum_{s=1}^{S} \Big(\prod_{i=1}^{|D_s|} \Lambda_{s,i}^{(\kappa)} - \| \Delta \rho_s^{(\kappa)} \|_2^2 \Big) \Big\}$$

and the volumes of the ellipsoids $\Delta X_r^{(\kappa)}$ and $\Delta E_s^{(\kappa)}$

$$(R''_{Det}) \qquad \text{Maximize} \quad \sum_{\kappa=1}^{T} \Big\{ \sum_{r=1}^{R} \Big(\big[\mathcal{V}_r^{(\kappa)} \big]^2 - \| \Delta \mu_r^{(\kappa)} \|_2^2 \Big) + \sum_{s=1}^{S} \Big(\big[\mathcal{W}_s^{(\kappa)} \big]^2 - \| \Delta \rho_s^{(\kappa)} \|_2^2 \Big) \Big\},$$

where

$$\mathcal{V}_r^{(\kappa)} := \pi^{\frac{2}{|C_r|}} \, \Gamma\Big(\frac{|C_r|}{2} + 1 \Big) \operatorname{vol}\big(\Delta X_r^{(\kappa)} \big),$$
$$\mathcal{W}_s^{(\kappa)} := \pi^{\frac{2}{|D_s|}} \, \Gamma\Big(\frac{|D_s|}{2} + 1 \Big) \operatorname{vol}\big(\Delta E_s^{(\kappa)} \big).$$

4.4 The Diameter Criterion

The diameter of the ellipsoids $\Delta X_r^{(\kappa)}$ and $\Delta E_s^{(\kappa)}$ can be used to introduce the following regression model:

$$(R_{Dia}) \qquad \text{Maximize} \quad \sum_{\kappa=1}^{T} \Big\{ \sum_{r=1}^{R} \Big(\operatorname{diam}\big(\mathcal{E}(0, \Sigma_r^{(\kappa)}) \big) - \| \Delta \mu_r^{(\kappa)} \|_2^2 \Big) + \sum_{s=1}^{S} \Big(\operatorname{diam}\big(\mathcal{E}(0, \Pi_s^{(\kappa)}) \big) - \| \Delta \rho_s^{(\kappa)} \|_2^2 \Big) \Big\}.$$

An equivalent formulation of (R_{Dia}) can be given in terms of the eigenvalues of $\Sigma_r^{(\kappa)}$ and $\Pi_s^{(\kappa)}$:

$$(R'_{Dia}) \qquad \text{Maximize} \quad \sum_{\kappa=1}^{T} \Big\{ \sum_{r=1}^{R} \Big(2 \cdot \sqrt{\lambda_r^{(\kappa)}} - \| \Delta\mu_r^{(\kappa)} \|_2^2 \Big) + \sum_{s=1}^{S} \Big(2 \cdot \sqrt{\Lambda_s^{(\kappa)}} - \| \Delta\rho_s^{(\kappa)} \|_2^2 \Big) \Big\}$$

with $\lambda_r^{(\kappa)} := \max\{\lambda_{r,j}^{(\kappa)} \mid j = 1,\ldots,|C_r|\}$ and $\Lambda_s^{(\kappa)} := \max\{\Lambda_{s,i}^{(\kappa)} \mid i = 1,\ldots,|D_s|\}$. As the objective function of (R'_{Dia}) is nonsmooth with well-understood max-type functions [79, 80, 81] but not Lipschitz-continuous, we also introduce the additional regression problem

$$(R''_{Dia}) \qquad \text{Maximize} \quad \sum_{\kappa=1}^{T} \Big\{ \sum_{r=1}^{R} \Big(\lambda_r^{(\kappa)} - \| \Delta\mu_r^{(\kappa)} \|_2^2 \Big) + \sum_{s=1}^{S} \Big(\Lambda_s^{(\kappa)} - \| \Delta\rho_s^{(\kappa)} \|_2^2 \Big) \Big\}$$

as an alternative proposal.

4.5 Optimization Methods

The regression models of the previous subsections depend on the configuration matrices $\Sigma_r^{(\kappa)}$ and $\Pi_s^{(\kappa)}$ of the ellipsoids $\Delta X_r^{(\kappa)}$ and $\Delta E_s^{(\kappa)}$. Semidefinite programming [18] can be applied, because the objective functions of these volume-related programming problems depend on, e.g., the determinant or eigenvalues of symmetric positive semidefinite matrices. However, in order to obtain positive semidefinite representable objective functions [14], some regression models have to be slightly modified. For example, the objective function of the regression model (R_{Det}) depends directly on the determinant of the configuration matrices. Unfortunately, det (M) considered as a function of symmetric positive semidefinite $n \times n$-matrices M (short: $M \succcurlyeq 0$) is neither a convex nor a concave function of M (if $n \geq 2$). However, if p is a rational number with $0 \leq p \leq \frac{1}{n}$, then

$$f(M) = \begin{cases} -\det^p(M) & , M \succcurlyeq 0 \\ \infty & , \text{otherwise} \end{cases}$$

is positive semidefinite representable ([14], p. 81). Therefore, we introduce the regression model

$$(\widetilde{R}_{Det}) \qquad \text{Maximize} \quad \sum_{\kappa=1}^{T} \Big\{ -\sum_{r=1}^{R} \Big(\det^p(\Delta\Sigma_r^{(\kappa)}) + \| \Delta\mu_r^{(\kappa)} \|_2^2 \Big) - \sum_{s=1}^{S} \Big(\det^q(\Delta\Pi_s^{(\kappa)}) + \| \Delta\rho_s^{(\kappa)} \|_2^2 \Big) \Big\},$$

where the rational numbers p, q fulfill the conditions $0 \leq p \leq \frac{1}{|C_r|}$ and $0 \leq q \leq \frac{1}{|D_s|}$. As $\det(M) = \prod_{i=1}^{n} \lambda_i(M)$, where $\lambda_i(M)$ are the eigenvalues of M, we can replace (R'_{Det}) by

$$(\widetilde{R}'_{Det}) \qquad \text{Maximize} \quad \sum_{\kappa=1}^{T} \Bigg\{ -\sum_{r=1}^{R} \Bigg(\Bigg(\prod_{j=1}^{|C_r|} \lambda_{r,j}^{(\kappa)} \Bigg)^p + \| \Delta\mu_r^{(\kappa)} \|_2^2 \Bigg) - \sum_{s=1}^{S} \Bigg(\Bigg(\prod_{i=1}^{|D_s|} \Lambda_{s,i}^{(\kappa)} \Bigg)^q + \| \Delta\rho_s^{(\kappa)} \|_2^2 \Bigg) \Bigg\}$$

and instead of (R''_{Det}) we suggest

$$(\widetilde{R}''_{Det}) \qquad \text{Maximize} \quad \sum_{\kappa=1}^{T} \Bigg\{ \sum_{r=1}^{R} \Big(\big[\mathcal{V}_r^{(\kappa)}\big]^{2p} - \| \Delta\mu_r^{(\kappa)} \|_2^2 \Big) + \sum_{s=1}^{S} \Big(\big[\mathcal{W}_s^{(\kappa)}\big]^{2q} - \| \Delta\rho_s^{(\kappa)} \|_2^2 \Big) \Bigg\}.$$

In case of positive definite configuration matrices $\Delta\Sigma_r^{(\kappa)}$ and $\Delta\Pi_s^{(\kappa)}$ negative powers of the determinant can be used. If p is a positive rational, the function

$$f(M) = \begin{cases} \det^{-p}(M) & , M \succ 0 \\ \infty & , \text{otherwise} \end{cases}$$

of the symmetric $n \times n$-matrix M is positive semidefinite representable ([14], p. 83). Here, $M \succ 0$ means that M is positive semidefinite. Now, with two positive rationals p, q we obtain the additional regression model

$$(R'''_{Det}) \qquad \text{Maximize} \quad \sum_{\kappa=1}^{T} \Bigg\{ \sum_{r=1}^{R} \Big(\det^{-p}\big(\Delta\Sigma_r^{(\kappa)}\big) - \| \Delta\mu_r^{(\kappa)} \|_2^2 \Big) + \sum_{s=1}^{S} \Big(\det^{-q}\big(\Delta\Pi_s^{(\kappa)}\big) - \| \Delta\rho_s^{(\kappa)} \|_2^2 \Big) \Bigg\}.$$

The regression model (R''_{Dia}) directly depends on the largest eigenvalues of the configuration matrices $\Delta\Sigma_r^{(\kappa)}$ and $\Delta\Pi_s^{(\kappa)}$ and, thus, on positive semidefinite representable functions ([14], p. 78). In (R'_{Tr}), sums of all eigenvalues of the configuration matrices $\Delta\Sigma_r^{(\kappa)}$ and $\Delta\Pi_s^{(\kappa)}$ are considered, which can also be regarded as positive semidefinite representable functions ([14], p. 80). In general, *interior point methods* can applied which have a moderate complexity [50, 51, 52, 54]. Alternatively, for regression problems with sums of eigenvalues or maximal eigenvalues in the objective function, asscociated *bilevel problems* can be considered which could be solved by *gradient methods*. In fact, in [53] structural frontiers of conic programming are discussed with other optimization methods compared, and future applications in machine learning and data mining prepared.

5 Mixed Integer Regression Problem

As nowadays high-throughput technologies are available, regulatory networks are huge and for practical reasons we have to rarefy them by diminishing the number of branches. Here, upper bounds on the indegrees of nodes are introduced firstly. That means, the number of clusters regulating a specific target or environmental cluster in our network has to be bounded. We use *binary constraints* to decide whether or not there is a connection between two clusters of data and by this we obtain a *mixed-integer optimization problem*. As these constraints are very strict and as they can even destroy our regulatory network, we pass to continuous constraints and introduce a further relaxation in terms of a *continuous optimization problem*.

Given two clusters A, B we use the notation $A \sim B$ if cluster A is regulated by cluster B and $A \not\sim B$ if cluster A is not regulated by cluster B. Now, we define the Boolean matrices

$$\chi_{jr}^{TT} = \begin{cases} 1 & \text{, if } C_j \sim C_r \\ 0 & \text{, if } C_j \not\sim C_r, \end{cases} \qquad \chi_{js}^{TE} = \begin{cases} 1 & \text{, if } C_j \sim D_s \\ 0 & \text{, if } C_j \not\sim D_s, \end{cases}$$

$$\chi_{is}^{EE} = \begin{cases} 1 & \text{, if } D_i \sim D_s \\ 0 & \text{, if } D_i \not\sim D_s, \end{cases} \qquad \chi_{ir}^{ET} = \begin{cases} 1 & \text{, if } D_i \sim C_r \\ 0 & \text{, if } D_i \not\sim C_r, \end{cases}$$

indicating whether or not pairs of clusters in our regulatory network are directly related. If two clusters are not related, the corresponding parts of the matrices A^{TT}, A^{TE}, A^{EE}, A^{ET} and vectors V^{TT}, V^{TE}, V^{EE}, V^{ET} have zero entries.

For $j \in \{1, \ldots, R\}$ we define the *indegree* of cluster C_j in our regulatory network with respect to the target clusters and environmental clusters by

$$\deg(C_j)^{TT} := \sum_{r=1}^{R} \chi_{jr}^{TT} \quad \text{and} \quad \deg(C_j)^{TE} := \sum_{s=1}^{S} \chi_{js}^{TE},$$

respectively. That means, the indegrees $\deg(C_j)^{TT}$ and $\deg(C_j)^{TE}$ count the number of target and environmental clusters which regulate cluster C_j. Similarly, for $i \in \{1, \ldots, S\}$ the *indegree* of cluster D_i with respect to the environmental clusters and the target clusters is given by

$$\deg(D_i)^{EE} := \sum_{s=1}^{S} \chi_{is}^{EE} \quad \text{and} \quad \deg(D_i)^{ET} := \sum_{r=1}^{R} \chi_{ir}^{ET}.$$

Now, the indegrees $\deg(D_i)^{EE}$ and $\deg(D_i)^{ET}$ count the number of environmental and target clusters which regulate cluster D_i.

For network rarefication we introduce upper bounds on the indegrees. The values of these bounds depend on any a priori information available and they have to be given by the practitioner. Including these additional constraints, we obtain the following *mixed integer optimization problem*:

$$(RMI) \quad \begin{cases} \text{Maximize} \sum_{\kappa=1}^{T} \Big\{ \sum_{r=1}^{R} \| \Delta X_r^{(\kappa)} \|_* - \| \Delta \mu_r^{(\kappa)} \|_2^2 \\ \qquad + \sum_{s=1}^{S} \| \Delta E_s^{(\kappa)} \|_* - \| \Delta \rho_s^{(\kappa)} \|_2^2 \Big\} \\ \text{subject to } \deg(C_j)^{TT} \le \alpha_j^{TT},\ j = 1, \ldots, R \\ \qquad \deg(C_j)^{TE} \le \alpha_j^{TE},\ j = 1, \ldots, R \\ \qquad \deg(D_i)^{EE} \le \alpha_i^{EE},\ i = 1, \ldots, S \\ \qquad \deg(D_i)^{ET} \le \alpha_i^{ET},\ i = 1, \ldots, S. \end{cases}$$

We note that our network rarefication can also be achieved by bounding the outdegrees of the nodes. Such an approach was utilized in [82, 83, 84] in order to obtain a more flexible representation of gene-environment networks with respect to uncertain states in terms of intervals and parallelpipes.

The topology of the network may have significant consequences on error and attack tolerance of the regulatory system [3,20]. These generic properties of complex networks refer to robustness against local failures and the vulnerability to the removal of a few nodes that play a vital role in maintaining the network connectivity. In general, two major classes of complex networks can be divided: *homogenous networks* and *inhomogeneous* or *scale-free networks* [46]. These networks are characterized by the *connectivity distribution* $P(k)$, giving the probability that a node in the network is connected to k other nodes. In homogeneous networks, $P(k)$ peaks at an average $\langle k \rangle$ and decays exponentially for large k, whereas in scale-free networks the probability decays as a power law $P(k) \sim k^{-\gamma}$, i.e., it is free of a characteristic scale. In homogenous networks, like the random graph models of Erdös and Rényi [16,23], each node has approximately the same number of links. In contrast, in scale-free networks, like metabolic networks [37], some highly connected nodes are statistically significant and although they can be considered as robust and demonstrate a high tolerance against (random) failures, they are highly vulnerable against attacks.

The binary constraints of (RMI) are very strict and if the constraints are not appropriate, important branches of the regulatory network could be deleted. For this reason, we use continuous optimization for a relaxation of (RMI) by replacing the binary variables χ_{jr}^{TT}, χ_{js}^{TE}, χ_{is}^{EE} and χ_{ir}^{ET} with real variables $P_{jr}^{TT}, P_{js}^{TE}, P_{is}^{EE}, P_{ir}^{ET} \in [0,1]$, which is also interpretable as probabilities (we refer to [65] for optimization models with probabilistic constraints). These variables should linearly depend on the corresponding elements of $\Gamma_{jr}^{TT}, \Gamma_{js}^{TE}, \Gamma_{is}^{EE}, \Gamma_{ir}^{ET}$ and $\Phi_j^{TT}, \Phi_j^{TE}, \Phi_i^{EE}, \Phi_i^{ET}$.

The real-valued *indegree* of cluster C_j in our regulatory network with respect to the target clusters and environmental clusters are now defined by

$$\deg(C_j)^{TT} := \sum_{r=1}^{R} P_{jr}^{TT}(\Gamma_{jr}^{TT}, \Phi_j^{TT}) \quad \text{and} \quad \deg(C_j)^{TE} := \sum_{s=1}^{S} P_{js}^{TE}(\Gamma_{js}^{TE}, \Phi_j^{TE}),$$

respectively. Similarly, the real-valued *indegree* of cluster D_i with respect to the environmental clusters and the target clusters is given by

$$\deg(D_i)^{EE} := \sum_{s=1}^{S} P_{is}^{EE}(\Gamma_{is}^{EE}, \Phi_i^{EE}) \quad \text{and} \quad \deg(D_i)^{ET} := \sum_{r=1}^{R} P_{ir}^{ET}(\Gamma_{ir}^{ET}, \Phi_i^{ET}).$$

Now, we replace the binary constraints of (RMI) with continuous constraints and obtain the following optimization problem:

$$(RC) \begin{cases} \text{Maximize} \sum_{\kappa=1}^{T} \Big\{ \sum_{r=1}^{R} \| \Delta X_r^{(\kappa)} \|_* - \| \Delta \mu_r^{(\kappa)} \|_2^2 \\ \qquad + \sum_{s=1}^{S} \| \Delta E_s^{(\kappa)} \|_* - \| \Delta \rho_s^{(\kappa)} \|_2^2 \Big\} \\ \\ \text{subject to} \sum_{r=1}^{R} P_{jr}^{TT}(\Gamma_{jr}^{TT}, \Phi_j^{TT}) \leq \alpha_j^{TT}, \; j = 1, \ldots, R \\ \sum_{s=1}^{S} P_{js}^{TE}(\Gamma_{js}^{TE}, \Phi_j^{TE}) \leq \alpha_j^{TE}, \; j = 1, \ldots, R \\ \sum_{s=1}^{S} P_{is}^{EE}(\Gamma_{is}^{EE}, \Phi_i^{EE}) \leq \alpha_i^{EE}, \; i = 1, \ldots, S \\ \sum_{r=1}^{R} P_{ir}^{ET}(\Gamma_{ir}^{ET}, \Phi_i^{ET}) \leq \alpha_i^{ET}, \; i = 1, \ldots, S. \end{cases}$$

REMARK. We point out that the methods introduced are particularly applicable in the financial sector, e.g., in the modeling of stochastic differential equations and, as a very new contribution, the optimization of the statistical ROC curve for an improved classification and prediction of credit default [86]. Here, we point out a new view onto credits given by the study of our paper. All the interaction among the items that we investigate can be regarded as a "credit" taken or given, as a measurement which asks for an appropriate response, such as an equivalent effect (maybe, plus a gain) in future. There are consumptions of various kinds, medical treatments, expenditures in education, science and the improvements in environmental protection. The realization of their purposes has to be priced, discounted and compared, the degrees of these achievements can be enforced by penalty terms in our models of optimization and dynamics. This new view is subject of our future studies.

6 Conclusion

In this paper, we analyzed a time-discrete model of target-environment networks under ellipsoidal uncertainty. We introduced the power of modern optimization by means of semidefinite programming and the efficiency of interior point methods for the modeling of our regression problem and nonsmooth optimization that we use a priori for clustering our items. This pioneering approach offers a new view on parameter estimation and optimization of TE-regulatory systems depending on various kinds of errors, where the dynamics of clusters of targets and environmental items and their mutual effects are determined by corresponding clusters of parameters. Our research includes clustering theory which we support by statistical investigations about the number of clusters and their stability and by means of statistical learning we find the clusters with the help of nonsmooth optimization. The representation of the dynamic states in terms of ellipsoids was motivated by our and our colleagues' studies on gene-environment networks and eco-finance networks, where errors and uncertainty are modeled by intervals [92, 94, 95]. Here, we extended the interval model by a representation of errors in terms of ellipsoids what refers to stochastic dependencies between the various target and environmental items. These uncertainty sets are directly related to covariance matrices and they provide good approximations of convex sets. In particular, models based on Gaussian random noise refer to the ellipsoidal approach. However, Gaussian random distributions are often used as simplifications and in many applications non-Gaussian probability distributions have to be applied. Therefore, we will further extend our models based on ellipsoidal calculus and, by this, in future works we will turn to a more set-theoretic representation of errors and uncertainty based on semi-algebraic sets. We will combine this new perception with refined optimization methods and by this we will offer a further avenue for the analysis of TE-regulatory systems, particularly with regard to applications and real-world data. Furthermore, we propose that collaborative game theory under uncertainty which was recently modeled with the help of intervals [4, 5, 6, 7] could become refined by our ellipsoidal calculus, herewith allowing a great wealth of dependencies and subcoalitions preassigned.

References

1. Akhmet, M.U., Gebert, J., Öktem, H., Pickl, S.W., Weber, G.-W.: An improved algorithm for analytical modeling and anticipation of gene expression patterns. Journal of Computational Technologies 10(4), 3–20 (2005)
2. Akume, D., Weber, G.-W.: Cluster algorithms: theory and methods. Journal of Computational Technologies 7(1), 15–27 (2002)
3. Albert, R., Jeong, H., Barabási, A.-L.: Error and attack tolerance of complex networks. Nature 406, 378–381 (2000)
4. Alparslan Gök, S.Z.: Cooperative interval games. PhD Thesis at Institute of Applied Mathematics of METU, Ankara (2009)
5. Alparslan Gök, S.Z., Branzei, R., Tijs, S.: Convex interval games. Journal of Applied Mathematics and Decision Sciences 2009, 14, article ID 342089 (2009), doi:10.1155/2009/342089
6. Alparslan Gök, S.Z., Branzei, R., Tijs, S.: Airport interval games and their Shapley value. Operations Research and Decisions 2, 9–18 (2009)
7. Alparslan Gök, S.Z., Miquel, S., Tijs, S.: Cooperation under interval uncertainty. Math. Methods Oper. Res. 69, 99–109 (2009)
8. Aster, A., Borchers, B., Thurber, C.: Parameter estimation and inverse problems. Academic Press, London (2004)

9. Bagirov, A.M., Ugon, J.: Piecewise partially separable functions and a derivative-free algorithm for large scale nonsmooth optimization. J. Global Optim. 35, 163–195 (2006)
10. Bagirov, A.M., Yearwood, J.: A new nonsmooth optimization algorithm for minimum sum-of-squares clustering problems. European J. Oper. Res. 170(2), 578–596 (2006)
11. Barzily, Z., Volkovich, Z.V., Akteke-Öztürk, B., Weber, G.-W.: Cluster stability using minimal spanning trees. In: ISI Proceedings of 20th Mini-EURO Conference Continuous Optimization and Knowledge-Based Technologies, Neringa, Lithuania, May 20-23, 2008, pp. 248–252 (2008)
12. Barzily, Z., Volkovich, Z.V., Akteke-Öztürk, B., Weber, G.-W.: On a minimal spanning tree approach in the cluster validation problem. In: Dzemyda, G., Miettinen, K., Sakalauskas, L (guest eds.) To appear in the special issue of INFORMATICA at the occasion of 20th Mini-EURO Conference Continuous Optimization and Knowledge Based Technologies, Neringa, Lithuania, May 20-23 (2008)
13. Benedetti, R.: Real algebraic and semi-algebraic sets. In: Hermann (ed.) des Sciences et des Arts, Paris (1990)
14. Ben-Tal, A.: Conic and robust optimization. Lecture notes (2002), `http://iew3.technion.ac.il/Home/Users/morbt.phtml`
15. Bochnak, J., Coste, M., Roy, M.-F.: Real algebraic geometry. Springer, Heidelberg (1998)
16. Bollobás, B.: Random graphs. Academic, London (1985)
17. Borenstein, E., Feldman, M.W.: Topological signatures of species interactions in metabolic networks. J. Comput. Biol. 16(2), 191–200 (2009), doi:10.1089/cmb.2008.06TT
18. Boyd, S., Vandenberghe, L.: Convex Optimization. Cambridge University Press, Cambridge (2004)
19. Chen, T., He, H.L., Church, G.M.: Modeling gene expression with differential equations. In: Proc. Pacific Symposium on Biocomputing, pp. 29–40 (1999)
20. Crucitti, P., Latore, V., Marchiori, M., Rapisarda, A.: Error and attack tolerance of complex networks. Physica A 340, 388–394 (2004)
21. Durieu, P., Walter, É., Polyak, B.: Multi-input multi-output ellipsoidal state bounding. J. Optim. Theory Appl. 111(2), 273–303 (2001)
22. Elishakoff, I.: Whys and Hows in Uncertainty Modelling: Probability, Fuzziness and Anti-Optimization. Springer, Heidelberg (1999)
23. Erdös, P., Rényi, A.: On the evolution of random graphs. Publ. Math. Inst. Hung. Acad. Sci. 5, 17–60 (1960)
24. Ergenç, T., Weber, G.-W.: Modeling and prediction of gene-expression patterns reconsidered with Runge-Kutta discretization. Journal of Computational Technologies 9(6), 40–48 (2004); special issue at the occasion of seventieth birthday of Prof. Dr. Karl Roesner, TU Darmstadt
25. Gebert, J., Lätsch, M., Pickl, S.W., Radde, N., Weber, G.-W., Wünschiers, R.: Genetic networks and anticipation of gene expression patterns. In: Computing Anticipatory Systems: CASYS(92)03 – Sixth International Conference, AIP Conference Proceedings, vol. 718, pp. 474–485 (2004)
26. Gebert, J., Lätsch, M., Pickl, S.W., Weber, G.-W., Wünschiers, R.: An algorithm to analyze stability of gene-expression pattern. In: Anthony, M., Boros, E., Hammer, P.L., Kogan, A. (guest eds.) Special issue Discrete Mathematics and Data Mining II of Discrete Appl. Math.,vol. 154(7), pp. 1140–1156.

27. Gebert, J., Lätsch, M., Quek, E.M.P., Weber, G.-W.: Analyzing and optimizing genetic network structure via path-finding. Journal of Computational Technologies 9(3), 3–12 (2004)
28. Gebert, J., Öktem, H., Pickl, S.W., Radde, N., Weber, G.-W., Yılmaz, F.B.: Inference of gene expression patterns by using a hybrid system formulation – an algorithmic approach to local state transition matrices. In: Lasker, G.E., Dubois, D.M. (eds.) Anticipative and predictive models in systems science I, IIAS (International Institute for Advanced Studies) in Windsor, Ontario, pp. 63–66 (2004)
29. Gebert, J., Radde, N., Weber, G.-W.: Modelling gene regulatory networks with piecewise linear differential equations. To appear in the special issue (feature cluster) Challenges of Continuous Optimization in Theory and Applications of European J. Oper. Res (2006)
30. Gökmen, A., Kayalgil, S., Weber, G.-W., Gökmen, I., Ecevit, M., Sürmeli, A., Bali, T., Ecevit, Y., Gökmen, H., DeTombe, D.J.: Balaban Valley Project: Improving the Quality of Life in Rural Area in Turkey. International Scientific Journal of Methods and Models of Complexity 7(1) (2004)
31. Hardt, R.M., Lambrechts, P., Turchin, V., Volić, I.: Real homotopy theory of semi-algebraic sets (2008), eprint arXiv 0806, 476
32. Harris, J.R., Nystad, W., Magnus, P.: Using genes and environments to define asthma and related phenotypes: applications to multivariate data. Clinical and Experimental Allergy 28(1), 43–45 (1998)
33. Hastie, T., Tibshirani, R.: Discriminant adaptive nearest neighbor classification. IEEE Transactions on Pattern Analysis and Machine Intelligence 18(6), 607–616 (1996)
34. Hastie, T., Tibshirani, R., Friedman, J.: The elements of statistical learning. Springer, Heidelberg (2001)
35. Hoon, M.D., Imoto, S., Kobayashi, K., Ogasawara, N., Miyano, S.: Inferring gene regulatory networks from time-ordered gene expression data of Bacillus subtilis using differential equations. In: Proc. Pacific Symposium on Biocomputing, pp. 17–28 (2003)
36. Işcanoğlu, A., Weber, G.-W., Taylan, P.: Predicting default probabilities with generalized additive models for emerging markets. Graduate Summer School on New Advances in Statistics, METU (2007) (invited lecture)
37. Jeong, H., Tombor, B., Albert, R., Oltvai, Z.N., Barabási, A.-L.: The large-scale organization of metabolic networks. Nature 407, 651–654 (2000)
38. Jong, H.D.: Modeling and simulation of genetic regulatory systems: a literature review. J. Comput. Biol. 9, 103–129 (2002)
39. Krabs, W.: Mathematical modelling, Teubner, Stuttgart (1997)
40. Krabs, W.: Dynamische Systeme: Steuerbarkeit und chaotisches Verhalten, Teubner, Stuttgart (1998)
41. Krabs, W., Pickl, S.: A game-theoretic treatment of a time-discrete emission reduction model. Int. Game Theory Rev. 6(1), 21–34 (2004)
42. Kropat, E., Pickl, S., Rössler, A., Weber, G.-W.: On theoretical and practical relations between discrete optimization and nonlinear optimization. Special issue Colloquy Optimization – Structure and Stability of Dynamical Systems (at the occasion of the colloquy with the same name, Cologne, October 2000) of Journal of Computational Technologies, 7 (special Issue), pp. 27–62 (2002)
43. Kropat, E., Weber, G.-W., Akteke-Öztürk, B.: Eco-Finance networks under uncertainty. In: Herskovits, J., Canelas, A., Cortes, H., Aroztegui, M. (eds.) Proceedings of the International Conference on Engineering, EngOpt 2008, Rio de Janeiro, Brazil (2008), ISBN 978857650156-5, CD
44. Kurzhanski, A.B., Vályi, I.: Ellipsoidal calculus for estimation and control. Birkhäuser (1997)
45. Kurzhanski, A.A., Varaiya, P.: Ellipsoidal toolbox manual, EECS Department, University of California, Berkeley (2008)

46. Li, L., Alderson, D., Tanaka, R., Doyle, J.C., Willinger, W.: Towards a Theory of Scale-Free Graphs: Definition, Properties, and Implications (Extended Version). Technical Report CIT-CDS-04-006, Engineering & Applied Sciences Division California Institute of Technology, Pasadena, CA, USA (2005)
47. Li, Y.F., Venkatesh, S., Li, D.: Modeling global emissions and residues of pesticided. Environmental Modeling and Assessment 9, 237–243 (2004)
48. Liu, Q., Yang, J., Chen, Z., Yang, M.Q., Sung, A.H., Huang, X.: Supervised learning-based tagSNP selection for genome-wide disease classifications. BMC Genomics 9, 1 (2007)
49. Lorenz, R., Boyd, S.: An ellipsoidal approximation to the Hadamard product of ellipsoids. In: Proceedings IEEE Conference on Acoustics, Speech, and Signal Processing (ICASSP), pp. 1193–1196 (2002)
50. Nemirovski, A.: Five lectures on modern convex optimization. C.O.R.E. Summer School on Modern Convex Optimization (2002), `http://iew3.technion.ac.il/Labs/Opt/opt/LN/Final.pdf`
51. Nemirovski, A.: Lectures on modern convex optimization. Israel Institute of Technology (2002), `http://iew3.technion.ac.il/Labs/Opt/opt/LN/Final.pdf`
52. Nemirovski, A.: Interior point polynomial time algorithms in convex programming, lecture Notes (2004), `https://itweb.isye.gatech.edu`
53. Nemirovski, A.: Modern convex optimization. In: PASCAL Workshop, Thurnau, March 16-18 (2005)
54. Nesterov, Y.E., Nemirovskii, A.S.: Interior point polynomial algorithms in convex programming. SIAM, Philadelphia (1994)
55. Özöğür, S.: Mathematical modelling of enzymatic reactions, simulation and parameter estimation. MSc. thesis at Institute of Applied Mathematics, METU, Ankara (2005)
56. Özögür-Akyüz, S., Akteke-Öztürk, B., Tchemisova, T., Weber, G.-W.: New optimization methods in data mining. To appear in the proceedings of International Conference Operations Research (OR 2008), Augsburg, Germany, September 3-5, Springer, Heidelberg (2008)
57. Özöğür, S., Sağdıçoğlu Celep, A.G., Karasözen, B., Yıldırım, N., Weber, G.-W.: Dynamical modelling of enzymatic reactions, simulation and parameter estimation with genetic algorithms. In: HIBIT – Proceedings of International Symposium on Health Informatics and Bioinformatics, Antalya, Turkey, pp. 78–84 (2005)
58. Partner, M., Kashtan, N., Alon, U.: Environmental variability and modularity of bacterial metabolic networks. BMC Evolutionary Biology 7, 169 (2007), doi:10.1186/1471-2148-7-169
59. Pickl, S.: Der τ-value als Kontrollparameter - Modellierung und Analyse eines Joint-Implementation Programmes mithilfe der dynamischen kooperativen Spieltheorie und der diskreten Optimierung. Thesis, Darmstadt University of Technology, Department of Mathematics (1998)
60. Pickl, S.: An iterative solution to the nonlinear time-discrete TEM model - the occurence of chaos and a control theoretic algorithmic approach. In: AIP Conference Proceedings, vol. 627(1), pp. 196–205 (2002)
61. Pickl, S.: An algorithmic solution for an optimal decision making process within emission trading markets. In: Proceedings of the DIMACS-LAMSADE Workshop on Computer Science and Decision Theory, Annales du Lamsade No. 3, Laboratoire d'Analyse et Modélisation de Systémes pour l'Aide a la Décision
62. Pickl, S., Weber, G.-W.: Optimization of a time-discrete nonlinear dynamical system from a problem of ecology - an analytical and numerical approach. Journal of Computational Technologies 6(1), 43–52 (2001)
63. Riener, C., Theobald, T.: Positive Polynome und semidefinite Optimierung. Jahresbericht der DMV - JB 100. Band, Heft 2, 57–76 (2008)

64. Ros, L., Sabater, A., Thomas, F.: An ellipsoidal calculus based on propagation and fusion. IEEE Transactions on Systems, Man and Cybernetics, Part B: Cybernetics 32(4), 430–442 (2002)
65. Shapiro, A., Dentcheva, D., Ruszczyński, A.: Lectures on stochastic programming: modeling and theory. SIAM, Philadelphia (2009)
66. Taştan, M.: Analysis and prediction of gene expression patterns by dynamical systems, and by a combinatorial algorithm, Institute of Applied Mathematics, METU, MSc Thesis (2005)
67. Taştan, M., Ergenç, T., Pickl, S.W., Weber, G.-W.: Stability analysis of gene expression patterns by dynamical systems and a combinatorial algorithm. In: HIBIT – Proceedings of International Symposium on Health Informatics and Bioinformatics, Antalya, Turkey, pp. 67–75 (2005)
68. Taştan, M., Pickl, S.W., Weber, G.-W.: Mathematical modeling and stability analysis of gene-expression patterns in an extended space and with Runge-Kutta discretization. In: Proceedings of Operations Research, Bremen, September 2005, pp. 443–450. Springer, Heidelberg (2005)
69. Taylan, P., Weber, G.-W.: New approaches to regression in financial mathematics by additive models. Journal of Computational Technologies 12(2), 3–22 (2007)
70. Taylan, P., Weber, G.-W., Beck, A.: New approaches to regression by generalized additive models and continuous optimization for modern applications in finance, science and techology. In: Rubinov, A., Burachik, B., Yang, X. (guest eds.) (The special issue in honour) Optimization, vol. 56(5-6), pp. 1–24 (2007), doi: http://dx.doi.org/doi:10.1080/02331930701618740
71. Taylan, P., Weber, G.-W., Kropat, E.: Approximation of stochastic differential equations by additive models using splines and conic programming. To appear in International Journal of Computing Anticipatory Systems 20-21-22; Dubois, D.M. (ed.) At the occasion of CASYS 2007, Eighth International Conference on Computing Anticipatory Systems, Liege, Belgium, August 6-11, 2007 (2008), ISSN 1373-5411
72. Taylan, P., Weber, G.-W., Liu, L., Yerlikaya, F.: On foundation of parameter estimation for generalized partial linear models with B-Splines and continuous optimization. Computers and Mathematics with Applications (CAMWA) 60(1), 134–143 (2010)
73. Taylan, P., Weber, G.-W., Yerlikaya, F.: Continuous optimization applied in MARS for modern applications in finance, science and technology. In: The ISI Proceedings of 20th Mini-EURO Conference Continuous Optimization and Knowledge-Based Technologies, Neringa, Lithuania, May 20-23, pp. 317–322 (2008)
74. Taylan, P., Weber, G.-W., Yerlikaya, F.: A new approach to multivariate adaptive regression spline by using Tikhonov regularization and continuous optimization. TOP (the Operational Research Journal of SEIO (Spanish Statistics and Operations Research Society) 18(2), 377–395 (2010)
75. Uğur, Ö., Pickl, S.W., Weber, G.-W., Wünschiers, R.: An algorithmic approach to analyze genetic networks and biological energy production: an Introduction and contribution where OR meets biology. Optimization 58(1), 1–22 (2009)
76. Uğur, Ö., Weber, G.-W.: Optimization and dynamics of gene-environment networks with intervals. In: The special issue at the occasion of the 5th Ballarat Workshop on Global and Non-Smooth Optimization: Theory, Methods and Applications, November 28-30; J. Ind. Manag. Optim. 3(2), 357–379 (2006)
77. Vazhentsev, A.Y.: On internal ellipsoidal approximations for problems of control synthesis with bounded coordinates. J. Comput. System Sci. Int. 39(3), 399 (2000)

78. Volkovich, Z., Barzily, Z., Weber, G.-W., Toledano-Kitai, D.: Cluster stability estimation based on a minimal spanning trees approach. In: Hakim, A.H., Vasant, P. (Guest eds.) Proceedings of the Second Global Conference on Power Control and Optimization, AIP Conference Proceedings 1159, Bali, Indonesia, June 1-3. Subseries: Mathematical and Statistical Physics, pp. 299–305 (August 2009), ISBN: 978-0-7354-0696-4
79. Weber, G.-W.: Charakterisierung struktureller Stabilität in der nichtlinearen Optimierung. In: Bock, H.H., Jongen, H.T., Plesken, W. (eds.) Aachener Beiträge zur Mathematik 5, Augustinus publishing house (now: Mainz publishing house), Aachen (1992)
80. Weber, G.-W.: Minimization of a max-type function: Characterization of structural stability. In: Guddat, J., Jongen, H.T., Kummer, B., Nožička, F. (eds.) Parametric Optimization and Related Topics III, pp. 519–538. Peter Lang publishing house, Frankfurt a.M. (1993)
81. Weber, G.-W.: Generalized semi-infinite optimization and related topics. In: Hofmannn, K.H., Wille, R. (eds.) Research and Exposition in Mathematics 29, Lemgo, Heldermann Publishing House (2003)
82. Weber, G.-W., Alparslan-Gök, S.Z., Dikmen, N.: Environmental and life sciences: gene-environment networks - optimization, games and control - a survey on recent achievements. The Special Issue of Journal of Organisational Transformation and Social Change 5(3), 197–233 (2008); Guest editor: DeTombe, D.
83. Weber, G.-W., Alparslan-Gök, S.Z., Söyler, B.: A new mathematical approach in environmental and life sciences: gene-environment networks and their dynamics. Environmental Modeling & Assessment 14(2), 267–288 (2007)
84. Weber, G.-W., Kropat, E., Akteke-Öztürk, B., Görgülü, Z.-K.: A survey on OR and mathematical methods applied on gene-environment networks. Central European Journal of Operations Research (CEJOR) 17(3), 315–341 (2009); Dlouhy, M., Pickl, P., Rauner, M., Leopold-Wildburger, U. (Guest eds.): CEJOR special issue at the occasion of EURO XXII 2007, Prague, Czech Republic, July 8-11 (2007)
85. Weber, G.-W., Kropat, E., Tezel, A., Belen, S.: Optimization applied on regulatory and eco-finance networks - survey and new developments. Pacific Journal of Optimization 6(2), 319–340 (2010); Fukushima, M., Kelley, C.T., Qi, L., Sun J., Ye, Y. (Guest eds.): Special issue in memory of Professor Alexander Rubinov
86. Weber, G.-W., Kürüm, E., Yildirak, K.: A classification problem of credit risk rating investigated and solved by optimization of the ROC curve. To appear in CEJOR (Central European Journal of Operations Research) special issue at the occasion of EURO XXIV 2010, Lisbon (2010), doi:10.1007/s10100-011-0224-5
87. Weber, G.-W., Özögür-Akyüz, S., Kropat, E.: A review on data mining and continuous optimization applications in computational biology and medicine. Embryo Today, Birth Defects Research (Part C) 87, 165–181 (2009)
88. Weber, G.-W., Taylan, P., Alparslan-Gök, S.-Z., Özöğür, S., Akteke-Öztürk, B.: Optimization of gene-environment networks in the presence of errors and uncertainty with Chebychev approximation. TOP, the Operational Research Journal of SEIO (Spanish Statistics and Operations Research Society) 16(2), 284–318 (2008)
89. Weber, G.-W., Tezel, A.: On generalized semi-infinite optimization of genetic networks. TOP 15(1), 65–77 (2007)
90. Weber, G.-W., Tezel, A., Taylan, P., Soyler, A., Çetin, M.: Mathematical contributions to dynamics and optimization of gene-environment networks. Optimization 57(2), 353–377 (2008); Pallaschke, D., Stein, O. (Guest eds.): Special Issue: In Celebration of Prof. Dr. Hubertus Th. Jongen's 60th Birthday
91. Weber, G.-W., Uğur, Ö., Taylan, P., Tezel, A.: On optimization, dynamics and uncertainty: a tutorial for gene-environment networks. The special issue Networks in Computational Biology of Discrete Applied Mathematics 157(10), 2494–2513 (2009)

92. Yerlikaya, F.: A new contribution to nonlinear robust regression and classification with mars and its applications to data mining for quality control in manufacturing. Thesis, Middle East Technical University, Ankara, Turkey (2008)
93. Yerlikaya, F., Weber, G.-W., Batmas, I., Köksal, G., Taylan, P.: MARS Algoritmasínda Tikhonov düzenlemesi ve çok amaçli optimizasyon kullanimi. In: The Proceedings of Operational Research and Industrial Engineering Annual Conference (YA/EM 2008), Galatasaray University, Istanbul, Turkey (2008)
94. Yılmaz, F.B.: A mathematical modeling and approximation of gene expression patterns by linear and quadratic regulatory relations and analysis of gene networks, Institute of Applied Mathematics, METU, MSc Thesis (2004)
95. Yılmaz, F.B., Öktem, H., Weber, G.-W.: Mathematical modeling and approximation of gene expression patterns and gene networks. In: Fleuren, F., den Hertog, D., Kort, P.(eds.): Operations Research Proceedings, pp. 280–287 (2005)

Chapter 4
A Visual Environment for Designing and Running Data Mining Workflows in the Knowledge Grid

Eugenio Cesario[1], Marco Lackovic[2], Domenico Talia[1,2], and Paolo Trunfio[2]

[1] ICAR-CNR
[2] DEIS, University of Calabria
Via P. Bucci 41c, 87036 Rende, Italy
cesario@icar.cnr.it,
{mlackovic,talia,trunfio}@deis.unical.it

Abstract. Data mining tasks are often composed by multiple stages that may be linked each other to form various execution flows. Moreover, data mining tasks are often distributed since they involve data and tools located over geographically distributed environments, like the Grid. Therefore, it is fundamental to exploit effective formalisms, such as workflows, to model data mining tasks that are both multi-staged and distributed. The goal of this work is defining a workflow formalism and providing a visual software environment, named DIS3GNO, to design and execute distributed data mining tasks over the Knowledge Grid, a service-oriented framework for distributed data mining on the Grid. DIS3GNO supports all the phases of a distributed data mining task, including composition, execution, and results visualization. The paper provides a description of DIS3GNO, some relevant use cases implemented by it, and a performance evaluation of the system.

1 Introduction

Data mining techniques and systems are widely used in many scientific and business scenarios to infer useful knowledge from the increasing amount of available data. Data mining tasks and knowledge discovery in databases (KDD) processes are often composed of multiple stages (e.g., data extraction, data filtering, data analysis, results evaluation) that may be linked each other by different dependencies to form various execution flows. Moreover, data mining tasks are often distributed since they involve data and tools located over geographically distributed environments, like computational Grids. Therefore, it is fundamental to provide formalisms and environments to design and execute data mining tasks that are both multi-staged and distributed.

Workflows are commonly-used formalisms to represent data and execution flows associated with complex data mining tasks. A data mining workflow is a graph in which nodes typically represent data sources, filtering tools, data

D.E. Holmes, L.C. Jain (Eds.): Data Mining: Found. & Intell. Paradigms, ISRL 24, pp. 57–75.
springerlink.com

mining algorithms, and visualizers, and edges represent execution dependencies among nodes. An important benefit of workflows is that, once defined, they can be stored and retrieved for modifications and/or re-execution: this allows users to define typical data mining patterns and reuse them in different contexts. The goal of this work is designing a high-level workflow formalism and implementing a visual software environment to design and execute distributed data mining tasks as workflows of services over the Knowledge Grid [1].

The Knowledge Grid is a software system providing services and mechanisms to execute distributed data mining tasks or KDD processes in a Grid environment. The workflow concept plays a fundamental role in the Knowledge Grid at different levels of abstraction. A client application submits a distributed data mining task to the Knowledge Grid by describing it through an XML workflow formalism named *conceptual model*. The conceptual model describes data and tools to be used, without specifying information about their location or implementation.

The Knowledge Grid creates an execution plan for the workflow on the basis of the conceptual model and executes it by using the resources effectively available. To understand this logic, the Knowledge Grid follows a two-step approach: it initially models an *abstract execution plan* that in a second step is resolved into a *concrete execution plan*. The abstract execution plan may not contain specific information about the involved Grid resources (e.g., the actual site where a data mining tool will be executed), while in the concrete execution plan all the resources must be actually specified, by finding a mapping between requested resources and available ones in the distributed computing infrastructure.

The aim of the high-level workflow formalism proposed in this work is to allow domain-expert users (i.e., data analysts) to design a distributed data mining task without specific expertise about Grid programming. A visual software environment, named DIS3GNO, has been implemented to allow a user to: *i*) compose a distributed data mining workflow; *ii*) execute the workflow onto the Knowledge Grid; *iii*) visualize the results of the data mining task. DIS3GNO performs the mapping of the user-defined workflow to the conceptual model and submits it to the Knowledge Grid services, managing the overall computation in a way that is transparent to the user.

The remainder of this paper is organized as follows. Section 2 provides an overview of the Knowledge Grid architecture and implementation. Section 3 describes the main components of the proposed workflow formalism for distributed data mining. Section 4 presents the DIS3GNO system. Section 5 describes how a data mining workflow is executed in the Knowledge Grid. Section 6 presents some uses cases and a performance evaluation of the system. Section 7 discusses related work. Finally, Section 8 concludes the paper.

2 The Knowledge Grid

The Knowledge Grid is a software framework to support the execution of distributed data mining tasks in a Grid environment [1]. The framework supports data mining on the Grid by providing mechanisms and services for publishing and searching data-mining related resources (data sources, data mining tools, etc.), creating and executing distributed data mining processes, and managing data mining results.

The Knowledge Grid services are organized in two hierarchical layers: the *core layer* and the *high-level layer*, as shown in Fig. 1. The design idea is that client applications directly interact with high-level services that, in order to satisfy client requests, invoke suitable operations exported by the core-level services. In turn, core-level services perform their operations by invoking basic services provided by available Grid environments running on the specific host, as well as by interacting with other core-level services.

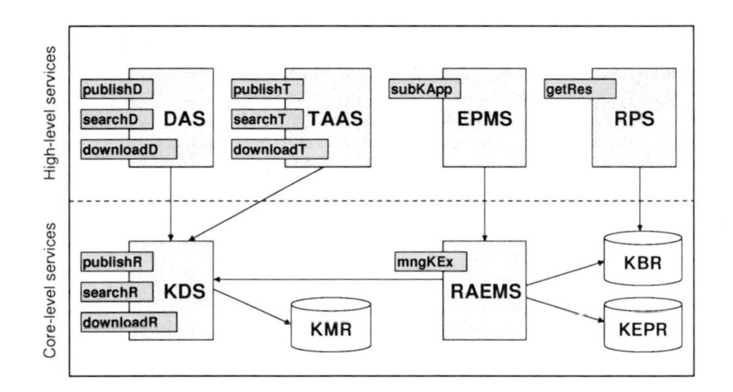

Fig. 1. Knowledge Grid layered services

The high-level layer includes the following services:

- *Data Access Service (DAS)*, which provides operations for publishing, searching and downloading data to be mined (`publishData`, `searchData`, and `downloadData` operations);
- *Tools and Algorithms Access Service (TAAS)*, which is responsible for publishing, searching and downloading tools and algorithms for data extraction, pre-processing and mining (`publishTool`, `searchTool`, and `downloadTool` operations);
- *Execution Plan Management Service (EPMS)*, which receives a conceptual model of the data mining task through the `submitKApplication` operation, translates it into an abstract execution plan, and passes it to the RAEMS service (see below).
- *Results Presentation Service (RPS)*, which allows to retrieve the results (i.e., the inferred models) of previous data mining computations through the `getResults` operation.

The core-level layer includes two services:

- *Knowledge Directory Service (KDS)*, which is responsible for managing metadata about the Knowledge Grid resources (data, tools and algorithms). It provides three operations (`publishResource`, `searchResource`, and `downloadResource`) to publish, search and download resource metadata, which are stored in a *Knowledge Metadata Repository* (*KMR*) as XML documents (details about structure and use of metadata in the Knowledge Grid can be found in [2]).

- *Resource Allocation and Execution Management Service* (*RAEMS*), which starting from an abstract execution plan (received through the `manageKApplication` operation) generates a concrete execution plan and manages its execution. Generated execution plans are stored in a *Knowledge Execution Plan Repository* (*KEPR*), while the results are stored in a *Knowledge Base Repository* (*KBR*).

All the Knowledge Grid services have been implemented as Web services that comply with the Web Services Resource Framework (WSRF) family of standards, as described in a previous work [3]. In particular, we used the WSRF library provided by Globus Toolkit 4 [4], as well as some basic Grid services (e.g., reliable file transfer, authentication and authorization) provided by the same toolkit.

3 Workflow Components

As mentioned earlier, we use workflows as a structured way to model and express the variety of constraints and implications of complex data mining applications.

In DIS3GNO a workflow is represented as a directed acyclic graph whose nodes represent resources and whose edges represent the dependencies among the resources.

Fig. 2. Nodes types

The types of resources which can be present in a data mining workflow (graphically depicted by the icons in Fig. 2) are:

- *Dataset*, representing a dataset;
- *Tool*, representing a tool to perform any kind of operation which may be applied to a dataset (data mining, filtering, splitting, etc.) or to a model (e.g., voting operations);
- *Model*, represents a knowledge model (e.g., a decision tree or a set of association rules), that is the result produced by a data mining tool.

Each node contains a description of a resource as a set of properties which provide information about its features and actual use. This description may be full or partial: in other words, it is both possible to specify a particular resource and its location in the Grid, or just a few of its properties, leaving to the system the task to find a resource matching the specified characteristics and its location. In the former case we will refer to the resource as *concrete*, in the latter one as *abstract*.

For example, in the case of a data mining tool, one could be interested in any algorithm, located in any node of the Grid, provided it is a decision tree classification algorithm able to handle arff files, or could want specifically the algorithm named *NaiveBayes* located in a specified host. Once the workflow will be executed, the Knowledge Grid middleware will find, as explained in Section 2, a concrete resource matching the metadata, whether they are completely or partially specified. Clearly only dataset and tool nodes can be either concrete or abstract, the model node can't be abstract as it represents the result of a computation. The model node has only one property, the *location*, which if left empty will be implicitly set to the same location of the tool node in input.

When a particular resource property is entered, a label is attached below to the corresponding icon, as shown in the example in Fig. 3. The property chosen as the label is the one considered most representative for the resource, i.e. the *Name* for the dataset and tool nodes and the *Location* for the model node.

Fig. 3. Nodes labels

In order to ease the workflow composition and to allow a user to monitor its execution, each resource icon bears a symbol representing the status in which the corresponding resource is at a given time. When the resource status changes, as consequence of the occurrence of certain events, its status symbol changes accordingly. The resource states can be divided in two categories: the *composition-time* and the *run-time* states.

The *composition-time* states (shown in Table 1), useful during the workflow composition phase, are:

1. *No information provided* = no parameter has been specified in the resource properties;
2. *Abstract resource* = the resource is defined through constraints about its features, but it is not known a priori; the *S* in the icon stands for *search*, meaning that the resource has to be searched in the Grid;
3. *Concrete resource* = the resource is specifically defined through its KDS URL; the *K* in the icon stands for *KDS URL*;

4. *Location set* = a location for the model has been specifically set (this status is pertinent to the model node only);

Table 1. Nodes composition-time states

Symbol	Meaning
	No information provided
	Abstract resource
	Concrete resource
	Location set

Table 2. Nodes run-time states

Symbol	Meaning
	Matching resource found
	Running
	Resource not found
	Execution failed
	Task completed successfully

The *run-time* states (shown in Table 2), useful during the workflow execution phase, are:

1. *Matching resource found* = a concrete resource has been found matching the metadata;
2. *Running* = the resource is being executed/managed.
3. *Resource not found* = the system hasn't found a resource matching the metadata;
4. *Execution failed* = some error has occurred during the management of the corresponding resource;
5. *Task completed successfully* = the corresponding resource has successfully fulfilled its task;

Each resource may be in one of these run-time states only in a specific phase of the workflow execution: i.e. state 1 and 2 only during the execution, state 3 and 4 during or after the execution, state 5 only after the execution.

The nodes may be connected with each other through edges, establishing specific dependency relationships among them. All the possible connections are show in Table 3; those not present in Table 3 are not allowed and the graphical user interface ensures a user is prevented to create them.

When an edge is being created between two nodes a label is automatically attached to it representing the kind of relationship between the two nodes. In most of the cases this relationship is strict but in one case (dataset-tool connection) requires further input from a user to be specified.

The possible edge labels are:

- *dataset*: indicates that the input or output of a tool node is a dataset;
- *train*: indicates that the input of a tool node has to be considered a training set;

Table 3. Nodes connections

First resource	Second resource	Label	Meaning	Graphical representation
dataset	dataset	transfer	Explicit file transfer	transfer
dataset	tool	dataset, train, test	Type of input for a tool node	?
tool	dataset	dataset	Dataset produced by a tool	dataset
tool	model	model	Model produced by a DM algorithm	model
model	tool	model	Model received by a tool	model
model	model	transfer	Explicit transfer of a model	transfer

- *test*: indicates that the input of a tool node has to be considered a test set;
- *transfer*: indicates an explicit transfer of a dataset, or a result of a computation, from one Grid node to another;
- *model*: indicates a result of a computation of a data mining algorithm.

4 The DIS3GNO System

DIS3GNO represents the user front-end for two main Knowledge Grid functionalities:

- *Metadata management.* DIS3GNO provides an interface to publish and search metadata about data and tools, through the interaction with the DAS and TAAS services.
- *Execution management.* DIS3GNO provides an environment to design and execute distributed data mining applications as workflows, through the interaction with the EPMS service.

The DIS3GNO GUI, depicted in Fig. 4, has been designed to reflect this two-fold functionality. In particular, it provides a panel (on the left) dedicated to publish and search resource metadata, and a panel (on the right) to compose and execute data mining workflows.

In the top-left corner of the window there is a menu used for opening, saving and creating new workflows, viewing and modifying some program settings and viewing the previously computed text results present in the local file system. Below the menu bar there is a toolbar containing some buttons for the execution control (starting/stopping the execution and resetting the nodes states) and

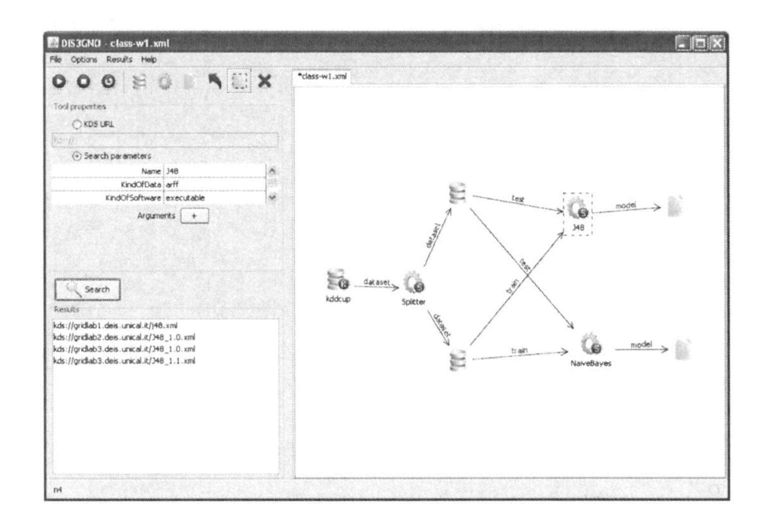

Fig. 4. A screenshot of the DIS3GNO GUI

other for the workflow editing (creation of nodes representing datasets, tools or viewers, creation of edges, selection of multiple nodes and deletion of nodes or edges).

To outline the main functionalities of DIS3GNO, we briefly describe how it is used to compose and run a data mining workflow. By exploiting the DIS3GNO GUI, a user can compose a workflow in a very simple way. First, she starts by selecting from the toolbar the type of resource to be inserted in the workflow (a dataset, a tool or a model node) and drags it into the workflow composition panel. Such operation should be repeated as many times as needed to insert all the required application nodes. Then, she has to insert suitable edges by setting, for each one, the specific dependency relationship between the nodes (as described in Section 3 and summarized in Table 3). Typically, most nodes in a workflow represent abstract resources. In other terms, a user initially concentrates on the application logic, without focusing on the actual datasets or data mining tool to be used.

The simple workflow in Fig. 4 includes a concrete resource (the kddcup dataset) and three abstract resources: a *Splitter* tool and an instance of *J48* and *NaiveBayes*. As described in the previous section, the *S* in the icon of such nodes means that the corresponding resources are defined through constraints about their features. To specify the constraints for a given resource, a user selects the corresponding node in the workflow and fills a set of properties shown on the left panel. For example, in Fig. 4, the node associated with the J48 node has been selected (as highlighted by the dashed box) and some of its properties have been specified in the *Tool properties* panel that is shown on the left.

Once the properties of a resource have been specified, a user can press the *Search* button to obtain the list of all resources that currently match those properties. The results of such search (a list of KDS URLs) are shown in the bottom of the left panel. Given such list of matching resources, a user may decide to select a specific resource, or to leave the system doing so at run time. The workflow can be submitted to the EPMS service by pressing the *Run* button in the toolbar. As a first action, if a user credentials are not available or have expired, a Grid Proxy Initialization window is loaded (see Fig. 5). After that, the workflow execution actually starts and proceeds as detailed in the next section.

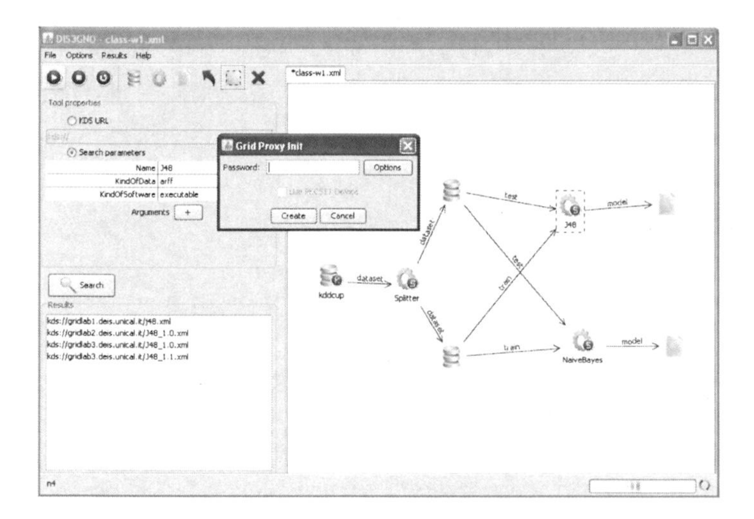

Fig. 5. Proxy initialization at workflow submission

During the workflow execution, the runtime status of the computation is shown to the user. As described in the previous section, this is done by labelling each node of the workflow with a symbol associated with the current status of the corresponding resource. After completion, the user can visualize an inferred model by selecting the corresponding node in the workflow. For example, Fig. 6 shows the model generated by the J48 algorithm.

5 Execution Management

As described earlier (see Section 1), starting from the data mining workflow designed by a user, DIS3GNO generates an XML representation of the data mining task referred to as *conceptual model*. DIS3GNO passes the *conceptual model* to a given EPMS, which is in charge of transforming it into an *abstract execution plan* for subsequent processing by the RAEMS. The RAEMS receives the abstract execution plan and creates a *concrete execution plan*. In order to carry out such a task, the RAEMS needs to evaluate and resolve a set of resources, by contacting the KDS and choosing the most appropriate ones. As soon as the RAEMS has built the concrete execution plan, it is in charge of coordinating its

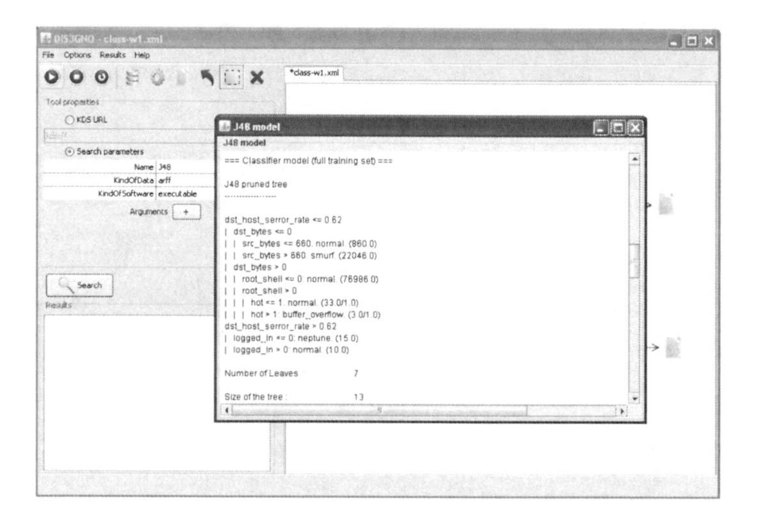

Fig. 6. Results visualization after workflow completion

execution. The status of the computation is notified to the EPMS, which in turn forwards the notifications to the DIS3GNO system for visualization to the user, as discussed in Section 4.

Fig. 7 describes the interactions that occur when an invocation of the EPMS is performed. In particular, the figure outlines the sequence of invocations to others services, and the interchanges with them when a data mining workflow is submitted for allocation and execution. To this purpose, the EPMS exposes the `submitKApplication` operation, through which it receives a conceptual model of the application to be executed (step 1).

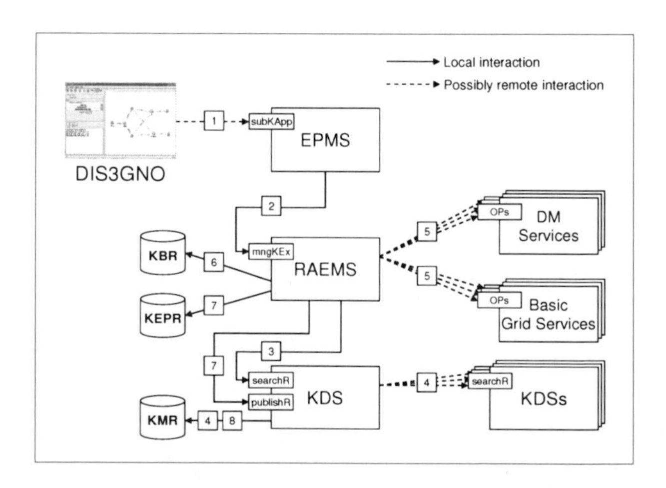

Fig. 7. Execution management

The basic role of the EPMS is to transform the conceptual model into an abstract execution plan for subsequent processing by the RAEMS. An abstract execution plan is a more formal representation of the structure of the application. Generally, it does not contain information on the physical Grid resources to be used, but rather constraints about them.

The RAEMS exports the `manageKExecution` operation, which is invoked by the EPMS and receives the abstract execution plan (step 2). First of all, the RAEMS queries the local KDS (through the `searchResource` operation) to obtain information about the resources needed to instantiate the abstract execution plan (step 3). Note that the KDS performs the searching both accessing the local Knowledge Metadata Repository (KMR) and querying all the reachable remote KDSs (step 4). To reach as many remote KDSs as needed, an unstructured peer-to-peer overlay is built among Knowledge Grid nodes. To this end, each node possesses a configurable set of neighboring nodes to which forward a query.

After the instantiated execution plan is obtained, the RAEMS coordinates the actual execution of the overall computation. To this purpose, the RAEMS invokes the appropriate data mining services (DM Services) and basic Grid services (e.g., file transfer services), as specified by the instantiated execution plan (step 5). The results of the computation are stored by the RAEMS into the Knowledge Base Repository (KBR) (step 6), while the execution plan is stored into the Knowledge Execution Plan Repository (KEPR) (step 7). To make available the results stored in the KBR, it is necessary to publish results metadata into the KMR. To this end, the RAEMS invokes the `publishResource` operation of the local KDS (steps 7 and 8).

6 Use Cases and Performance

In this section we present two examples of distributed data mining workflows designed and executed on a Grid using the DIS3GNO system. The first workflow is a parameter sweeping application in which a dataset is processed using multiple instances of the same classification algorithm with different parameters, with the goal of finding the best classifier based on some accuracy parameters. In the second workflow, a dataset is analyzed using different classification algorithms. The resulting classification models are combined through voting to derive a global model that is more accurate than the single ones. Both of these workflows have been executed on a Grid composed of several machines to evaluated the effectiveness of the systems as well as its performance in terms of scalability.

6.1 Parameter Sweeping Workflow

We used DIS3GNO to compose an application in which a given dataset is analyzed by running multiple instances of the same classification algorithm, with the goal of obtaining multiple classification models from the same data source.

The dataset *covertype*[1] from the UCI KDD archive, has been used as data source. The dataset contains information about forest cover type for a large number of sites in the United States. Each dataset instance, corresponding to a site observation, is described by 54 attributes that give information about the main features of a site (e.g., elevation, aspect, slope, etc.). The 55th attribute contains the cover type, represented as an integer in the range 1 to 7. The original dataset is made of 581,012 instances and is stored in a file having a size of 72MB. From this dataset we extracted three datasets with 72500, 145000 and 290000 instances and a file size of 9 MB, 18 MB and 36 MB respectively. Then we used DIS3GNO to perform a classification analysis on each of those datasets.

DIS3GNO has been used to run an application in which 8 independent instances of the J48 algorithm perform a different classification task on the covertype data set. In particular, each J48 instance has been asked to classify data using a different value of confidence, ranging from 0.15 to 0.50. The same application has been executed using a number of computing nodes ranging from 1 to 8 to evaluate the speedup of the system.

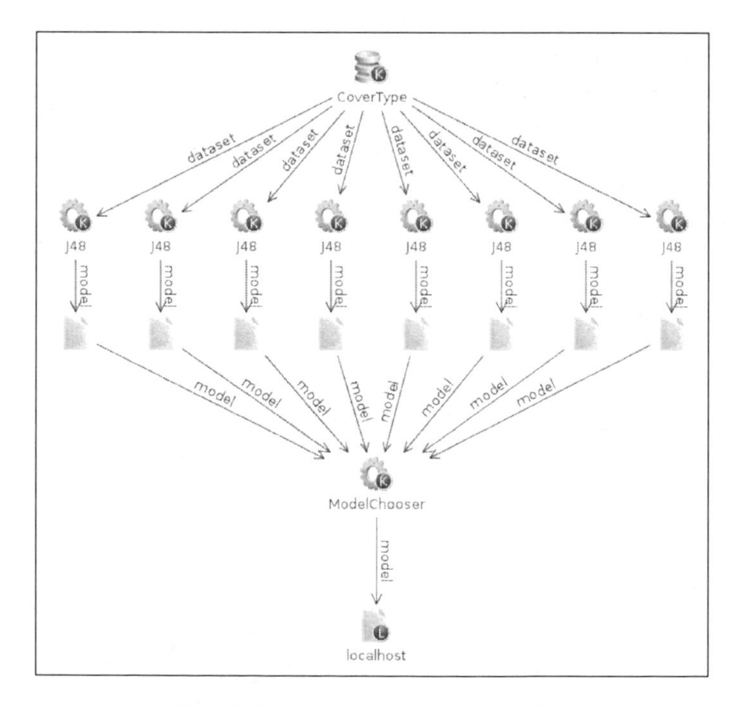

Fig. 8. Parameter sweeping workflow

The workflow corresponding to the application is shown in Fig. 8. It includes a dataset node (representing the covertype dataset) connected to 8 tool nodes, each one associated with an instance of the J48 classification algorithm with a

[1] http://kdd.ics.uci.edu/databases/covertype/covertype.html

different value of confidence (ranging from 0.15 to 0.50). These nodes are in turn connected to another tool node, associated with a model chooser which selects the best classification model among those learnt by the J48 instances. Finally, the node associated with the model chooser is connected to a viewer node having the location set to localhost; this enforces the model to be transferred to the client host for its visualization.

The workflow has been executed using a number of computing nodes ranging from 1 to 8 for each of the three datasets (9 MB, 18 MB and 36 MB) in order to evaluate the speedup of the system. Table 4 reports the execution times of the application when 1, 2, 4 and 8 computing nodes are used. The 8 classification tasks that constitute the overall application are indicated as $DM_1..DM_8$, corresponding to the tasks of running J48 with a confidence value of 0.15, 0.20, 0.25, 0.30, 0.35, 0.40, 0.45, and 0.50, respectively. The table shows how the classification tasks are assigned to the computing nodes (denoted as $N_1..N_8$), as well as the execution times for each dataset size.

Table 4. Task assignments and execution times for the parameter sweeping workflow (times expressed as hh:mm:ss)

No of nodes	Task assignments (Node ← Tasks)	Exec. time 9 MB	Exec. time 18 MB	Exec. time 36 MB
1	$N_1 \leftarrow DM_1, ..., DM_8$	2:43:47	7:03:46	20:36:23
2	$N_1 \leftarrow DM_1, DM_3, DM_5, DM_7$ $N_2 \leftarrow DM_2, DM_4, DM_6, DM_8$	1:55:19	4:51:24	14:14:40
4	$N_1 \leftarrow DM_1, DM_5$ $N_2 \leftarrow DM_2, DM_6$ $N_3 \leftarrow DM_3, DM_7$ $N_4 \leftarrow DM_4, DM_8$	58:30	2:26:48	7:08:16
8	$N_i \leftarrow DM_i$ for $1 \leq i \leq 8$	32:35	1:21:32	3:52:32

When the workflow is executed on more than one node, the execution time includes the overhead due to file transfers. For example, in our network scenario, the transfer of a 36 MB dataset from the user node to a computing node takes on average 15 seconds. This value is small as compared to the amount of time required to run a classification algorithm on the same dataset, which takes between 2.5 and 3.9 hours depending on the computing node. The overall execution time also includes the amount of time needed to invoke all the involved services (i.e., EPMS, RAEMS, KDS) as required by the workflow. However, such an amount of time (approximatively 2 minutes) is negligible as compared to the total execution time.

For the 36 MB dataset, the total execution time decreases from more than 20 hours obtained using 1 computing node, to less than 4 hours obtained with 8 nodes. The achieved execution speedup ranged from 1.45 using 2 nodes, to 5.32 using 8 nodes. Similar trends have been registered with the other two datasets. The execution times and speedup values for different number of nodes and dataset sizes are shown in Fig. 9.

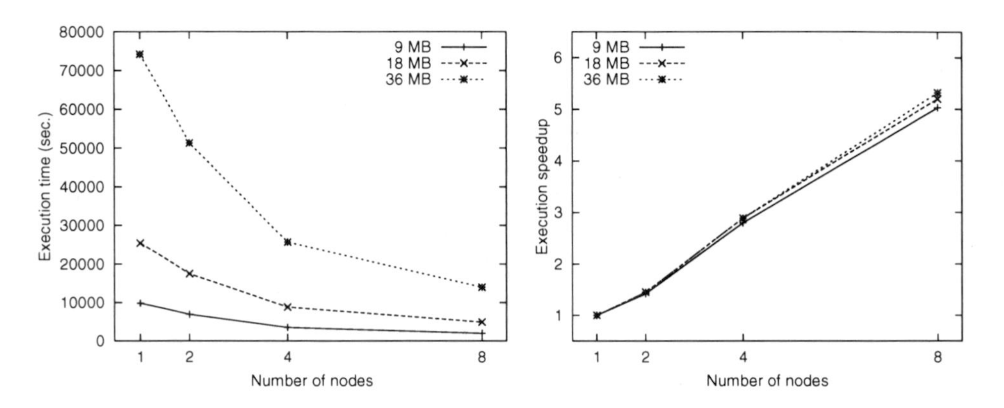

Fig. 9. Execution times and speedup values for different numbers of nodes and dataset sizes, for the parameter sweeping workflow

6.2 Ensemble Learning Workflow

Ensemble learning is a machine learning paradigm where multiple learners are trained to solve the same problem. In contrast to ordinary machine learning approaches which try to learn one model from training data, ensemble methods build a set of models and combine them to obtain the final model [5]. In a classification scenario, an ensemble method constructs a set of *base classifiers* from training data and performs classification by taking a vote on the predictions made by each classifier. As proven by mathematical analysis, ensemble classifiers tend to perform better (in terms of error rate) than any single classifier [6].

The DIS3GNO system has been exploited to design a workflow implementing an ensemble learning application which analyzes a given dataset using different classifiers and performs a voting on the models inferred by them.

As input dataset we used *kddcup99*[2]. This data set, used for the KDD'99 Competition, contains a wide set of data produced during seven weeks of monitoring in a military network environment subject to simulated intrusions. We extracted three data sets from it, with 940000, 1315000 and 1692000 instances and a size of 100 MB, 140 MB and 180 MB.

DIS3GNO has been used to split the dataset into two parts: a test set (1/3 of the original dataset) and a training set (2/3 of the original dataset). The latter has been processed using four classifiers: ConjuctiveRule, NaiveBayes, RandomForest and J48. The models generated by the four classifiers are then collected to a node where they are given to a voter component; the classification is performed and evaluated on the test set by taking a vote, for each instance, on the

[2] http://kdd.ics.uci.edu/databases/kddcup99/kddcup99.html

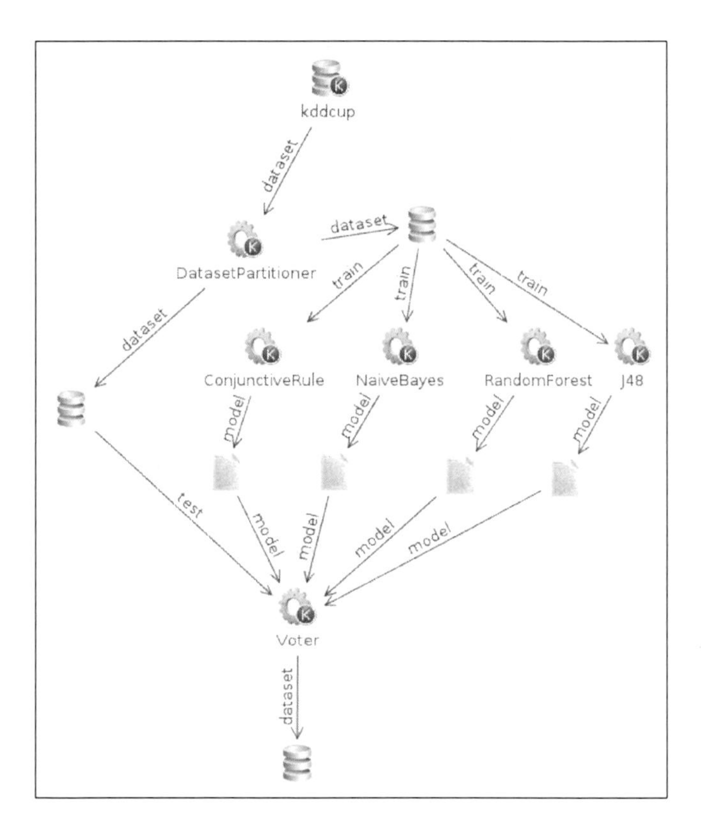

Fig. 10. Ensemble learning workflow

predictions made by each classifier. The same workflow has been executed, for each of the three datasets, using a number of computing nodes ranging from 1 to 4 (excluding the node where we performed the voting operation) to evaluate the speedup of the system.

The workflow corresponding to the application is shown in Fig. 10. It includes a dataset node representing the kddcup dataset, connected to a tool node associated with a dataset partitioner, from which a test set and a training set are obtained, as detailed above. The training set is connected to four tool nodes, associated with the classification algorithms mentioned earlier. The four models generated by such algorithms are connected to a tool node associated with a voter which assigns to each istance of the test set a class obtained through a voting operation.

Table 5 reports the execution times of the application when 1, 2 and 4 computing nodes are used. The four tasks are indicated as $DM_1..DM_4$, corresponding ConjuctiveRule, NaiveBayes, RandomForest and J48 respectively. The table shows how the tasks are assigned to the computing nodes, as well as the execution times for each dataset size.

Table 5. Task assignments and execution times for the ensemble learning workflow

No of nodes	Task assignments (Node ← Tasks)	Exec. time 100 MB	Exec. time 140 MB	Exec. time 180 MB
1	$N_1 \leftarrow DM_1, ..., DM_4$	1:30:50	2:31:14	3:34:27
2	$N_1 \leftarrow DM_1, DM_3$ $N_2 \leftarrow DM_2, DM_4$	1:03:47	1:37:05	2:07:05
4	$N_1 \leftarrow DM_i$ for $1 \leq i \leq 4$	46:16	1:13:47	1:37:23

The execution times and speedup values for different number of nodes and dataset sizes are represented in Fig. 11. In this case, the speedup is lower than that obtained with the parameter sweeping workflow. This is due to the fact that the four algorithms used require very different amounts of time to complete their execution on a given dataset. In fact, the overall execution time is bound to the execution time of the slowest algorithm, thus limiting the speedup. However, the absolute amount of time saved by running the application on a distributed environment is still significant, particularly for the largest dataset when four computing nodes are used.

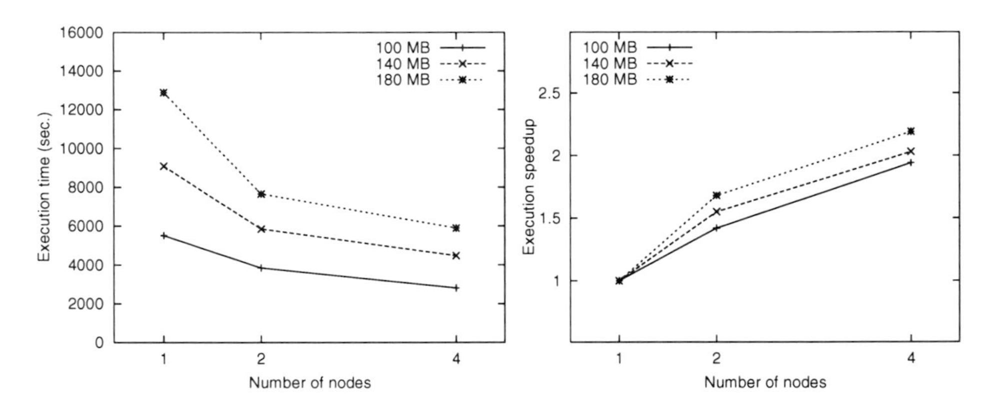

Fig. 11. Execution times and speedup values for different numbers of nodes and dataset sizes, for the ensemble learning workflow

7 Related Work

Other workflow systems, although most of them not specifically designed for distributed data mining applications, have been proposed for Grid environments; among them the most popular ones are Askalon [7], Kepler [8], Pegasus [9], Taverna [10], Triana [11], Weka4WS [12].

ASKALON [7] is an Application Development and Runtime Environment for the Grid. Developed at the University of Innsbruck, Austria, it uses a custom language called AGWL for describing Grid workflow applications at a high level of abstraction. It has a SOA-based runtime environment with stateful services and uses the Globus Toolkit as Grid platform.

Kepler [8] provides a graphical user interface and a run-time engine that can execute workflows (with an emphasis on ecology and geology) either from within the graphical interface or from a command line. It is developed and maintained by a team consisting of several key institutions at the University of California, USA. Kepler works based on the concept of *directors*, which dictate the models of execution used within a workflow. It is a java-based application that is maintained for the Windows, OSX, and Linux operating systems and freely available under the BSD License.

The Pegasus [9] project, developed at the University of Southern California, USA, encompasses a set of technologies to execute workflow-based applications in a number of different environments, i.e., desktops, campus clusters, Grids, and Clouds. The worfklow management system of Pegasus can manage the execution of complex workflows on distributed resources and it is provided with a sophisticated error recovery system.

Taverna [10] is an open source tool for designing and executing workflows, developed at the University of Manchester, UK. Its own workflow definition language is characterized by an implicit iteration mechanism (single node implicit parallelism). The Taverna team has primarily focused on supporting the Life Sciences community (biology, chemistry and medical imaging) although does not provide any analytical or data services itself. It supports different types of Web services, including WSDL-based, Soaplab, BioMoby and BioMart services.

Triana [11] is a problem solving environment, developed at Cardiff University, UK, that combines a visual interface with data analysis tools. It can connect heterogeneous tools (e.g. Web services, Java units, JXTA services) on one workflow. Triana uses its own custom workflow language, although can use other external workflow language representations such as BPEL4WS [13] which are available through *pluggable* language readers and writers. Triana comes with a wide variety of built-in tools for signal-analysis, image-manipulation, desk-top publishing, etc.

Weka4WS [12] is a framework developed at the University of Calabria, Italy, to extend the widely used Weka toolkit for supporting distributed data mining on Grid environments. Weka4WS has been designed by using the Web Services Resource Framework (WSRF) as enabling technology. In particular, it has been developed by using the WSRF Java library provided by Globus Toolkit 4.0.

Differently from most of the system described above, DIS3GNO has been specifically developed to support distributed data mining application design. Also compared to the other systems that are data-mining oriented (e.g., Weka4WS), DIS3GNO provides additional features for metadata management, supports abstract resources and runtime matching, and allows an easier use of third-party algorithms.

8 Conclusions

Workflows are effective formalisms to represent data and execution flows associated with complex data mining tasks. The DIS3GNO system described in this chapter provides a set of visual facilities to design and execute distributed data mining workflows in Grids.

The DIS3GNO GUI operates as an intermediary between the final user and the Knowledge Grid, a service-oriented system for high-performance distributed KDD. All the Knowledge Grid services for metadata and execution management are accessed transparently by DIS3GNO, thus allowing the domain experts to compose and run complex data mining application without worrying about the underlying infrastructure details.

The experimental evaluation conducted by executing some typical data mining patterns has demonstrated the effectiveness of the DIS3GNO system to support data mining workflows design and execution in distributed Grid environments.

References

1. Cannataro, M., Talia, D.: The Knowledge Grid. Communitations of the ACM 46(1), 89–93 (2003)
2. Mastroianni, C., Talia, D., Trunfio, P.: Metadata for Managing Grid Resources in Data Mining Applications. Journal of Grid Computing 2(1), 85–102 (2004)
3. Congiusta, A., Talia, D., Trunfio, P.: Distributed data mining services leveraging WSRF. Future Generation Computer Systems 23(1), 34–41 (2007)
4. Foster, I.: Globus Toolkit Version 4: Software for service-oriented systems. In: Conf. on Network and Parallel Computing, pp. 2–13 (2005)
5. Zhou, Z.H.: Semi-supervised learning by disagreement. In: 4th IEEE International Conference on Granular Computing, p. 93 (2008)
6. Tan, P.N., Steinbach, M., Kumar, V.: Introduction to Data Mining. Addison-Wesley, Reading (2006)
7. Fahringer, T., Jugravu, A., Pllana, S., Prodan, R., Seragiotto, C. Jr., Truong, H.L.: ASKALON: A Tool Set for Cluster and Grid Computing. Concurrency and Computation: Practice & Experience 17(2-4) (2005)
8. Altintas, I., Berkley, C., Jaeger, E., Jones, M., Ludascher, B., Mock, S.: Kepler: an extensible system for design and execution of scientific workflows. In: 16th International Conference on Scientific and Statistical Database Management (2004)
9. Deelman, E., Blythe, J., Gil, Y., Kesselman, C., Mehta, G., Patil, S., Su, M.-H., Vahi, K., Livny, M.: Pegasus: Mapping Scientific Workflows onto the Grid. In: Across Grids Conference (2004)
10. Hull, D., Wolstencroft, K., Stevens, R., Goble, C., Pocock, M., Li, P., Oinn, T.: Taverna: a tool for building and running workflows of services. Nucleic Acids Research 34(Web Server issue), 729–732 (2006)

11. Shields, M., Taylor, I.: Programming Scientific and Distributed Workflow with Triana Services. In: Workflow in Grid Systems Workshop in GGF 2010 (2004)
12. Lackovic, M., Talia, D., Trunfio, P.: A Framework for Composing Knowledge Discovery Workflows in Grids. In: Abraham, A., Hassanien, A., Carvalho, A., Snel, V. (eds.) Foundations of Computational Intelligence, Data Mining Theoretical Foundations and Applications. SCI. Springer, Heidelberg (2009)
13. BPEL4WS. Business Process Execution Language for Web Services. See, http://www.ibm.com/developerworks/library/specification/ws-bpel/

Chapter 5
Formal Framework for the Study of Algorithmic Properties of Objective Interestingness Measures

Yannick Le Bras[1,3], Philippe Lenca[1,3], and Stéphane Lallich[2]

[1] Institut Telecom; Telecom Bretagne; UMR CNRS 3192 Lab-STICC
Technopôle Brest-Iroise - CS 83818 - 29238 Brest Cedex 3 - France
{yannick.lebras,philippe.lenca}@telecom-bretagne.eu
[2] Université de Lyon, Laboratoire ERIC, Lyon 2, France
stephane.lallich@univ-lyon2.fr
[3] Université européenne de Bretagne, France

Abstract. Association Rules Discovery is an increasing subdomain of Datamining. Many works have focused on the extraction and the evaluation of the association rules, leading to many technical improvments on the algorithms, and many different measures. But few number of them have tried to merge the both. We introduce here a formal framework for the study of association rules and interestingness measures that allows an analytic study of these objects. This framework is based on the contingency table of a rule and let us make a link between analytic properties of the measures and algorithmic properties. We give as example the case of three algorithmic properties for the extraction of association rules that were generalized and applied with the help of this framework. These properties allow a pruning of the search space based on a large number of measures and without any support constraint.

1 Introduction

Association Rules Discovery is an important task of Knowledge Discovery consisting of extracting patterns from databases of the form $\mathtt{A} \rightarrow \mathtt{B}$. Such rule $\mathtt{A} \rightarrow \mathtt{B}$ is based on an itemset $\mathtt{AB}$ and characterizes the co-occurrence of itemsets $\mathtt{A}$ and $\mathtt{B}$. The first step of the association rules discovery process is to extract all frequent itemsets. This step benefits from an efficient heuristic that allows the algorithm to efficiently prune the search space, and is at the heart of the APRIORI algorithm [3]. This heuristic says that the higher you go in the itemsets lattice, the less the itemsets are frequent. The algorithm APRIORI uses this heuristic to extract the frequent itemsets with respect to a given threshold: if one itemset is encountered that does not have a frequency higher than the given threshold *minsupp*, then none of its children has an higher frequency than *minsupp*. This heuristic is called the *antimonotony* property of the SUPPORT, where the SUPPORT of an itemset $\mathtt{I}$ is an equivalent term for its frequency and is defined by the proportion of transactions containing $\mathtt{I}$ in the whole database. The second

D.E. Holmes, L.C. Jain (Eds.): Data Mining: Found. & Intell. Paradigms, ISRL 24, pp. 77–98.
springerlink.com

step consists of generating all association rules from the frequent itemsets, and of selecting those having a CONFIDENCE value higher than a given threshold *minconf*. The CONFIDENCE of a rule $A \rightarrow B$ is the proportion of rules containing B in the set of rules containing A. At the moment, this step can only be exhaustive. Because of these thresholds, the APRIORI-like algorithms miss many rules, especially the rules that have a low SUPPORT and an high CONFIDENCE i.e. *nuggets of knowledge*: rules concerning rare diseases, very particular cases... In addition, choosing an high CONFIDENCE threshold favors rules $A \rightarrow B$ having a very frequent consequent B: for example since bread is present in many market transactions, a rule with bread in consequent is not really interesting. As a consequence, in order to filter the large final set of rules one has to use a post-process, for instance with additional measures of interest. For a while only few works were interested in finding other algorithmic properties but it becomes nowadays of great importance.

Since the origin of the field of association rules discovery, many works have focused on trying to accelerate the mining phase. In fact, mining association rules is a very costly task of datamining, and becomes always harder with the actual databases, which are larger each day. Since the first definition of APRIORI algorithm [3], many efforts have been made to decrease the computation time, by changing the data structure [16] or optimizing the implementations [6]. As time goes by, the originally used SUPPORT/CONFIDENCE's couple came out as inadequate, and others measures where used (at the best of our knowledge, the more advanced inventory, with 69 measures, can be found in [15]), but none of them could be used at the heart of the algorithms. Indeed, whatever the measure, one had to first mine frequent itemsets, and then generate interesting rules, whilst assuming a large number of possible rules.

Consequently, it appeared that no measure presents an algorithmic advantage, and in order to distinguish one from each other, specific properties of variation and behavior were studied. This led to complex models and studies, and approximate formulations. In this domain, there was a real lack of a general framework to study interestingness measures.

In this context and after many years of technical improvements, the first algorithms based on algorithmic properties of measures arrived. Three of them, which we considered as particularly interesting, have attracted our attention. The reason is that they allow a pruning of the search space in the manner of the SUPPORT. The first two works are exclusively based on CONFIDENCE. [32] discovered a generalization of CONFIDENCE for itemsets that has the same antimonotny property as the SUPPORT. Although losing many rules, the main advantage of this new measure was that it allowed the reuse of all the technical improvements made around APRIORI. As for [40], they described an algorithmic property of CONFIDENCE for classification rules, i.e. rules with a predetermined target item. Unlike antimonotonicity, this property allows a top-down pruning of the search space. The main advantage is that this pruning strategy finds nuggets of knowledge, i.e. rules with high CONFIDENCE and low SUPPORT. Finally, [29] introduced the notion of optimal rule sets and proposed an efficient algorithm to mine them. This work was a great step forward since the underlying algorithmic property can be applied to a larger set of measures.

In our view, these works are very encouraging, particularly the one of [29]. Since it can apply to many measures, it was natural for us to try to extend this list. However, an arduous case-by-case analysis appeared to us as inadmissible, and the fact that the same property can be applied to many measures persuaded us that this had to see with intrinsic properties of the measures. To work with this assumption, we present here a framework for the analytical study of measures, that can take into account any parameterization of the measure. In fact, many works have focused on the behavior of measures with the variation of examples, but some have shown the importance of the behavior of a measure against the counter examples, or of its relation with CONFIDENCE. Our framework allows us to choose any of these points of view.

This chapter presents a survey of our works in this domain. We first draw the scientific landscape of our work, then we describe in depth the relevant framework and finally present its applications in the domain of pruning strategies. For more precisions, references and complete proofs, we suggest that the interested reader has a look at [22,24,25,23].

In the following, the notations will be precisely detailed. In broad strokes, $\mathtt{I}$ is an item (or valuated attribute), $\mathtt{A}$ is an attribute, $\mathtt{T}$ is a transaction, $\mathtt{X}$, $\mathtt{Y}$, $\mathtt{Z}$ stand for itemsets (or sets of valuated attributes), $\mathbb{P}$ is the classical symbol for probabilities, and we denote by p_x the value of $\mathbb{P}(\mathtt{X})$.

2 Scientific Landscape

Before introducing our formal framework, let first describe the scientific landscape of our works. The following parts refer to the domain of association rule mining and evaluation in the datamining task. Therefore, many concepts have to be described, namely the concepts of *database*, *association rule* and *evaluation*. We will describe them in the preceding order.

Table 1.

	$\mathtt{I}_1$	$\mathtt{I}_2$	$\mathtt{I}_3$	$\mathtt{I}_4$	$\mathtt{I}_5$	$\mathtt{I}_6$	$\mathtt{I}_7$
$\mathtt{T}_1$	1	1	0	1	1	0	1
$\mathtt{T}_2$	0	1	0	1	1	1	0
$\mathtt{T}_3$	1	0	1	0	0	0	1
$\mathtt{T}_4$	1	1	1	0	1	1	1
$\mathtt{T}_5$	0	1	0	0	0	1	1
$\mathtt{T}_6$	0	0	1	1	1	0	1

2.1 Database

A Database is described by a set of items $I = \{\mathtt{I}_1, \ldots, \mathtt{I}_n\}$, a set of transactions $T = \{\mathtt{T}_1, \ldots, \mathtt{T}_m\}$ and a binary relation $\mathcal{R}$ over $T \times I$. It can be viewed as a matrix

Table 2. Example of a categorical database

WORKCLASS	EDUCATION	MARITAL-STATUS	OCCUPATION	RELATIONSHIP	INCOME
State-gov	Bachelors	Never-married	Adm-clerical	Not-in-family	≤50K
Self-emp-not-inc	Bachelors	Married-civ-spouse	Exec-managerial	Husband	≤50K
Private	HS-grad	Divorced	Handlers-cleaners	Not-in-family	≤50K
Private	11th	Married-civ-spouse	Handlers-cleaners	Husband	≤50K
Private	Bachelors	Married-civ-spouse	Prof-specialty	Wife	≤50K
Private	Masters	Married-civ-spouse	Exec-managerial	Wife	≤50K
Private	9th	Married-spouse-absent	Other-service	Not-in-family	≤50K
Self-emp-not-inc	HS-grad	Married-civ-spouse	Exec-managerial	Husband	>50K

as shown Table 1: If $\mathtt{T}_p\mathcal{R}\mathtt{I}_q$ then the element (p, q) of the matrix is 1, else 0. This formalism stands for *the transaction number p contains the item q*. Equivalently, one can see a transaction T_p as the itemset of all items in relation with T_p. For example, in Table 1, $\mathtt{T}_3 = \{\mathtt{I}_1, \mathtt{I}_3, \mathtt{I}_7\}$. This kind of database is a binary database, and describes the presence/absence of an item in the transactions. For example, it can describe the presence of products in a market basket, or the presence/absence of symptoms in a medical database.

However, many of the actual databases (see for example [4]) have categorical or numerical attributes, instead of simple items. Our works focus on binary databases and categorical databases. In case of numerical attributes, we first apply discretization algorithms to obtain categorical attributes. As such, let us focus on categorical databases. A categorical database is described by a set of attributes $A = \{\mathtt{A}_1, \ldots, \mathtt{A}_n\}$, for each attribute $\mathtt{A}_i$ a set of values $\mathcal{V}\mathtt{A}_i = \{a_1^{(i)}, \ldots, a_{n_i}^{(i)}\}$, a set of transactions $T = \{\mathtt{T}_1, \ldots, \mathtt{T}_m\}$ and a function f over $T \times A$ such that $f(\mathtt{T}_p, \mathtt{A}_q) \in \mathcal{V}\mathtt{A}_q$, meaning that in transaction $\mathtt{T}_p$, the value of $\mathtt{A}_q$ is $a_k^{(q)} \in \mathcal{V}\mathtt{A}_q$. Table 2 shows an example of categorical database extracted from the well known Census Database. In this example, we have an attribute EDUCATION whose values are $\mathcal{V}$EDUCATION= {bachelors,HS-grad,11th,Masters,9th}. It is important to notice that a categorical database can be simply binarized by creating one attribute for each couple $(\mathtt{A}_i, a_p^{(i)})$. One major drawback of this method is the large increase of size when each attribute has a large number of values. However, it let us use the simple word *database* for either of those two types of databases, binary or categorical.

Databases are collected in many different manners, and for many different reasons and applications. Our works focus on the observation of co-appearance of items or attributes in the data. In this context, we call *itemset* a set of items, or a set of valuated attributes. This task makes a distinction between two sorts of databases: databases without mining constraints, and classification databases. The latter are databases with a so called class attribute, used for prediction tasks. As an example, the attribute INCOME in the Census database is a class attribute. This can be used as target in decision tree building for example. Databases without a class attribute are *without mining constraints*, and can be used to observe association between attributes, such as setting up aisle end displays in a market basket database for example.

2.2 Association Rules

As mentioned above, we focus here on the observation of co-appearance of items or attributes in a given database $\mathcal{DB}$. More precisely, we are interested in *association rules*. An association rule is an object of the form $\mathtt{X} \stackrel{\mathcal{DB}}{\rightarrow} \mathtt{Y}$ where:

- $\mathtt{X}$ and $\mathtt{Y}$ are non-empty itemsets,
- $\mathtt{X} \cap \mathtt{Y} = \emptyset$,
- $\mathtt{X}$ (resp. $\mathtt{Y}$) is called antecedent (resp. consequent) of the rule,

When no ambiguity is possible, we only write $\mathtt{X} \rightarrow \mathtt{Y}$.

The literal translation of an association rule $\mathtt{X} \stackrel{\mathcal{DB}}{\rightarrow} \mathtt{Y}$ could be *"if one can find* $\mathtt{X}$ *in a transaction of database* $\mathcal{DB}$*, then he would probably find* $\mathtt{Y}$ *too"*. The big deal with association rules is to quantify this *probably*. Historically, this has been done by using two measures, SUPPORT (*supp*) and CONFIDENCE (*conf*). The SUPPORT is the probability of appearance of the itemset $\mathtt{XY}$ in the whole database and is the expression of the frequency of the itemset, while CONFIDENCE is the probability of appearance of the itemset $\mathtt{XY}$ in the set of transactions containing $\mathtt{X}$ and expresses the dependence of $\mathtt{Y}$ on $\mathtt{X}$. In terms of probabilities,SUPPORT can be noted as $\mathbb{P}_{\mathcal{DB}}(\mathtt{XY})$ and CONFIDENCE as $\mathbb{P}_{\mathcal{DB}}(\mathtt{Y}|\mathtt{X})$. As an example, in table 2, the rule r={OCCUPATION=Exec-managerial→INCOME ≤50K } has values $supp(r) = 2/8$ and $conf(r) = 2/3$.

Generally, association rules are defined with respect to a given SUPPORT threshold, say *minsupp*, and a given CONFIDENCE threshold, *minconf*. The first algorithms for mining association rules were AIS and APRIORI. APRIORI was the first real stride in the domain of association rule mining, since it used an algorithmic property of the SUPPORT, called antimonotony. To understand its relevance, it is important to understand that mining association rules is a hard task, due to the large number of possibilities. In fact, if $\mathcal{DB}$ is a database with n items and m transactions, the number of possible itemsets is 2^n, and the number of association rules that can be derived from these itemsets is 3^n. Furthermore, it has been proved that the underlying decision problem is NP-Complete. So, there is no efficient implementation of an association rule mining algorithm. The only possibility to mine association rules, given *minsupp* and *minconf*, is to use heuristics. That's the advantage of antimonotonic property of the SUPPORT: It allows to prune the search space by using a specific heuristic. We give here its definition:

$$\text{if } supp(\mathtt{X}) \leq minsupp, \text{ then for any } \mathtt{I} \notin \mathtt{X},\ supp(\mathtt{XI}) \leq minsupp.$$

The main idea is, when mining all itemsets such that $supp(\mathtt{X}) \geq minsupp$, that this property directs the search by avoiding it for useless cases. This property made the search more effective, but since its introduction, the only technical progresses made were to increase the speed of implementations. In particular, the search for confident rules (those with $conf(\mathtt{X} \rightarrow \mathtt{Y}) \geq minconf$) is always done exhaustively in a distinct phase, by checking, for each frequent itemset, all possibly derived rules. Moreover, the legitimacy of the couple SUPPORT/CONFIDENCE

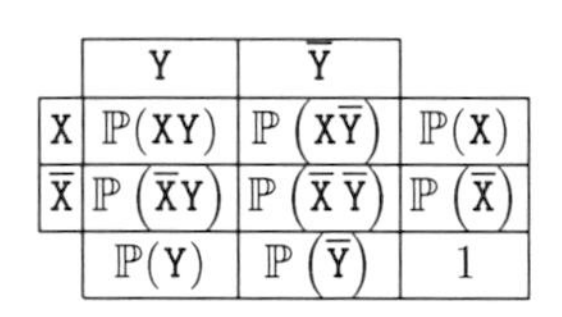

	Y	$\overline{\text{Y}}$	
X	$\mathbb{P}(\text{XY})$	$\mathbb{P}(\text{X}\overline{\text{Y}})$	$\mathbb{P}(\text{X})$
$\overline{\text{X}}$	$\mathbb{P}(\overline{\text{X}}\text{Y})$	$\mathbb{P}(\overline{\text{X}}\,\overline{\text{Y}})$	$\mathbb{P}(\overline{\text{X}})$
	$\mathbb{P}(\text{Y})$	$\mathbb{P}(\overline{\text{Y}})$	1

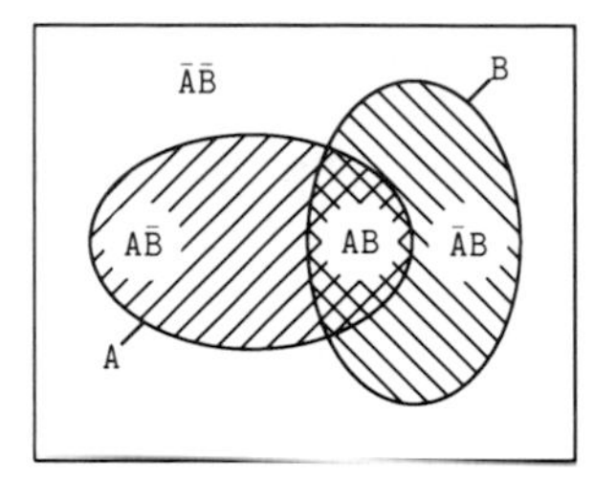

Fig. 1. Contingency table of X and Y, as table and as graphic

Table 3. A set of 38 measures

measure	expression	reference
IWD	$\left(\left(\frac{p_{xy}}{p_x \times p_y}\right)^k - 1\right) \times p_{xy}^m$	[14]
CONFIDENCE	$\frac{p_{xy}}{p_x}$	[10]
ADDED VALUE	$p_{y\|x} - p_y$	[]
CONTRAMIN	$\frac{2p_{xy} - p_x}{p_y}$	[5]
CONVICTION	$\frac{p_x p_{\bar{y}}}{p_{x\bar{y}}}$	[8]
COSINE	$\frac{p_{xy}}{\sqrt{p_x p_y}}$	[35]
COVERAGE	p_x	[]
BAYESIAN FACTOR	$\frac{p_{x\|y}}{p_{x\|\bar{y}}}$	[19]
COLLECTIVE STRENGTH	$\frac{p_{xy} + p_{\bar{x}\bar{y}}}{p_x \times p_y + p_{\bar{x}} \times p_{\bar{y}}} \times \frac{p_{\bar{x}} \times p_y + p_x \times p_{\bar{y}}}{p_{\bar{x}y} + p_{x\bar{y}}}$	[1]
INFORMATION GAIN	$\log \frac{p_{xy}}{p_x p_y}$	[9]
GINI INDEX	$\frac{1}{p_x} \times ({p_{xy}}^2 + {p_{x\bar{y}}}^2) + \frac{1}{p_{\bar{x}}} \times ({p_{\bar{x}y}}^2 + {p_{\bar{x}\bar{y}}}^2) - {p_y}^2 - {p_{\bar{y}}}^2$	[13]
IMPLICATION INDEX	$\sqrt{n}\frac{p_{xy} - p_x p_y}{\sqrt{p_x p_{\bar{y}}}}$	[28]
INTEREST	$\|p_{xy} - p_x p_y\|$	[]
J1-MEASURE	$p_{xy} \times \log \frac{p_{xy}}{p_x p_y}$	[41]
JACCARD	$\frac{\mathbb{P}(A \cap B)}{\mathbb{P}(A \cup B)}$	[18]
J-MEASURE	$p_{xy} \times \log \frac{p_{xy}}{p_x p_y} + p_{x\bar{y}} \times \log \frac{p_{x\bar{y}}}{p_x p_{\bar{y}}}$	[37]
KAPPA	$2\frac{p_{xy} - p_x p_y}{p_x p_{\bar{y}} + p_y p_{\bar{x}}}$	[11]
KLOSGEN	$\sqrt{p_{xy}} \times (p_{y\|x} - p_y)$	[20]
LEVERAGE	$p_{xy} - p_x p_y$	[34]
LIFT	$\frac{p_{xy}}{p_x p_y}$	[7]
LOEVINGER	$\frac{p_{y\|x} - p_y}{1 - p_y}$	[31]
ODDS RATIO	$\frac{p_{xy} p_{\bar{x}\bar{y}}}{p_{x\bar{y}} p_{\bar{x}y}}$	[45]
ONE WAY SUPPORT	$p_{y\|x} \times \log \frac{p_{xy}}{p_x p_y}$	[43]
PEARSON	$\frac{p_{xy} - p_x p_y}{\sqrt{p_x p_y p_{\bar{x}} p_{\bar{y}}}}$	[33]
PIATETSKY-SHAPIRO	$n \times (p_{xy} - p_x p_y)$	[34]
PRECISION	$p_{xy} + p_{\bar{x}\bar{y}}$	[]
PREVALENCE	p_y	[]
YULE'S Q	$\frac{p_{xy} \times p_{\bar{x}\bar{y}} - p_{x\bar{y}} \times p_{\bar{x}y}}{p_{xy} \times p_{\bar{x}\bar{y}} + p_{x\bar{y}} \times p_{\bar{x}y}}$	[45]
RECALL	$\frac{p_{xy}}{p_y}$	[10]
RELATIVE RISK	$\frac{p_{y\|x}}{p_{y\|\bar{x}}}$	[]
SEBAG-SHOENAUER	$\frac{p_{xy}}{p_{x\bar{y}}}$	[36]
SPECIFICITY	$p_{\bar{y}\|\bar{x}}$	[]
RELATIVE SPE.	$p_{\bar{y}\|\bar{x}} - p_{\bar{y}}$	[21]
SUPPORT	p_{xy}	[2]
EX COUNTEREX RATE	$1 - \frac{p_{x\bar{y}}}{p_{xy}}$	[]
SYM ADDED VALUE	$\max(p_{y\|x} - p_y, p_{x\|y} - p_x)$	[39]
YULE'S Y	$\frac{\sqrt{p_{xy} \times p_{\bar{x}\bar{y}}} - \sqrt{p_{x\bar{y}} \times p_{\bar{x}y}}}{\sqrt{p_{xy} \times p_{\bar{x}\bar{y}}} + \sqrt{p_{x\bar{y}} \times p_{\bar{x}y}}}$	[45]
ZHANG	$\frac{p_{xy} - p_x p_y}{\max(p_{xy} p_{\bar{y}}, p_y p_{x\bar{y}})}$	[46]

for mining association rules has been questioned many times. As an example, the case of nuggets of knowledge, with rules having very low SUPPORT and high CONFIDENCE, was pointed out. With APRIORI implementations, these rules can only be traversed by setting up a very low SUPPORT threshold, which makes the search exhaustive. But the problem is not only quantitative, but qualitative too. Association rules mined with the SUPPORT/CONFIDENCE framework are not always pertinent, because these measures don't always represent the real interest of the user.

2.3 Interestingness Measures

One way for solving the qualitative issue is to use other measures, called *interestingness measures*, to quantify the interest of a rule. Interestingness measures are functions associating a real number to association rules, qualifying thus the interest of the rule for the user. As a direct consequence, the number of interestingness measures is as large as the number of application domains, users... and is a real problem for their study. Moreover, there exists two types of interestingness measures: subjective and objective interestingness measures. The former are measures based on expert's knowledge, which means that the expert has a real role in the evaluation process. Consequently, the number of presented rules can only be very restricted. The latter are measures based only on the contingency table (figure 1) that is on statistical properties of the rule. They only need numeric calculations and no intervention of the expert.Thus, they can easily be implemented in the post-analysis like CONFIDENCE, but this analysis can once again only be exhaustive.

Interestingness Measures can have many origins. As examples, SUPPORT and CONFIDENCE come from probabilities theory, the measure of JACCARD, defined as $\frac{|\mathtt{X} \cup \mathtt{Y}|}{|\mathtt{X} \cap \mathtt{Y}|}$ comes from sets theory, or ONE WAY SUPPORT, $\frac{\mathbb{P}(\mathtt{XY})}{\mathbb{P}(\mathtt{X})} \log \frac{\mathbb{P}(\mathtt{XY})}{\mathbb{P}(\mathtt{X})\mathbb{P}(\mathtt{Y})}$, comes from information theory. The rule

$$r = \{\text{OCCUPATION} = \text{Exec-managerial} \rightarrow \text{INCOME} \leq 50K\}$$

from preceding section has values $Jacc(r) = 1/4$ and $OWS(r) = -0.68$. That is, two measures give very different values to the same rule. The set of objective measures is very large, but there are some rules based on common sense for the definition of a measure. [34] for example gave some recommendations for a measure μ that were mainly followed at this time:

- $\mu = 0$ if $\mathbb{P}(\mathtt{XY}) = \mathbb{P}(\mathtt{X})\mathbb{P}(\mathtt{Y})$. If X and Y are statistically independent, the rule is not interesting.
- μ monotonically increases with $\mathbb{P}(\mathtt{XY})$ when other parameters remain the same.
- μ monotonically decreases with $\mathbb{P}(\mathtt{X})$ (or $\mathbb{P}(\mathtt{Y})$) when other parameters remain the same.

Interesting surveys can be found [12,27,38,15], but if one wants to introduce the measures in an algorithm as a heuristic, an exhaustive study does not seem to be reasonable. Moreover, one measure may not be sufficient, and some users may want to aggregate different measures. This widely increases the number of possibilities. The best way to study interestingness measures is to introduce a specific framework that would allow an automatic study of interestingness measures.

3 A Framework for the Study of Measures

We propose here to introduce a formal framework that will enable an analytic study of interestingness measures. We only focus on objective interestingness measures. Such measures can be expressed with the help of the contingency table in relative frequencies, and consequently with three parameters. The study of their variations with respect to these variables will allow us to create a link between the measures and their algorithmic properties, but they require the description of a domain of definition in order to study only real cases.

3.1 Adapted Functions of Measure

We here rely on an idea introduced by [17] for describing interestingness measures in an analytical way. Our main contribution is to allow the use of the framework in many situations by considering the contingency table. We will describe here this idea, but at first, some notions need to be introduced.

Contingency Tables. We already discussed this tool above, but we give here more precisions on its specifics. Let $\mathtt{X}$ and $\mathtt{Y}$ be two itemsets on the database $\mathcal{DB}$. The contingency table in relative joint frequencies of $\mathtt{X}$ and $\mathtt{Y}$ gives information about the simultaneous presence of these itemsets (figure 1). The contingency table has 3 degrees of freedom: one needs at least 3 of its values to describe it, and 3 values are enough to find all other values. For example, the contingency table is fully described by the two marginal frequencies $supp(\mathtt{X})$ and $supp(\mathtt{Y})$ and the joint frequency $supp(\mathtt{XY})$. An association rule on a given database is described by two itemsets. One can also speak about the contingency table of an association rule, which leads us to the notion of descriptor system. For practical purpose, the study of interestingness measures is focused on one particular cell of the contingency table: The Piatetsky-Shapiro recommendations focus on the examples rate of the rules, *i.e.* $supp(\mathtt{XY})$, but the interestingness measures were also studied by considering the counter-examples rate of the rules for robustness [26], or their relation to CONFIDENCE. To consider all these possibilities, we introduced the notion of *descriptor system*.

Definition 1. *We call* descriptor system *of the contingency table a triplet of functions* (f, g, h) *over the association rules which fully describes the contingency table of association rules.*

The meaning of this definition is that, given a descriptor system (f, g, h), any cell of the contingency table, as an example $\mathbb{P}(\mathtt{XY})$, can be described as a function of the descriptor system, *i.e.* $\mathbb{P}(\mathtt{XY}) = u(f(\mathtt{X} \rightarrow \mathtt{Y}), g(\mathtt{X} \rightarrow \mathtt{Y}), h(\mathtt{X} \rightarrow \mathtt{Y}))$. The functions of the descriptor system can be elements of the contingency table, but not exclusively. We give here an example, using the CONFIDENCE, to give a better understanding.

Example 1. We define the following functions:

$$conf(\mathtt{X} \rightarrow \mathtt{Y}) = \frac{supp(\mathtt{XY})}{supp(\mathtt{X})}; \; ant(\mathtt{X} \rightarrow \mathtt{Y}) = supp(\mathtt{X}); \; cons(\mathtt{X} \rightarrow \mathtt{Y}) = supp(\mathtt{Y})$$

The triplet $(conf, ant, cons)$ is a descriptor system of the contingency table.

The same stands for the functions $ex(\mathtt{X} \rightarrow \mathtt{Y}) = supp(\mathtt{XY})$ and $c\text{-}ex(\mathtt{X} \rightarrow \mathtt{Y}) = supp(\mathtt{X\bar{Y}})$: the triplets $(ex, ant, cons)$ and $(c\text{-}ex, ant, cons)$ are descriptor systems.

There exists a large number of measures [39,12,44,27], but most of them can be expressed with the contingency table and thus considered as 3 variables functions (a descriptor system of the contingency table). In the following, we only focus on this kind of measures.

Minimal Joint Domain. As we want to use descriptor systems to analytically study the measures, we will study the three variables function mentioned above. For example, we want to study their variations. The question is: why study the variations at a point that will never be reached by a rule. For instance, if we want to study the variations of the function $x \mapsto x^2$ on real positive values (the function increases), it's useless to study the variations (decreasing) for negative values, since it would introduce noise in our thinking. A descriptor system $d = (f, g, h)$ of the contingency table is a triplet of variables over the space of association rules, and an interestingness measure μ can be written with the help of a function ϕ_μ of this triplet. If we want to do an analytic study of this function, we need only to restrict the analysis to the joint variation domain of the triplet. Moreover, the study will provide no sense out of this domain, where the points match no real situation. Thus, the joint variation domain D_d must be such that:

- if r is a rule, then $(f(r), g(r), h(r)) \in D_d$
- if $(x, y, z) \in D_d$ then there exists a database $\mathcal{DB}$ and a rule r on $\mathcal{DB}$ such that $(f(r), g(r), h(r)) = (x, y, z)$.

Then the joint variation domain is complete and minimal.

If d is a descriptor system of the contingency table, the joint variation domain associated with this system is defined by the constraints laid down by the values of d between themselves. Table 4 shows different variation domains, Figure 2 shows their appearance, and we give here a simple proof for the domain associated to CONFIDENCE.

Table 4. Joint Variation Domain for 3 parameterizations

CONFIDENCE

$$D_{conf} = \left\{ \begin{pmatrix} c \\ y \\ z \end{pmatrix} \in \mathbb{Q}^3 | \begin{array}{ccc} 0 & < y < & 1 \\ 0 & < z < & 1 \\ \max\{0, 1 - \frac{1-z}{y}\} & \leq c \leq & \min\{1, \frac{z}{y}\} \end{array} \right\}$$

Counterexamples

$$D_{c-ex} = \left\{ \begin{pmatrix} \bar{x} \\ y \\ z \end{pmatrix} \in \mathbb{Q}^3 | \begin{array}{ccc} 0 & < y < & 1 \\ 0 & < z < & 1 \\ \max\{0, y - z\} & \leq \bar{x} \leq & \min\{y, 1 - z\} \end{array} \right\}$$

Examples

$$D_{ex} = \left\{ \begin{pmatrix} x \\ y \\ z \end{pmatrix} \in \mathbb{Q}^3 | \begin{array}{ccc} 0 & < y < & 1 \\ 0 & < z < & 1 \\ \max\{0, 1 - y - z\} & \leq x \leq & \min\{y, z\} \end{array} \right\}$$

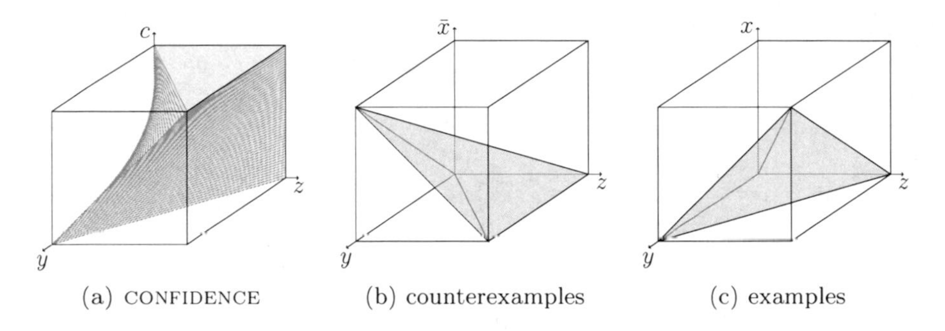

(a) CONFIDENCE (b) counterexamples (c) examples

Fig. 2. Joint Variation Domain for 3 parameterizations

Proof. The proof we give here is the proof of the inclusion of D_{conf} in the adapted domain associated to the CONFIDENCE. We will prove that any point (c, y, z) of D_{conf} is the projection of a rule r such that:

$$(conf(r), ant(r), cons(r)) = (c, y, z)$$

Consider an element (c, y, z) of D_{conf}, we need to construct a database $\mathcal{DB}$ containing an association rule $\mathtt{X} \rightarrow \mathtt{Y}$, such that $\mu(\mathtt{X} \rightarrow \mathtt{Y})$ equals to $\phi_\mu(c, y, z)$. Our database should then verify the following equalities:

$$conf(\mathtt{X} \rightarrow \mathtt{Y}) = c,\ supp(\mathtt{X}) = y,\ supp(\mathtt{Y}) = z. \quad (1)$$

Since c, y and z are rational numbers, we define n as an integer such that $(c \times y \times n, y \times n, z \times n) \in \mathbb{N}^3$. The constraints of the domain D_{conf} (see Table 4 assure that $0 \leq (1 - c) \times y \times n \leq y \times n \leq y \times n \times (1 - c) + z \times n \leq n$ holds, and we can thus construct the database of table 5, satisfying the equalities 1. Then, the inclusion is verified, since there is a database $\mathcal{DB}$ containing a rule r verifying equation 1. That is, any point of D_{conf} is associated to a rule. □

Table 5. Database for the domain D_{conf}

X (brace over the first columns)

	1		$(1-c) \times y \times n$			$y \times n$			$((1-c) \times y + z) \times n$			n
X	1	···	···	···	···	1	0	···	···	···	···	0
Y	0	···	0	1	···	···	···	···	1	0	···	0

Y (brace under the middle columns)

Finally, we have identified the joint variation domain of the descriptor system d_{conf}: It is exactly D_{conf}. The same method is used to prove similar results for D_{ex} and D_{c-ex}.

Now, it clearly appears that to do an analytic study of an interestingness measure, three things have to be focused carefully. One first has to exactly define the interesting parameters for this study (this is our notion of descriptor system), then the measure has to be expressed as a function of these parameters (this is our function Φ_μ of three variables), and finally, the variation domain of the variables of this function has to be exactly defined, as minimal and complete (this is what we called minimal joint domain of d, or d-adapted domain). To aggregate all of these concepts, we introduce the unified notion of d-adapted function of measure.

Definition 2. *We call the couple (ϕ_μ, D_d), made from this function and the joint variation domain (associated to a specific descriptor system), the d-*adapted function of measure *of the measure μ.*

It is important to see that the form of the functional part of this function of measure depends on the descriptor system chosen. However, when this system is fixed, the adapted function of measure is uniquely defined. In the following, we voluntarily omit to mention the chosen descriptor system if there is no possibility of ambiguity.

3.2 Expression of a Set of Measures

As stressed above, most of the objective interestingness measures are functions of the contingency table. For example, the measure of SEBAG SHOENAUER is known as $\frac{\mathbb{P}(XY)}{\mathbb{P}(X\bar{Y})}$ (the quotient of number of examples by the number of counterexamples). The D_{ex}-adapted function of measure for SEBAG SHOENAUER is then $\frac{x}{y-x}$, the D_{c-ex}-adapted function of measure is $\frac{y-x}{x}$ and finally the D_{conf}-adapted function of measure is $\frac{1-c}{c}$. Table 6 gives the expression of a non-exhaustive set of objective measures in the 3 different adapted domains mentioned above. We now benefit from an analytical framework for studying interestingness measures. With the help of the adapted functions of measure, we shall study them rigorously like any analytic function. One of the most important criteria is the study of variations. Indeed, many works have focused on the variations of measures with one particular value of the contingency table. For instance, Piatetsky-Shapiro introduced recommendations based on the variations of measures when some parameters where fixed. This can be translated in our framework. The 3 recommendations of Piatetsky-Shapiro become:

Let μ be a measure and (Φ_μ, D_{ex}) its adapted function of measure.

- $\Phi_\mu(y \times z, y, z) = 0$,
- $\partial_1\Phi_\mu$ shall be positive,
- $\partial_2\Phi_\mu$ and $\partial_3\Phi_\mu$ shall be negative.

We show here the importance of adapted domain. Let's take the case of specificity Measure: in D_{ex}, we have $\partial_2\Phi_{spe}(x, y, z) = -\frac{z-x}{(1-y)^2}$. This could be positive, if $z - x < 0$, but since we are on D_{ex}, the constraints assume that $x \leq z$. We can prove in the same manner that the specificity measure respects all the

Table 6. Expression of the measures in 3 different adapted domains

name	examples	counterexamples	CONFIDENCE
IWD	$\left(\left(\frac{x}{y\times z}\right)^k-1\right)\times x^m$	$\left(\left(\frac{y-\bar{x}}{y\times z}\right)^k-1\right)\times (y-\bar{x})^m$	$\left(\left(\frac{c}{z}\right)^k-1\right)\times (c\times y)^m$
CONFIDENCE	$\frac{x}{y}$	$\frac{y-\bar{x}}{y}$	c
ADDED VALUE	$\frac{x}{y}-z$	$1-z-\frac{\bar{x}}{y}$	$c-z$
CONTRAMIN	$\frac{2x-y}{z}$	$\frac{y-2\bar{x}}{z}$	$y\times\frac{2c-1}{z}$
CONVICTION	$\frac{y\times(1-z)}{y-x}$	$\frac{y\times(1-z)}{\bar{x}}$	$\frac{1-z}{1-c}$
COSINE	$\frac{x}{\sqrt{y\times z}}$	$\frac{y-\bar{x}}{\sqrt{y\times z}}$	$c\times\sqrt{\frac{y}{z}}$
COVERAGE	y	y	y
BAYESIAN FACTOR	$\frac{x\times(1-z)}{z\times(y-x)}$	$\frac{(y-\bar{x})\times(1-z)}{z\times\bar{x}}$	$\frac{c\times(1-z)}{z\times(1-c)}$
COLLECTIVE STRENGTH	$\frac{1+2x-y-z}{y\times z+(1-y)\times(1-z)}\times\frac{y\times(1-z)+z\times(1-y)}{y+z-2x}$	$\frac{1+y-z-2\bar{x}}{y\times z+(1-y)\times(1-z)}\times\frac{y\times(1-z)+z\times(1-y)}{2\bar{x}+z-y}$	$\frac{1+2c\times y-y-z}{y\times z+(1-y)\times(1-z)}\times\frac{y\times(1-z)+z\times(1-y)}{y+z-2c\times y}$
INFORMATION GAIN	$\log\frac{x}{y\times z}$	$\log\frac{y-\bar{x}}{y\times z}$	$\log c\times z$
GINI INDEX	$\frac{1}{y}\times(x^2+(y-x)^2)+\frac{1}{1-y}\times((z-x)^2+(1-y-(z-x))^2)-z^2-(1-z)^2$	$\frac{1}{y}\times((y-\bar{x})^2+\bar{x}^2)+\frac{1}{1-y}\times((z-y+\bar{x})^2+(1-z-\bar{x})^2)-z^2-(1-z)^2$	$y\times(c^2+(1-c)^2)+\frac{1}{1-y}\times((z-c\times y)^2+(1-z-(1-c)\times y)^2)-z^2-(1-z)^2$
IMPLICATION INDEX	$\sqrt{n}\frac{x-y\times z}{\sqrt{y\times(1-z)}}$	$\sqrt{n}\frac{y\times(1-z)-\bar{x}}{\sqrt{y\times(1-z)}}$	$(c-z)\times\sqrt{\frac{ny}{z}}$
INTEREST	$\lvert x-y\times z\rvert$	$\lvert y\times(1-z)-\bar{x}\rvert$	$\lvert y\times(c-z)\rvert$
J1-MEASURE	$x\times\log\frac{x}{y\times z}$	$(y-\bar{x})\times\log\frac{y-\bar{x}}{y\times z}$	$c\times y\times\log\frac{c}{z}$
JACCARD	$\frac{x}{y+z-x}$	$\frac{y-\bar{x}}{z+\bar{x}}$	$\frac{c}{1-c+\frac{z}{y}}$
J-MEASURE	$x\times\log\frac{x}{y\times z}+(y-x)\times\log\frac{y-x}{y\times(1-z)}$	$(y-\bar{x})\times\log\frac{y-\bar{x}}{y\times z}+\bar{x}\times\log\frac{\bar{x}}{y\times(1-z)}$	$c\times y\times\log\frac{c}{z}+y\times(1-c)\times\log\frac{1-c}{1-z}$
KAPPA	$2\frac{x-y\times z}{y+z-2y\times z}$	$2\frac{y\times(1-z)-\bar{x}}{y+z-2y\times z}$	$2\frac{y\times(c-z)}{y+z-2y\times z}$
KLOSGEN	$\sqrt{x}\times(\frac{x}{y}-z)$	$\sqrt{y-\bar{x}}\times(1-z-\frac{\bar{x}}{y})$	$\sqrt{c\times y}\times(c-z)$
LEVERAGE	$x-y\times z$	$y\times(1-z)-\bar{x}$	$y\times(c-z)$
LIFT	$\frac{x}{y\times z}$	$\frac{y-\bar{x}}{y\times z}$	$\frac{c}{z}$
LOEVINGER	$1-\frac{y-x}{y\times(1-z)}$	$1-\frac{\bar{x}}{y\times(1-z)}$	$1-\frac{1-c}{1-z}$
ODDS RATIO	$1+\frac{x-y\times z}{(y-x)\times(z-x)}$	$1+\frac{y\times(1-z)-\bar{x}}{\bar{x}\times(z-y+\bar{x})}$	$1+\frac{c-z}{(1-c)\times(z-c\times y)}$
ONE WAY SUPPORT	$\frac{x}{y}\times\log\frac{x}{y\times z}$	$\frac{y-\bar{x}}{y}\times\log\frac{y-\bar{x}}{y\times z}$	$c\times\log\frac{c}{z}$
PEARSON	$\frac{x-y\times z}{\sqrt{y\times z\times(1-y)\times(1-z)}}$	$\frac{y\times(1-z)-\bar{x}}{\sqrt{y\times z\times(1-y)\times(1-z)}}$	$\frac{y\times(c-z)}{\sqrt{y\times z\times(1-y)\times(1-z)}}$
PIATETSKY-SHAPIRO	$n\times(x-y\times z)$	$n\times(y\times(1-z)-\bar{x})$	$n\times y\times(c-z)$
PRECISION	$2x+1-y-z$	$y-z-2\bar{x}+1$	$y\times(2c-1)+1-z$
PREVALENCE	z	z	z
YULE'S Q	$\frac{x\times(1+x-y-z)-(y-x)\times(z-x)}{x\times(1+x-y-z)+(y-x)\times(z-x)}$	$\frac{(y-\bar{x})\times(1-\bar{x}-z)-\bar{x}\times(z-y+\bar{x})}{(y-\bar{x})\times(1-\bar{x}-z)+\bar{x}\times(z-y+\bar{x})}$	$\frac{c\times(1-y\times(1-c)-z)-(1-c)\times(z-c\times y)}{c\times(1-y\times(1-c)-z)+(1-c)\times(z-c\times y)}$
RECALL	$\frac{x}{z}$	$\frac{y-\bar{x}}{z}$	$\frac{y}{z}\times(1-c)$
RELATIVE RISK	$\frac{x}{y}\times\frac{1-y}{z-x}$	$\frac{y-\bar{x}}{y}\times\frac{1-y}{z-y+\bar{x}}$	$c\times\frac{1-y}{z-c\times y}$
SEBAG-SHOENAUER	$\frac{x}{y-x}$	$\frac{y-\bar{x}}{\bar{x}}$	$\frac{1-c}{c}$
SPECIFICITY	$1-\frac{z-x}{1-y}$	$\frac{1-z-\bar{x}}{1-y}$	$1-\frac{z-c\times y}{1-y}$
RELATIVE SPE.	$y-\frac{z-x}{1-y}$	$y-\frac{z-y+\bar{x}}{1-y}$	$y-\frac{z-c\times y}{1-y}$
SUPPORT	x	$y-\bar{x}$	$c\times y$
EX COUNTEREX RATE	$1-\frac{y-x}{x}$	$1-\frac{\bar{x}}{y-\bar{x}}$	$1-\frac{c}{1-c}$
SYM ADDED VALUE	$\max(\frac{x}{y}-z,\frac{x}{z}-y)$	$\max(1-z-\frac{\bar{x}}{y},\frac{y-\bar{x}}{z}-y)$	$\max(c-z,y\times(\frac{c}{z}-1))$
YULE'S Y	$\frac{\sqrt{x\times(1+x-y-z)}-\sqrt{(y-x)\times(z-x)}}{\sqrt{x\times(1+x-y-z)}+\sqrt{(y-x)\times(z-x)}}$	$\frac{\sqrt{(y-\bar{x})\times(1-\bar{x}-z)}-\sqrt{\bar{x}\times(z-y+\bar{x})}}{\sqrt{(y-\bar{x})\times(1-\bar{x}-z)}+\sqrt{\bar{x}\times(z-y+\bar{x})}}$	$\frac{\sqrt{c\times(1-y\times(1-c)-z)}-\sqrt{(1-c)\times(z-c\times y)}}{\sqrt{c\times(1-y\times(1-c)-z)}+\sqrt{(1-c)\times(z-c\times y)}}$
ZHANG	$\frac{x-y\times z}{\max(x\times(1-z),z\times(y-x))}$	$\frac{y\times(1-z)-\bar{x}}{\max((y-\bar{x})\times(1-z),z\times\bar{x})}$	$\frac{c-z}{\max(c\times(1-z),z\times(1-c))}$

Piatetski-Shapiro recommendations except the first one, since we have $\Phi_{spe}(y\times z,y,z)=1-z$. This recommendation is the most discussed, and is not even respected by CONFIDENCE ($\Phi_{conf}(y\times z,y,z)=z$). The most important is that the independence ($\mathbb{P}(\mathtt{XY})=\mathbb{P}(\mathtt{X})\mathbb{P}(\mathtt{Y})$) must be locatable, no matter if 0, 1 (lift) or any other particular value.

We will apply our framework and the associated study of variations to different pruning strategies that we found in the literature. We will show that the study of the measure's variations can explain some behaviors with respect to an underlying pruning strategy.

4 Application to Pruning Strategies

The number of pruning strategies in the literature is quite low. Three of them received our full attention: the property of the measure of ALL-CONFIDENCE for itemsets [32], from which we define the notion of all-monotony [25], the property of Universal Existential Upward Closure for CONFIDENCE [40], from which we define a notion of General Universal Existential Upward Closure [23], and the property of optimal rules sets [29], from which we introduce the notion of optimonotony [22].

4.1 All-Monotony

As stressed above, APRIORI like algorithms have generated many technical improvements for minimizing time complexity. It's important to consider these improvement and to try to use them. [32] introduced in 2003 the notion of *all*-CONFIDENCE, which is a transformation of CONFIDENCE that allows the use of APRIORI-like algorithms to mine interesting itemsets. The definition of *all*-CONFIDENCE for a given itemset Z is the following:

$$all - conf(\mathtt{Z}) = \min_{\mathtt{XY}=\mathtt{Z}}\{conf(\mathtt{X} \rightarrow \mathtt{Y})\}$$

An itemset Z is then interesting with respect to a given threshold σ *iff* all derived rules are confident with respect to this same threshold. At first glance, filtering itemsets with this measure can seem to be very constraining, but [42] showed that this filter allows for the exclusion of *cross-support* itemsets, those itemsets composed from items whose SUPPORT values are very different. Another advantage of this measure of ALL-CONFIDENCE is that it possesses the same property of antimonotonicity as the SUPPORT, and we can then use all APRIORI-like algorithms by only changing the measure (or adding the ALL-CONFIDENCE). Thus, this kind of generalization of the CONFIDENCE measure seems to be a very powerful process, and it would be interesting to use it with other measures than CONFIDENCE. Our thought process is not to check each measure one by one, but to try to automate the process. In order to achieve this, we generalize the ALL-CONFIDENCE to any measure μ by defining the corresponding *all*-μ measure, and we describe a link between the variations of measure μ and the fact that the *all*-μ measure possesses the antimonotony property.

Definition 3. *Let μ be an objective interestingness measure and* Z *an itemset. We define the* all-μ *associated measure by:*

$$\text{all-}\mu(\mathtt{Z}) = \min_{\mathtt{XY}=\mathtt{Z}}\{\mu(\mathtt{X} \rightarrow \mathtt{Y})\}$$

If $\mu_{\min}$ is a given threshold, the itemset Z is *all-interesting* with respect to μ and $\mu_{\min}$ *iff* any rule derived from Z is interesting with respect to μ and $\mu_{\min}$. We have then generalized the notion of ALL-CONFIDENCE to any measure, but with no reason to have an antimonotone property like SUPPORT. This is the main point of our work: how to highlight those measures whose associated *all*-measure is antimonotone? For such a measure, we say that it has the "*all-monotony property*". In [24], we prove the following theorem:

Theorem 1. *Let μ be an interestingness measure for association rules and (Φ_μ, D_{ex}) an adapted function of measure of μ. If Φ_μ is strictly decreasing on the second (the antecedent) and the third (the consequent) variables then the measure μ does not have the* all-monotony *property.*

One interesting remark is that this theorem excludes all measures that strictly follow the recommendations of Piatetsky-Shapiro, especially the third point. Consequently, the number of measures possessing this all-monotony property is not very high.

However, we prove also that a special class of measures possess the all-monotony property, those measures being those that can be expressed as an increasing function of the CONFIDENCE. Even if they are not very numerous, this result is interesting as it allows the use of APRIORI-like algorithms with other measures than SUPPORT.

We give in table 7 a survey of all measures verifying any of the properties we are studying here, all-monotony and the two others (sections 4.2 and 4.3). This table shows that all-monotony is a very constraining property that does not apply to a large set of measures. However, it is not only limited to CONFIDENCE, contrary to what one might think, and it is of importance to know that many measures can't be used in a similar process.

4.2 Universal Existential Upward Closure

The property of antimonotonicity shared by the SUPPORT and the all-monotone measures defines a bottom-up algorithmic property for pruning the search space. One may start from the empty itemset to mine ever-widening itemsets. [40] discovered another property of pruning verified by the CONFIDENCE without any transformation. The property is named Universal Existential Upward Closure by its authors, and defines a top-down approach: we start with the transactions in the database to mine step-by-step more general rules. Unlike the ALL-CONFIDENCE, this property applies to association rules, and in particular to classification rules, those rules with a predetermined consequent item (a class item), in databases with categorical attributes. In the algorithm presented by the authors, there is no need of a SUPPORT threshold, which allows to find nuggets of knowledge that is itemsets with a low SUPPORT value and a high CONFIDENCE value.

Since we will focus on databases with categorical attributes, we first need to introduce some notations. We keep the notation $\mathtt{A}$ for a non-valuated attribute and we call $\mathcal{V}\mathtt{A}$ the set of values that $\mathtt{A}$ may take. An itemset $\mathtt{X} = x$ is made of a set of attributes $\mathtt{X} = \mathtt{A}_1 \ldots \mathtt{A}_n$ and a set of values $x = (a_1, \ldots, a_n) \in \mathcal{V}\mathtt{A}_1 \times \cdots \times \mathcal{V}\mathtt{A}_n$ meaning that in itemset $\mathtt{X} = x$, the attribute $\mathtt{A}_i$ takes the value $a_i \in \mathcal{V}\mathtt{A}_i$. We are here interested in rules of the form $\mathtt{X} = x \to \mathtt{C} = c$ where $\mathtt{C}$ is of length 1. For short, we can write $x \to c$. If $\mathtt{A}$ is an attribute, an $\mathtt{A}$-specialization of the rule $x \to c$ is a rule $\mathtt{XA} = (x, a) \to \mathtt{C} = c$.

The property of UEUC is defined by [40] as follows:

Property 1. For every attribute A not occurring in a rule $x \to c$, (i) some A-specialization of $x \to c$ has at least the CONFIDENCE of $x \to c$, (ii) if $x \to c$ is confident, so is some A-specialization of $x \to c$.

Principally, this property is due to a barycenter property of the conditional probabilities: Since the $\mathtt{A} = a_i$ constitute a partition, we have

$$\mathbb{P}(c|x) = \sum_{a_i \in \mathcal{V}\mathtt{A}} \mathbb{P}(a_i|x)\mathbb{P}(c|xa_i)$$

Thus, the CONFIDENCE of the rule $x \to c$ is a barycenter of the CONFIDENCEs of the rules $xa_i \to c$ that is a barycenter of the CONFIDENCEs of all its A-specializations, and then, some specializations have an higher CONFIDENCE, and some have a lower CONFIDENCE. As a result, a top-down strategy of pruning appears naturally, having the important advantage of getting rid of the SUPPORT constraint.

This approach is really promising since it let us mine association rules directly, relying only on the value of CONFIDENCE, without assuming anything on the SUPPORT value. It would be of interest to find other measures with this kind of property. This is the subject of [23], where we generalize the UEUC property to a General-UEUC (GUEUC) property for any measure and give some conditions of existence of this property.

Definition 4. *An interestingness measure μ verifies the* General UEUC *property* iff *for every attribute* A *not occurring in a rule r: $x \to c$, some* A*-specialization of r has at least the value taken by r on the measure μ.*

A consequence is that, for such a measure, if r is interesting (with respect to a given threshold), so is some A-specialization of r. Clearly, the CONFIDENCE has the GUEUC property, and our GUEUC property is a good generalization of the UEUC property. We introduced three conditions for the existence of the GUEUC property for a given measure μ.

Proposition 1 (Trivial sufficient condition for GUEUC). *Let μ be an interestingness measure for association rules and μ be an affine transformation of the* CONFIDENCE. *Then μ does verify the barycenter property (with the same weights as for* CONFIDENCE*) and thus μ has the GUEUC property.*

Proposition 2 (Sufficient condition for GUEUC). *Let μ be an interestingness measure for association rules and (Φ_μ, D_{conf}) an adapted function of measure of μ. Let Φ_μ verify the two following properties:*

(a) $\forall (y,z) \in \mathbb{Q}^2 \cap [0,1]^2$, *the function $c \mapsto \Phi_\mu(c,y,z)$, where c is such that $(c,y,z) \in D_{conf}$, is a monotone function (increasing or decreasing);*
(b) $\forall (c,z) \in \mathbb{Q}^2 \cap [0,1]^2$, *the function $y \mapsto \Phi_\mu(c,y,z)$, where y is such that $(c,y,z) \in D_{conf}$, is a decreasing function (in the broad meaning of that term).*

Then μ has the GUEUC property.

Proposition 3 (Necessary condition for GUEUC). *If μ is an interestingness measure that verifies the GUEUC property, and (Φ_μ, D_{conf}) its adapted function of measure, then for every $(c, y, z) \in D_{conf}$, we have*

$$\Phi_\mu(c, y, z) \leq \Phi_\mu(c, \frac{y}{2}, z). \quad (2)$$

These three propositions permit the filtration of the measures that have the GUEUC property and that can be used with the same top-down algorithm than CONFIDENCE. Once again, this result gives a necessary condition, and a sufficient condition, but does not present an equivalence. However, considering the set of measures in table 7, one can see that a large part of measures are categorized for this property. Only the measure of ONE WAY SUPPORT still remains unclassified. This property seems less restrictive than all-monotony, since more measures accept it. Hence, with these measures, nuggets of knowledge can be mined, with an efficient algorithm. Moreover, since the workable measures are numerous, the user can choose several of them and the algorithm can aggregate them in the pruning strategy, to return interesting rules with respect to every measure. However, the number of workable measures still remains restricted. The following property is even less restrictive, and can be applied to a large number of measures, proving that pushing the measure as deep as possible in the algorithms is possible.

4.3 Optimal Rule Discovery

The previous two pruning strategies were only based on CONFIDENCE originally. We proved that they could be applied to more measures, but the number of concerned measures remains very limited. In this context, the case of optimal rules discovery is a great step forward in association rules mining, focused on classification rules. It was initiated by Li [29] where the author proved that optimal rules went together with a pruning strategy that returned coherent results for 13 interestingness measures. An optimal rule with respect to a given interestingness measure is a rule that has an interest value higher than any of its more general rules. Li described a way of generating optimal rules sets by using an efficient pruning strategy. This pruning strategy is quite independent of the measure.

Theorem 2. *If supp*(`XI¬C`) = *supp*(`X¬C`), *then rule* `XI → C` *and all its more-specific rules will not occur in an optimal rule set defined by* CONFIDENCE, ODDS RATIO, LIFT *(*INTEREST *or* STRENGTH*)*, GAIN, ADDED-VALUE, KLOSGEN, CONVICTION, P-S *(or* LEVERAGE*)*, LAPLACE, COSINE, CERTAINTY FACTOR, *or* JACCARD.

As mentioned before, the pruning strategy is measure independent, but the output is an optimal rule set only when considering the measures cited in the theorem. The pruning strategy is, as for the antimonotonicity of the SUPPORT, a bottom-up approach. This theorem presents two direct corollaries, and the interested reader may find them in [29]. In [22], we introduce the optimonotone character of an interestingness measure, and the underlying optimonotony property of pruning.

Definition 5 (optimonotone measure). *A measure of interest μ is optimonotone if, given a rule* $\mathtt{X} \rightarrow \mathtt{C}$ *and a specification* $\mathtt{XI} \rightarrow \mathtt{C}$*, we have*

$$(supp(\mathtt{XI}\neg\mathtt{C}) = supp(\mathtt{X}\neg\mathtt{C}) \implies \mu(\mathtt{XI} \rightarrow \mathtt{C}) \leq \mu(\mathtt{X} \rightarrow \mathtt{C})).$$

As an example, one can prove that CONFIDENCE is an optimonotone measure. In fact, let suppose that $supp(\mathtt{XI}\neg\mathtt{C}) = supp(\mathtt{X}\neg\mathtt{C})$, we have:

$$\begin{aligned}
conf(\mathtt{XI} \rightarrow \mathtt{C}) &= \frac{supp(\mathtt{XIC})}{supp(\mathtt{XI})} \\
&= 1 - \frac{supp(\mathtt{XI}\neg\mathtt{C})}{supp(\mathtt{XI})} \\
&= 1 - \frac{supp(\mathtt{X}\neg\mathtt{C})}{supp(\mathtt{XI})} \\
&\leq 1 - \frac{supp(\mathtt{X}\neg\mathtt{C})}{supp(\mathtt{X})} \\
&\leq \frac{supp(\mathtt{XC})}{supp(\mathtt{X})} = conf(\mathtt{X} \rightarrow \mathtt{C})
\end{aligned}$$

The advantage of this optimonotone property of a measure is that we can extend the number of measures in the process initiated by Li. In fact, we can adapt it's main theorem by the following:

Theorem 3. *If* $supp(\mathtt{XI}\neg\mathtt{C}) = supp(\mathtt{X}\neg\mathtt{C})$*, then rule* $\mathtt{XI} \rightarrow \mathtt{C}$ *and all its more-specific rules will not occur in an optimal rule set defined by an optimonotone measure.*

Then, the output of Li's algorithm is coherent with any optimonotone measure, that is, the returned rule set is an optimal rule set when using an optimonotone measure. Since the framework of optimal rules and the underlying algorithm are efficient, it is interesting to know which measure is optimonotone. In order to achieve this, we introduced a necessary and sufficient condition of existence of this optimonotone character for a measure.

Proposition 4. *Let μ be an interestingness measure, and (Φ_μ, D_{c-ex}) its adapted function of measure. μ is optimonotone* iff *μ increases with the second variable (associated with* $supp(\mathtt{X})$*).*

With the help of this necessary and sufficient condition, we proved that at least 31 measures are optimonotone and can be used with the optimal rule discovery algorithm. We thus have more than doubled the number of measures considered by Li, in an automatic way, and proved moreover that the KLOSGEN measure, considered by Li as usable within its framework, was not optimonotone, and we presented a counter example to the use of KLOSGEN measure with optimal rule discovery algorithm. We present in the following part the table detailing the measures and their properties.

Table 7. Properties of the measures

measure	OM	AM	GUEUC	measure	OM	AM	GUEUC	measure	OM	AM	GUEUC
IWD	No	No	No	INTEREST	No		No	PRECISION	Yes	No	No
CONFIDENCE	Yes	Yes	Yes	J1-MEASURE	No	No	No	PREVALENCE	Yes		Yes
ADDED VALUE	Yes	No	Yes	JACCARD	Yes	No	No	YULE'S Q	Yes	No	No
CONTRAMIN	Yes	No	No	J-MEASURE	No	No	No	RECALL	Yes	Yes	No
CONVICTION	Yes	No	Yes	KAPPA	Yes	No	No	RELATIVE RISK	Yes	No	No
COSINE	Yes	No	No	KLOSGEN	No	No	No	SEBAG-SHOENAUER	Yes	Yes	Yes
COVERAGE	Yes		No	LEVERAGE	Yes	No	No	SPECIFICITY	Yes	No	No
BAYESIAN FACTOR	Yes	No	Yes	LIFT	Yes	No	Yes	RELATIVE SPE.	Yes		No
COLLECTIVE STRENGTH	Yes	No	No	LOEVINGER	Yes	No	Yes	SUPPORT	Yes		No
INFORMATION GAIN	Yes	No	Yes	ODDS RATIO	Yes	No	No	EX COUNTEREX RATE	Yes	Yes	Yes
GINI INDEX	No		No	ONE WAY SUPPORT	No	No		SYM ADDED VALUE	Yes	No	No
IMPLICATION INDEX	Yes	No	No	PEARSON	Yes	No	No	YULE'S Y	Yes	No	No
				PIATETSKY-SHAPIRO	Yes	No	No	ZHANG	Yes	No	Yes

4.4 Properties Verified by the Measures

Using our framework to find links between algorithmic and analytic properties of the measures allows us to fill in Table 7. The main interest of such a table is to present to the user efficient measures (in an algorithmic sense), or to present to the user the algorithm that can be used with the measure he choses, and thus the type of output he can obtain (optimal rules, interesting rules, or interesting itemsets). Since the size of databases ever-increasing, it is of importance to use such algorithmic properties, even if there is a loss of precision in the results in the sense that we do not get all the interesting rules, for example with optimal rules or all-interesting itemsets. The GUEUC property allows to find all interesting rules, but their number might be very high.

To summarize, 31 out of 38 measures are optimonotone, only 4 of them are all-monotone, and 11 have the GUEUC property. It has to be said that 6 measures are not classified for the all-monotone property, due to the default of necessary and sufficient condition. The same holds, but for only one measure in the case of the GUEUC property. The optimonotony works with a large number of measures, but it's important to moderate this result. In fact, even if optimal rules have been described as very useful rules by Li, in the sense that they are good rules for learning and classification [30], one has to remember that the set of optimal rules is a very small part of the set of interesting rules. With this property, there is a large loss of precision in the result, conversely to the GUEUC property. In the same way, the all-monotony property does not allow the rebuilding of the entire set of interesting rules. So, one has always to chose between precision of results and duration of calculation.

Conclusion

In this article, we introduced a formal framework for the study of association rules and interestingness measures. We show that a measure may only be described by a function and a variation domain. We detailed the case of three particular domains: examples, counterexamples and confidence. We expressed 31 measures in these 3 domains.

This framework lets us to study the measures in a analytical way, and allows particularly the study of their variations. With this help, we generalized three algorithmic properties (all-monotony, GUEUC and opti-monotony) and we gave sufficient and/or necessary conditions for a measure to have a particular property. These conditions allow the classification of the 31 measures between the three properties. These properties are thus operational properties of the measures and can be used as a powerful parameter during the choice of a measure by the user.

References

1. Aggarwal, C.C., Yu, P.S.: A new framework for itemset generation. In: 1998 ACM SIGMOD-SIGACT-SIGART Symposium on Principles of Database Systems, Seattle, Washington, United States, pp. 18–24. ACM Press, New York (1998)
2. Agrawal, R., Imieliski, T., Swami, A.: Mining association rules between sets of items in large databases. In: Buneman, P., Jajodia, S. (eds.) ACM SIGMOD International Conference on Management of Data, Washington, D.C., United States, pp. 207–216. ACM Press, New York (1993)
3. Agrawal, R., Srikant, R.: Fast algorithms for mining association rules in large databases. In: Bocca, J.B., Jarke, M., Zaniolo, C. (eds.) 20th International Conference on Very Large Data Bases, Santiago de Chile, Chile, pp. 478–499. Morgan Kaufmann, San Francisco (1994)
4. Asuncion, A., Newman, D.: UCI machine learning repository (2007), `http://www.ics.uci.edu/~mlearn/MLRepository.html`
5. Azé, J., Kodratoff, Y.: Evaluation de la résistance au bruit de quelques mesures d'extraction de règles d'association. In: Hérin, D., Zighed, D.A. (eds.) 2nd Extraction et Gestion des Connaissances Conference, Montpellier, France. Extraction des Connaissances et Apprentissage, vol. 1-4, pp. 143–154. Hermes Science Publications (January 2002)
6. Borgelt, C., Kruse, R.: Induction of association rules: Apriori implementation. In: 15th Conference on Computational Statistics, Berlin, Germany, pp. 395–400. Physika Verlag, Heidelberg (2002)
7. Brin, S., Motwani, R., Silverstein, C.: Beyond market baskets: Generalizing association rules to correlations. In: Peckham, J. (ed.) ACM SIGMOD International Conference on Management of Data, Tucson, Arizona, USA, pp. 265–276. ACM Press, New York (1997)
8. Brin, S., Motwani, R., Ullman, J.D., Tsur, S.: Dynamic itemset counting and implication rules for market basket data. In: Peckham, J. (ed.) ACM SIGMOD International Conference on Management of Data, Tucson, Arizona, USA, pp. 255–264. ACM Press, New York (1997)
9. Church, K.W., Hanks, P.: Word association norms, mutual information, and lexicography. Computational Linguistics 16(1), 22–29 (1990)
10. Cleverdon, C.W., Mills, J., Keen, M.: Factors determining the performance of indexing systems. In: ASLIB Cranfield Project, Cranfield (1966)
11. Cohen, J.: A coefficient of agreement for nominal scales. Educational and Psychological Measurement 20(1), 37–46 (1960)
12. Geng, L., Hamilton, H.J.: Interestingness measures for data mining: A survey. ACM Computing Surveys 38(3, article 9) (2006)

13. Gini, C.: Measurement of inequality and incomes. The Economic Journal 31, 124–126 (1921)
14. Gray, B., Orlowska, M.E.: CCAIIA: Clustering categorical attributes into interesting accociation rules. In: Wu, X., Ramamohanarao, K., Korb, K.B. (eds.) PAKDD 1998. LNCS, vol. 1394, pp. 132–143. Springer, Heidelberg (1998)
15. Guillaume, S., Grissa, D., Nguifo, E.M.: Propriété des mesures d'intérêt pour l'extraction des règles. In: 6th Workshop on Qualité des Données et des Connaissances, in Conjunction With the 10th Extraction et Gestion des Connaissances Conference, Hammamet, Tunisie, pp. 15–28 (2010)
16. Han, J., Pei, J., Yin, Y.: Mining frequent patterns without candidate generation. In: Chen, W., Naughton, J.F., Bernstein, P.A. (eds.) ACM SIGMOD International Conference on Management of Data, pp. 1–12. ACM Press, New York (2000)
17. Hébert, C., Crémilleux, B.: Optimized rule mining through a unified framework for interestingness measures. In: Tjoa, A.M., Trujillo, J. (eds.) DaWaK 2006. LNCS, vol. 4081, pp. 238–247. Springer, Heidelberg (2006)
18. Jaccard, P.: Étude comparative de la distribution florale dans une portion des Alpes et du Jura. Bulletin de la Société Vaudoise des Sciences Naturelles 37, 547–579 (1901)
19. Jeffreys, H.: Some tests of significance, treated by the theory of probability. Proceedings of the Cambridge Philosophical Society 31, 203–222 (1935)
20. Klösgen, W.: Problems for knowledge discovery in databases and their treatment in the statistics interpreter EXPLORA. International Journal of Intelligent Systems 7, 649–673 (1992)
21. Lavrač, N., Flach, P.A., Zupan, B.: Rule evaluation measures: A unifying view. In: Džeroski, S., Flach, P.A. (eds.) ILP 1999. LNCS (LNAI), vol. 1634, pp. 174–185. Springer, Heidelberg (1999)
22. Le Bras, Y., Lenca, P., Lallich, S.: On optimal rule mining: A framework and a necessary and sufficient condition of antimonotonicity. In: Theeramunkong, T., Kijsirikul, B., Cercone, N., Ho, T.-B. (eds.) PAKDD 2009. LNCS, vol. 5476, pp. 705–712. Springer, Heidelberg (2009)
23. Le Bras, Y., Lenca, P., Lallich, S.: Mining interesting rules without support requirement: a general universal existential upward closure property. Annals of Information Systems 8(part 2), 75–98 (2010); 8232
24. Le Bras, Y., Lenca, P., Lallich, S., Moga, S.: Généralisation de la propriété de monotonie de la all-confidence pour l'extraction de motifs intéressants non fréquents. In: 5th Workshop on Qualité des Données et des Connaissances, in Conjunction With the 9th Extraction et Gestion des Connaissances Conference, Strasbourg, France, pp. 17–24 (January 2009)
25. Le Bras, Y., Lenca, P., Moga, S., Lallich, S.: All-monotony: A generalization of the all-confidence antimonotony. In: 4th International Conference on Machine Learning and Applications, pp. 759–764 (2009)
26. Le Bras, Y., Meyer, P., Lenca, P., Lallich, S.: A robustness measure of association rules. In: 13rd European Conference on Principles of Data Mining and Knowledge Discovery, Barcelona, Spain (2010)
27. Lenca, P., Meyer, P., Vaillant, B., Lallich, S.: On selecting interestingness measures for association rules: user oriented description and multiple criteria decision aid. European Journal of Operational Research 184(2), 610–626 (2008)
28. Lerman, I.C., Gras, R., Rostam, H.: Elaboration d'un indice d'implication pour les données binaires, I et II. Mathématiques et Sciences Humaines (74,75), 5–35, 5–47 (1981)

29. Li, J.: On optimal rule discovery. IEEE Transaction on Knowledge and Data Engineering 18(4), 460–471 (2006)
30. Li, J.: Robust rule-based prediction. IEEE Transaction on Knowledge and Data Engineering 18(8), 1043–1054 (2006)
31. Loevinger, J.: A systemic approach to the construction and evaluation of tests of ability. Psychological monographs 61(4) (1947)
32. Omiecinski, E.: Alternative interest measures for mining associations in databases. IEEE Transaction on Knowledge and Data Engineering 15(1), 57–69 (2003)
33. Pearson, K.: Mathematical contributions to the theory of evolution. III. regression, heredity, and panmixia. Philosophical Transactions of the Royal Society of London. Series A, Containing Papers of a Mathematical or Physical Character 187, 253–318 (1896)
34. Piatetsky-Shapiro, G.: Discovery, analysis, and presentation of strong rules. In: Knowledge Discovery in Databases, pp. 229–248. AAAI/MIT Press, Cambridge (1991)
35. Salton, G., McGill, M.J.: Introduction to Modern Retrieval. McGraw-Hill Book Company, New York (1983)
36. Sebag, M., Schoenauer, M.: Generation of rules with certainty and confidence factors from incomplete and incoherent learning bases. In: Boose, J., Gaines, B., Linster, M. (eds.) European Knowledge Acquisition Workshop, pp. 28.1–28.20. Gesellschaft für Mathematik und Datenverarbeitung mbH, Sankt Augustin, Germany (1988)
37. Smyth, P., Goodman, R.M.: Rule induction using information theory. In: Knowledge Discovery in Databases, pp. 159–176. AAAI/MIT Press, Cambridge (1991)
38. Suzuki, E.: Pitfalls for categorizations of objective interestingness measures for rule discovery. In: Gras, R., Suzuki, E., Guillet, F., Spagnolo, F. (eds.) Statistical Implicative Analysis, Theory and Applications, Studies in Computational Intelligence, vol. 127, pp. 383–395. Springer, Heidelberg (2008)
39. Tan, P.N., Kumar, V., Srivastava, J.: Selecting the right objective measure for association analysis. Information Systems 4(29), 293–313 (2004)
40. Wang, K., He, Y., Cheung, D.W.: Mining confident rules without support requirement. In: 10th International Conference on Information and Knowledge Management, Atlanta, Georgia, USA, pp. 89–96. ACM Press, New York (2001)
41. Wang, K., Tay, S.H.W., Liu, B.: Interestingness-based interval merger for numeric association rules. In: 4th ACM SIGKDD International Conference on Knowledge Discovery and Data Mining, New York, NY, USA, pp. 121–128. ACM Press, New York (1998)
42. Xiong, H., Tan, P.N., Kumar, V.: Mining strong affinity association patterns in data sets with skewed support distribution. In: 3rd IEEE International Conference on Data Mining, Melbourne, Florida, USA, pp. 387–394. IEEE Computer Society Press, Los Alamitos (2003)
43. Yao, J., Liu, H.: Searching multiple databases for interesting complexes. In: Lu, H., Motoda, H., Liu, H. (eds.) 1st Pacific-Asia Conference on Knowledge Discovery and Data Mining. KDD: Techniques and Applications, pp. 198–210. World Scientific Publishing Company, Singapore (1997)

44. Yao, Y., Chen, Y., Yang, X.D.: A measurement-theoretic foundation of rule interestingness evaluation. In: Lin, T.Y., Ohsuga, S., Liau, C.J., Hu, X. (eds.) Foundations and Novel Approaches in Data Mining. SCI, vol. 9, pp. 41–59. Springer, Heidelberg (2006)
45. Yule, G.U.: On the association of attributes in statistics: With illustrations from the material of the childhood society. Philosophical Transactions of the Royal Society of London. Series A, Containing Papers of a Mathematical or Physical Character 194, 257–319 (1900)
46. Zhang, T.: Association rules. In: Terano, T., Liu, H., Chen, A.L.P. (eds.) PAKDD 2000. LNCS, vol. 1805, pp. 245–256. Springer, Heidelberg (2000)

Chapter 6
Nonnegative Matrix Factorization: Models, Algorithms and Applications

Zhong-Yuan Zhang

School of Statistics, Central University of Finance and Economics, P.R. China
zhyuanzh@gmail.com

Abstract. In recent years, Nonnegative Matrix Factorization (NMF) has become a popular model in data mining society. NMF aims to extract hidden patterns from a series of high-dimensional vectors automatically, and has been applied for dimensional reduction, unsupervised learning (clustering, semi-supervised clustering and co-clustering, etc.) and prediction successfully. This chapter surveys NMF in terms of the model formulation and its variations and extensions, algorithms and applications, as well as its relations with K-means and Probabilistic Latent Semantic Indexing (PLSI). In summary, we draw the following conclusions: 1) NMF has a good interpretability due to its nonnegative constraints; 2) NMF is very flexible regarding the choices of its objective functions and the algorithms employed to solve it; 3) NMF has a variety of applications; 4) NMF has a solid theoretical foundation and a close relationship with the existing state-of-the-art unsupervised learning models. However, as a new and developing technology, there are still many interesting open issues remained unsolved and waiting for research from theoretical and algorithmic perspectives.

1 Introduction

Nonnegative Matrix Factorization (NMF,[1,2,3]) is evolved from Principal Component Analysis (PCA, [4,5]). PCA is one of the basic techniques for extracting the principal components (basic factors) from a series of vectors such that each vector is the linear combination of the components, in other words, PCA tries to give the best low dimensional representation with a common basis for a set of vectors. Formally, given a set of samples $\{x_i, i = 1, 2, \cdots, m\}$ in $\mathbb{R}^n$, PCA aims to provide the best linear approximation of the samples in a lower dimensional space, say $\mathbb{R}^k$. This problem can be represented as a nonlinear programming problem: $\min\limits_{\mu,\{\lambda_i\},V} \sum_{i=1}^{m} \|x_i - \mu - V\lambda_i\|_2^2$, where μ is column vector of size $n \times 1$, V is matrix of size $n \times k$ and column orthogonal ($V^T V = I$), and each λ_i, $i = 1, 2, \cdots, m$ is column vector of size $k \times 1$. Fixing μ and V, one can get the optimal solution of $\lambda_i = V^T(x_i - \bar{x})$, $i = 1, 2, \cdots, m$, where $\bar{x} = \sum\limits_i x_i/m$;

D.E. Holmes, L.C. Jain (Eds.): Data Mining: Found. & Intell. Paradigms, ISRL 24, pp. 99–134.
springerlink.com

similarly, fixing λ_i and V, one can get the optimal solution of $\mu = \bar{x}$. Hence the optimization problem can be re-written as:

$$\min_V \sum_{i=1}^{m} \|(x_i - \bar{x}) - VV^T(x_i - \bar{x})\|_2^2. \quad (1)$$

The optimization problem can be solved by Singular Value Decomposition (SVD) applied on the matrix X, each column of which is $x_i - \bar{x}$, such that $X = ASB^T$, where A is an $n \times m$ matrix satisfying $A^T A = I$, B is a $m \times m$ matrix satisfying $B^T B = I$ and S is a $m \times m$ diagonal matrix with diagonal elements $s_{11} \geqslant s_{22} \geqslant s_{33} \cdots s_{mm}$ (they are singular values of X). The first k columns of A constitute the matrix V in (1). The columns of V are called the principal components of X ([5]).

Note that there are both positive and negative elements in each of the principal components and also both positive and negative coefficients in linear combinations (i.e., λ_i, $i = 1, 2 \cdots, m$, has mixed signs). However the mixed signs contradict our experience and make it hard to explain the results. For example, the pixels in an image should be non-negative, hence the principal components with negative elements extracted from the images cannot be intuitively interpreted ([6]). In fact, in many applications such as image processing, biology or text mining, nonnegative data analysis is often important and nonnegative constraints on the wanted principal components (basis matrix) and coefficients (coding matrix) can improve the interpretability of the results. NMF is thus proposed to address this problem. In particular, NMF aims to find the non-negative basic representative factors which can be used for feature extraction, dimensional reduction, eliminating redundant information and discovering the hidden patterns behind a series of non-negative vectors.

Recent years, NMF has attracted considerable interests from research community. Various extensions are proposed to address the emerging challenges and have been successfully applied to the field of unsupervised learning in data mining including environmetrics ([3]), image processing ([1]) chemometrics ([7]), pattern recognition ([8]), multimedia data analysis ([9]), text mining ([10,11,12,13]) and bioinformatics ([14,15,16]), etc., and received lots of attention. In [17] it has been shown that when the least squares error is selected as the cost function, NMF is equivalent to the soft K-means model, which establishes the theoretical foundation of NMF used for data clustering. Besides the traditional least squares error (Frobenius norm), there are other divergence functions that can be used as the cost functions for NMF, such as K-L divergence and chi-square statistic ([2,18]). In [18] it has been shown that constrained NMF using with K-L divergence is equivalent to Probabilistic Latent Semantic Indexing, another unsupervised learning model popularly used in text analysis ([19,18]).

In this chapter, we give a systematic survey of Nonnegative Matrix Factorization, including the basic model, and its variations and extensions, the applications of NMF in text mining, image processing, bioinformatics, finance etc., and the relations with K-means and PLSI. This chapter will not cover all of the related works on NMF, but will try to address the most important ones that we are interested in.

The chapter is organized as follows: Section 2 gives the standard NMF model and several variations, Section 3 summarizes the divergence functions used in the standard NMF model and the algorithms employed for solving the model, Section 4 reviews some selected applications of NMF, Section 5 gives the theoretical analysis concerning the relations between NMF and the other two unsupervised learning models including K-means and Probabilistic Latent Semantic Indexing (PLSI), and Section 6 concludes.

2 Standard NMF and Variations

To easy explanation, Table 1 lists the notations used throughout the chapter.

Table 1. Notations used in this chapter

a_i	Column vector indexed by i;
A	Matrix;
A_{ij}	Element of the ith row and the jth column in matrix A;
$A_{:,j}$	The jth column of matrix A;
$A_{i,:}$	The ith row of matrix A;
$A \geqslant 0$	A is element-wise nonnegative, i.e., $A_{ij} \geqslant 0$ for all i and j;
A_+	Matrix A that satisfies $A \geqslant 0$;
$A_\pm$	Matrix A that has mixed signs, i.e., there is no restriction on the elements' signs of A;
$\frac{A.}{B}$	Matrix whose $(i,j)-th$ element is $\frac{A_{ij}}{B_{ij}}$;
$A^{(t)}$	The updated matrix A at the end of $t-$th iteration in the algorithm;
$A_{ij}^{(t)}$	The $(i,j)-th$ element of matrix $A^{(t)}$.

2.1 Standard NMF

Nonnegative Matrix Factorization (NMF) is one of the models that focus on the analysis of non-negative data matrices which are often originated from text mining, images processing and biology. Mathematically, NMF can be described as follows: given an $n \times m$ matrix X composed of non-negative elements, the task is to factorize X into a non-negative matrix F of size $n \times r$ and another non-negative matrix G of size $m \times r$ such that $X \approx FG^T$. r is preassigned and should satisfy $r \ll m, n$. It is usually formulated as an optimization:

$$\begin{aligned} \min_{F,G} \quad & J(X \| FG^T) \\ s.t. \quad & F \geqslant 0, G \geqslant 0, \end{aligned} \tag{2}$$

where $J(X\|FG^T)$ is some divergence function that measures dissimilarity between X and FG^T, and will be discussed in Sect. 3. Meanings of F and G can be explained variously in different fields or for different purposes and will be discussed in Sect. 4.

As we can see, all the elements of F and G are variables that need to be decided, hence this is a large scale optimization problem and the standard algorithms are not suitable, and one can observe that $J(X\|FG^T)$ is individually convex in F and in G, hence in general, most of the algorithms designed for NMF are iteratively and alternatively minimizing or decreasing F and G, which is summarized in Algorithm 1. The details will be discussed in Sect. 3.

Algorithm 1. Nonnegative Matrix Factorization (General Case)

Input: $F^{(0)}, G^{(0)}, t = 1$.
Output: F, G.
1: **while** 1 **do**
2: Fix $G^{(t-1)}$ and find $F^{(t)}$ such that $J(X\|F^{(t)}G^{(t-1)T}) \leqslant J(X\|F^{(t-1)}G^{(t-1)T})$;
3: Fix $F^{((t))}$ and find $G^{(t)}$ such that $J(X\|F^{(t)}G^{(t)T}) \leqslant J(X\|F^{(t)}G^{(t-1)T})$;
4: Test for convergence;
5: **if** Some convergence condition is satisfied **then**
6: $F = F^{(t)}$;
7: $G = G^{(t)}$;
8: **Break**
9: **end if**
10: $t = t + 1$;
11: **end while**

At last, we give an important property of NMF ([20,21]) to close this subsection. As we have mentioned above, the factors in Singular Value Decomposition (SVD): $X = ASB^T = A'B'^T$, where $A' = AS^{1/2}$ and $B' = BS^{1/2}$, typically contain mixed sign elements. And NMF differs from SVD due to the absence of cancellation of plus and minus signs. But what is the fundamental signature of this absence of cancellation? It is the *Boundedness Property*.

Theorem 1. *(Boundedness Property, [20,21]) Let* $0 \leqslant X \leqslant M$[1]*, where* M *is some positive constant, be the input data matrix.* F, G *are the nonnegative matrices satisfying*

$$X = FG^T. \tag{3}$$

There exists a diagonal matrix $D \geq 0$ *such that*

$$X = FG^T = (FD)(GD^{-1})^T = F^*G^{*T} \tag{4}$$

with

$$0 \leqslant F^*_{ij} \leqslant \sqrt{M},\ 0 \leqslant G^*_{ij} \leqslant \sqrt{M}. \tag{5}$$

If X *is symmetric and* $F = G^T$*, then* $G^* = G$.

Proof. See Appendix.

[1] $0 \leqslant X \leqslant M$ means $0 \leq X_{ij} \leqslant M$, $i = 1, 2, \cdots, n$, $j = 1, 2, \cdots, m$.

We note that SVD decomposition does not have the boundedness property. In this case, even if the input data are in the range of $0 \leq X_{ij} \leq M$, we can find some elements of A' and B' that are larger than $\sqrt{M}$.

In NMF, there is a scale flexibility, i.e., for any positive D, if (F, G) is a solution, so is (FD, GD^{-1}). This theorem assures the existence of an appropriate scale such that both F and G are bounded, i.e., their elements can not exceed the magnitude of the input data matrix. This ensures that F, G are in the same scale.

Consequently, we will briefly review the variations that are rooted from NMF and proposed from different perspectives. Note that only the motivations for the research and the model formulations are reviewed, their algorithms and the application results are omitted here due to space limitation. One can find more details in the corresponding references.

2.2 Semi-NMF ([22])

Semi-NMF is designed for the data matrix X that has mixed signs. In semi-NMF, G is restricted to be nonnegative while the other factor matrix F can have mixed signs, i.e., semi-NMF can take the following form[2]: $X_{\pm} \approx F_{\pm}G_{+}^{T}$. This model is motivated from the perspective of data clustering. When clustering the columns of data matrix X, the columns of F can be seen as the cluster centroids and the rows of G denote the cluster indicators, i.e., the column j of X belongs to cluster k if $k = \arg\max_p\{G_{jp}\}$. Hence the nonnegative constraint on F can be relaxed such that the approximation FG^T is tighter and the results are more interpretable. Naturally, semi-NMF can also take the form: $X_{\pm} \approx F_{+}G_{\pm}^{T}$ if we want to cluster the rows of matrix X.

2.3 Convex-NMF ([22])

Convex-NMF is also presented for reasons of interpretability. Since the factor F denotes the cluster centroids, the columns of F should lie within the column space of X, i.e., $F_{:,j}$, $j = 1, 2, \cdots, r$, can be represented as the convex combination of the columns of X: $F_{:,j} = \sum_{i=1}^{m} W_{ij}X_{:,i}$ or $F = XW$ with constraints $W \geqslant 0$ and $\sum_{i=1}^{m} W_{ij} = 1$, $j = 1, 2, \cdots, r$. Hence the model can take the following form: $X_{\pm} \approx X_{\pm}W_{+}G_{+}^{T}$. An interesting conclusion is that the convex-NMF factors F and G are naturally sparse.

2.4 Tri-NMF ([23])

Tri-NMF is presented to address the co-clustering problem (See Sect. 4.4), i.e., it presents a framework for clustering the rows and columns of the objective matrix X simultaneously. This model aims to find three factors F, S and G such that $X_{+} \approx F_{+}S_{+}G_{+}^{T}$ with constraints $F^TF = I$ and $G^TG = I$. F and G are the

[2] The subscripts $\pm$ and $+$ are used frequently to indicate the application scopes of the models.

membership indicator matrices of the rows and the columns of X respectively, and S is an additional degree of freedom which makes the approximation tighter.

2.5 Kernel NMF ([24])

For the element-wise mapping ϕ: $X_\pm \mapsto \phi(X_\pm) : \phi(X)_{ij} = \phi(X_{ij})$, kernel NMF is designed as: $\phi(X_\pm) \approx \phi(X_\pm)W_+G_+^T$, from which one can see that the kernel NMF is just an extension of the convex-NMF. Kernel-NMF is well-defined since $\|\phi(X) - \phi(X)WG^T\|^2 = \text{trace}(\phi^T(X)\phi(X) - 2\phi^T(X)\phi(X)WG^T + GW^T\phi^T(X)\phi(X)WG^T)$ only depends on the kernel $K = \phi^T(X)\phi(X)$. Note that the standard NMF or Semi-NMF does not have the kernel extension on $\phi(X)$ since, in that case, F and G will depend explicitly on the mapping $\phi(\cdot)$ which is unknown.

2.6 Local Nonnegative Matrix Factorization, LNMF ([25,26])

As we have mentioned above, NMF is presented as a "part of whole" factorization model and tries to mine localized part-based representation that can help to reveal low dimensional and more intuitive structures of observations. But it has been shown that NMF may give holistic representation instead of part-based representation ([25,27]). Hence many efforts have been done to improve the sparseness of NMF in order to identify more localized features that are building parts for the whole representation. Here we introduce several sparse variants of NMF, including LNMF, NNSC, SNMF, NMFSC, nsNMF, SNMF/R and SNMF/L, as the representative results on this aspect.

LNMF was presented by [25]. In simple terms, it imposes the sparseness constraints on G and locally constraints on F based on the following three considerations:

- Maximizing the sparseness in G;
- Maximizing the expressiveness of F;
- Maximizing the column orthogonality of F.

The objective function in the model of LNMF can take the following form: $\sum_{i,j}(X_{ij}\log\frac{X_{ij}}{(FG^T)_{ij}} - X_{ij} + (FG^T)_{ij}) + \alpha\sum_{i,j}(F^TF)_{ij} - \beta\sum_{i}(G^TG)_{ii}$.

2.7 Nonnegative Sparse Coding, NNSC ([28])

NNSC only maximizes the sparseness in G. The objective function to be minimized can be written as: $\|X - FG^T\|_F^2 + \lambda\sum_{i,j}G_{ij}$.

2.8 Spares Nonnegative Matrix Factorization, SNMF ([29,30,31])

The objective function in the above model of NNSC can be separated into a least squares error term $\|X - FG^T\|_F^2$ and an additional penalty term $\sum_{i,j}G_{ij}$.

Ref [29] replaced the least squares error term with the KL divergence to get the following new objective function: $\sum_{i,j}[X_{ij} \log \frac{X_{ij}}{(FG^T)_{ij}} - X_{ij} + (FG^T)_{ij}] + \lambda \sum_{i,j} G_{ij}$. Similarly, ref. [30] revised the penalty term to get another objective function:

$$\|X - FG^T\|_F^2 + \lambda \sum_{i,j} G_{ij}^2. \tag{6}$$

Furthermore, ref. [31] added an additional constraint on F, similar to that on G, into the objective function (6) to give the following CNMF model:

$$\min_{F\geqslant 0, G\geqslant 0} \|X - FG^T\|_F^2 + \alpha \sum_{i,j} F_{ij}^2 + \beta \sum_{i,j} G_{ij}^2.$$

2.9 Nonnegative Matrix Factorization with Sparseness Constraints, NMFSC ([32])

NMFSC employs the following measure to control the sparseness of F and G directly:

$$\mathrm{Sp}(a) = \frac{\sqrt{n} - \sum |a_j| / \sqrt{\sum a_j^2}}{\sqrt{n-1}}.$$

In other words, the model can be written as:

$$\begin{aligned} \min\ & \|X - FG^T\|_F^2 \\ s.t.\ & \mathrm{Sp}(F_{:,j}) = S_F, \\ & \mathrm{Sp}(G_{:,j}) = S_G, j = 1, 2, \cdots, r, \end{aligned}$$

where S_F and S_G are constants in [0,1], and it is easy to verify that the larger S_F and S_G, the more sparse F and G are.

2.10 Nonsmooth Nonnegative Matrix Factorization, nsNMF ([15])

nsNMF is also motivated by sparseness requirement of many applications and can be formulated as: $X = FSG^T$, where $S = (1-\theta)I + \frac{\theta}{k} II^T$ is a "smoothing" matrix, I is identity matrix and the parameter $\theta \in [0, 1]$ can indirectly control the sparseness of both the basis matrix F and the coding matrix G. One can observe that the larger the parameter θ, the more smooth (non-sparse) FS and GS are, in other words, each column of FS tends to be the constant vector with values equal to the average of the corresponding column of F as $\theta \to 1$. This is also the case for GS. But when updating G while fixing FS, the smoothness in FS will naturally enforce the sparseness in G and when updating F while fixing GS, the smoothness in GS will also enforce the sparseness in F. Hence F and G are enforced to be sparse iteratively. Note that $\theta = 0$ corresponds to the standard NMF.

2.11 Sparse NMFs: SNMF/R, SNMF/L ([33])

Sparse NMFs includes two formulations: SNMF/R for sparse G and SNMF/L for sparse F. SNMF/R is formulated as: $\min_{F\geqslant 0, G\geqslant 0} \|X - FG^T\|_F^2 + \eta \sum_{i,j} F_{ij}^2 + \beta \sum_i (\sum_j G_{ij})^2$ and SNMF/L is formulated as: $\min_{F\geqslant 0, G\geqslant 0} \|X - FG^T\|_F^2 + \eta \sum_{i,j} G_{ij}^2 + \alpha \sum_i (\sum_j F_{ij})^2$.

We note that there is still lack of systematic comparisons of the concordances and differences among the above seven sparse variants of NMF, which is an interesting topic.

2.12 CUR Decomposition ([34])

Instead of imposing the sparseness constraints on F and G, CUR decomposition constructs F from selected columns of X and G from selected rows of X respectively. In other words, the columns of F are composed of a small number of the columns in X and the columns of G are composed of a small number of the rows in X. The model can be formulated as follows: $X \approx FSG^T$[3], where S is introduced to make the approximation tighter, as its counterpart has done in Tri-NMF.

2.13 Binary Matrix Factorization, BMF ([20,21])

Binary Matrix Factorization (BMF) wants to factorize a binary matrix X (that is, elements of X are either 1 or 0) into two binary matrices F and G (thus conserving the most important integer property of the objective matrix X) satisfying $X \approx FG^T$. It has been shown that the bi-clustering problem (See Sect. 4.4) can be formulated as a BMF model ([21]). Unlike the greedy strategy-based models/algorithms, BMF are more likely to find the global optima. Experimental results on synthetic and real datasets demonstrate the advantages of BMF over existing bi-clustering methods. BMF will be further discussed in Sect. 4.

Table 2 summarizes the variations and extensions of NMF mentioned above.

3 Divergence Functions and Algorithms for NMF

In this part, we will review the divergence functions used for NMF and the algorithms employed for solving the model. We will consider several important divergence functions and the algorithmic extensions of NMF developed to accommodate these functions.

[3] In the original research, this model was presented as: $A \approx CUR$, which is the origin of the name CUR, and A may have mixed signs.

Table 2. Summary of different models based on NMF. Each row lists a variant and its associated constraints. $\pm$ means that the matrix in the corresponding column may have mixed signs, $+$ means that the matrix is nonnegative, $0-1$ means that the elements in the matrix can only be zero or one and I denotes identity matrix.

Models	Cost Function	X	F	S	G
NMF1 [1,2]	Least Squares Error	$+$	$+$	I	$+$
NMF2 [1,2]	K-L Divergence	$+$	$+$	I	$+$
Semi-NMF [22]	Least Squares Error	$\pm$	$\pm$	I	$+$
Convex-NMF [22]	Least Squares Error	$\pm$	$\pm$, $F_{:,j}$ is the convex combination of $\{X_{:,j}; j=1,\cdots,n\}$	I	$+$
Tri-NMF [23]	Least Squares Error	$+$	$+$, $F^TF=I$	$+$	$+$, $G^TG=I$
Symmetric-NMF [24]	Least Squares Error	$+$, symmetric	$+$, $F=G$	$+$	$+$
K-means [17]	Least Squares Error	$+$, symmetric	$+$, $F=G$	I	$+$, $G^TG=I$
PLSI[a] [18,19]	K-L Divergence	$\sum_{i,j} X_{ij}=1$	$\sum_i F_{ik}=1, i=1,\cdots m$	Diagonal, $\sum_k S_{kk}=1$	$\sum_j G_{jk}=1, j=1,\cdots n$
LNMF [25,26]	K-L Divergence with penalty terms[b]	$+$	$+$	I	$+$
NNSC [28]	Least Squares Error with penalty terms[c]	$+$	$+$	I	$+$
SNMF1 [29]	K-L Divergence with penalty terms[d]	$+$	$+$	I	$+$
SNMF2 [30]	Least Squares Error with penalty terms[e]	$+$	$+$	I	$+$
SNMF3 [31]	Least Squares Error with penalty terms[f]	$+$	$+$	I	$+$
NMFSC [32]	Least Squares Error	$+$	$+$, $\mathrm{Sp}(F_{:,j})=S_F$[g], $j=1,\cdots,k$	I	$+$, $\mathrm{Sp}(G_{:,j})=S_G$[h], $j=1,\cdots,k$
NMF/L [33]	Least Squares Error with penalty terms[i]	$+$	$+$	I	$+$
NMF/R [33]	Least Squares Error with penalty terms[j]	$+$	$+$	I	$+$
nsNMF [15]	K-L Divergence	$+$	$+$	$S=(1-\theta)I+\frac{\theta}{k}II^T$	$+$
CUR [34]	Least Squares Error	$+$	$+$[k]	$+$	$+$[l]
BMF [20,21]	Least Squares Error	$0-1$	$0-1$	I	$0-1$

[a] The relations between NMF and K-means, between NMF and PLSI will be reviewed in Sect. 5.

[b] $\sum_{i,j}(X_{ij}\log\frac{X_{ij}}{(FG^T)_{ij}} - X_{ij} + (FG^T)_{ij}) + \alpha\sum_{i,j}(F^TF)_{ij} - \beta\sum_i(G^TG)_{ii}$.

[c] $\|X-FG^T\|_F^2 + \lambda\sum_{i,j}G_{ij}$.

[d] $\sum_{i,j}[X_{ij}\log\frac{X_{ij}}{(FG^T)_{ij}} - X_{ij} + (FG^T)_{ij}] + \lambda\sum_{i,j}G_{ij}$.

[e] $\|X-FG^T\|_F^2 + \lambda\sum_{i,j}G_{ij}^2$.

[f] $\|X-FG^T\|_F^2 + \alpha\sum_{i,j}F_{ij}^2 + \beta\sum_{i,j}G_{ij}^2$.

[g] $\mathrm{Sp}(a) = (\sqrt{n} - \sum|a_j|/\sqrt{\sum a_j^2})/\sqrt{n-1}$, S_F is a constant.

[h] S_G is a constant.

[i] $\|X-FG^T\|_F^2 + \eta\|G\|_F^2 + \beta\sum_i\|F_{i,:}\|_1^2$.

[j] $\|X-FG^T\|_F^2 + \eta\|F\|_F^2 + \beta\sum_i\|G_{i,:}\|_1^2$.

[k] Columns of F are composed of a small number of columns in X.

[l] Columns of G are composed of a small number of rows in X.

3.1 Divergence Functions

One of the main advantages of NMF is its flexibility in the selection of the objective divergence functions. Here we will review several important divergence functions and the relations among them. These functions play important roles in solving NMF model, and may lead to different numerical performance. Hence research on the relations between the divergence functions and the appropriate applications is of great interest. Detailed theoretical analysis addressing this problem is in pressing need though some related numerical results have been given.

Csiszár's φ Divergence ([35]). The Csiszár's φ divergence is defined as: $D_\varphi(X||FG^T) = \sum_{i,j}(FG^T)_{ij}\varphi(\frac{X_{ij}}{(FG^T)_{ij}})$, where $X_{ij} \geqslant 0, (FG^T)_{ij} \geqslant 0$ and $\varphi : [0,\infty) \to (-\infty,\infty)$ is some convex function and continuous at point zero. Based on the flexibility of φ, the divergence has many instances. For example:

- $\varphi = (\sqrt{x}-1)^2$ corresponds to Hellinger divergence;
- $\varphi = (x-1)^2$ corresponds to Pearson's χ^2 divergence;
- $\varphi = x(x^{\alpha-1}-1)/(\alpha^2-\alpha)+(1-x)/\alpha$ corresponds to Amari's $\alpha-$divergence, which will be introduced later.

Note that though the selection of φ is flexible, Csiszár's φ divergence does not include the traditional least squares error: $D_{\mathrm{LSE}}(X\|FG^T) = \sum_{i,j}(X_{ij} - (FG^T)_{ij})^2$.

$\alpha-$Divergence, ([36,37,38,39]). The $\alpha-$divergence is defined as: $D_\alpha(X||FG^T) = \frac{1}{\alpha(1-\alpha)}\sum_{i,j}(\alpha X_{ij} + (1-\alpha)(FG^T)_{ij} - X_{ij}^{\alpha}(FG^T)_{ij}^{1-\alpha})$, where $\alpha \in (-\infty,\infty)$. Different selection of α may corresponds to different specific divergence. For example:

- $\lim_{\alpha\to 0} D_\alpha(X||FG^T)$ corresponds to K-L divergence $D_{\mathrm{KL}}(FG^T||X)$;
- $\alpha = \frac{1}{2}$ corresponds to Hellinger divergence;
- $\lim_{\alpha\to 1} D_\alpha(X||FG^T)$ corresponds to K-L divergence $D_{\mathrm{KL}}(X||FG^T)$;
- $\alpha = 2$ corresponds to Pearson's χ^2 divergence.

Since $\alpha-$divergence is a special case of Csiszár's φ divergence, as we have mentioned above, it does not include the least squares error either.

Bregman Divergence ([40]). The Bregman divergence can be defined as: $D_{\mathrm{Breg}}(X\|FG^T) = \sum_{i,j}\varphi(X_{ij}) - \varphi((FG^T)_{ij}) - \varphi'((FG^T)_{ij})(X_{ij} - (FG^T)_{ij})$, where $\varphi : S \subseteq \mathbb{R} \to \mathbb{R}$ is some strictly convex function that has continuous first derivative, and $(FG^T)_{ij} \in \mathrm{int}(S)$ (the interior of set S). Some instances of Bregman divergence are listed as follows:

- $\varphi = \frac{x^2}{2}$ corresponds to least squares error;
- $\varphi = x \log x$ corresponds to K-L divergence;
- $\varphi = -\log x$ corresponds to Itakura-Saito (IS) divergence.

$\beta-$Divergence ([41,39]). The $\beta-$divergence is defined as: $D_\beta(X||FG^T) = \sum_{i,j}(X_{ij}\frac{X_{ij}^\beta - (FG^T)_{ij}^\beta}{\beta} - \frac{X_{ij}^{\beta+1} - (FG^T)_{ij}^{\beta+1}}{\beta+1})$ where $\beta \neq 0, -1$. This divergence is also a big family including K-L divergence, least squares error, etc. Specifically:

- $\lim_{\beta\to 0} D_\beta(X||FG^T)$ corresponds to K-L divergence $D_{\text{KL}}(X||FG^T)$;
- $\beta = 1$ corresponds to least squares error $D_{\text{LSE}}(X||FG^T)$;
- $\lim_{\beta\to -1} D_\beta(X||FG^T)$ corresponds to Itakura-Saito (IS) divergence which will be introduced later.

Note that $\beta-$divergence $D_\beta(x\|y)$ can be got from $\alpha-$divergence $D_\alpha(x\|y)$ by nonlinear transformation: $x = x^{\beta+1}$, $y = y^{\beta+1}$ and supposing $\alpha = \frac{1}{\beta+1}$ ([42]).

Itakura-Saito (IS) Divergence ([43]). The Itakura-Saito divergence is defined as: $D_{\text{IS}}(X\|FG^T) = \sum_{i,j}(\frac{X_{ij}}{(FG^T)_{ij}} - \log\frac{X_{ij}}{(FG^T)_{ij}} - 1)$. Note that IS divergence is a special case of both the Bregman divergence ($\phi(x) = -\log x$) and the β-divergence ($\beta = -1$).

K-L Divergence ([2]). The K-L divergence is defined as: $D_{\text{KL}}(X\|FG^T) = \sum_{i,j}[X_{ij}\log\frac{X_{ij}}{(FG^T)_{ij}} - X_{ij} + (FG^T)_{ij}]$. As we have discussed above, the K-L divergence is a special case of $\alpha-$divergence, Bregman divergence and $\beta-$divergence.

Least Squares Error ([2]). The least squares error is defined as: $D_{\text{LSE}}(X\|FG^T) = \|X - FG^T\|_F^2 = \sum_{i,j}(X_{ij} - (FG^T)_{ij})^2$, which is a special case of Bregman divergence and $\beta-$divergence.

We summarize the different divergence functions and the corresponding multiplicative update rules (See Sect. 3.2) in Table 3. The other algorithms such as Newton algorithm or Quasi-Newton algorithm that are specially designed for some of the divergence functions will be reviewed in the next subsection.

3.2 Algorithms for NMF

The algorithm design for solving NMF is an important direction and several algorithms, according to different objective divergence functions and different

Table 3. Summary of the different divergence functions and the corresponding multiplicative update rules. Note that "Convergence" only says whether the update rules have been proven to be monotonically decreasing. Even if this is proven, the algorithm does not necessarily converge to a local minimum ([44]).

Divergence Function	Multiplicative Update Rules of F and G	Convergence	Comments
Csiszár's φ Divergence	—	—	—
α−Divergence	$F_{ik} := F_{ik}(\frac{((\frac{X}{FG^T})^\alpha G)_{ik}}{\sum_l G_{lk}})^{\frac{1}{\alpha}}$ $G_{ik} := G_{ik}(\frac{((\frac{X^T}{GF^T})^\alpha F)_{ik}}{\sum_l F_{lk}})^{\frac{1}{\alpha}}$	proved	special case of φ−divergence ($\varphi(x) = x(x^{\alpha-1} - 1)/(\alpha^2 - \alpha) + (1 - x)/\alpha$)
Bregman Divergence	$F_{ik} := F_{ik} \frac{\sum_j \nabla^2\phi(FG^T)_{ij} X_{ij} G_{jk}}{\sum_j \nabla^2\phi(FG^T)_{ij}(FG^T)_{ij} G_{jk}}$ $G_{ik} := G_{ik} \frac{\sum_j \nabla^2\phi(GF^T)_{ij} X_{ji} F_{jk}}{\sum_j \nabla^2\phi(GF^T)_{ij}(GF^T)_{ij} F_{jk}}$	proved	—
β−Divergence	$F_{ik} := F_{ik} \frac{\sum_j ((FG^T)_{ij}^{\beta-1} X_{ij}) G_{jk}}{\sum_j (FG^T)_{ij}^{\beta} G_{jk}}$ $G_{ik} := G_{ik} \frac{\sum_j ((FG^T)_{ji}^{\beta-1} X_{ji}) F_{jk}}{\sum_j (FG^T)_{ji}^{\beta} F_{jk}}$	proved when $0 \leqslant \beta \leqslant 1$ ([43])	—
Itakura-Saito (IS) Divergence	$F_{ik} := F_{ik} \frac{\sum_j \frac{X_{ij}}{(FG^T)_{ij}^2} G_{jk}}{\sum_j \frac{G_{jk}}{(FG^T)_{ij}}}$ $G_{ik} := G_{ik} \frac{\sum_j \frac{X_{ji}}{(FG^T)_{ji}^2} F_{jk}}{\sum_j \frac{F_{jk}}{(FG^T)_{ji}}}$	not proved	special case of Bregman divergence ($\varphi(x) = -\log x$) and β−divergence ($\beta = -1$)
K-L Divergence	$F_{ik} := \frac{F_{ik}}{\sum_j G_{jk}} \sum_j \frac{X_{ij}}{(FG^T)_{ij}} G_{jk}$ $G_{ik} := \frac{G_{ik}}{\sum_j F_{jk}} \sum_j \frac{X_{ji}}{(FG^T)_{ji}} F_{jk}$	proved	special case of α−divergence ($\alpha = 1$), Bregman divergence ($\varphi(x) = x \log x$) and β−divergence ($\beta = 0$)
Least Squares Error	$F_{ik} := F_{ik} \frac{(XG)_{ik}}{(FG^TG)_{ik}}$ $G_{ik} := G_{ik} \frac{(X^TF)_{ik}}{(GF^TF)_{ik}}$	proved	special case of Bregman divergence ($\varphi(x) = \frac{x^2}{2}$) and β−divergence ($\beta = 1$)

application purposes, have been proposed. In this part, we will briefly review the representative ones. Note that to simplify the complexity of the problem, we only consider the standard NMF model, i.e., only the optimization problem (2) is considered. The algorithms for its variations presented in Sect. 2 can be obtained by simple derivations and can be found in the corresponding literature.

Multiplicative Update Algorithm ([1,2]). The multiplicative update rules of NMF with its convergence proof (indeed, only the monotonic decreasing property is proved) was firstly presented by Lee & Seung ([1,2]). Because of the simplicity and effectiveness, it has become one of the most influential algorithms that are widely used in the data mining community. This algorithm is gradient-descent-based and similar to the Expectation Maximization Algorithm (EM). Specifically when the K-L divergence is selected as the objective function, the multiplicative update algorithms can be summarized as Algorithm 2. In addition, there are several interesting properties of the relations between the multiplicative update rules with K-L divergence and the EM algorithm employed in Probabilistic Latent Semantic Indexing (PLSI), which will be discussed in Sect. 5.

The update rules in line 2 and line 3 of Algorithm 2 vary with the user-selected objective functions and have been summarized in Table 3.

Algorithm 2. Nonnegative Matrix Factorization (K-L divergence, Multiplicative Update Rules)

Input: $F^{(0)}, G^{(0)}, t = 1$.
Output: F, G.
1: **while** 1 **do**
2: Update $F_{ik}^{(t)} := \frac{F_{ik}^{(t-1)}}{\sum_j G_{jk}^{(t-1)}} \sum_j \frac{X_{ij}}{(F^{(t-1)}G^{(t-1)T})_{ij}} G_{jk}^{(t-1)}$;
3: Update $G_{jk}^{(t)} := \frac{G_{jk}^{(t-1)}}{\sum_i F_{ik}^{(t)}} \sum_i \frac{X_{ij}}{(F^{(t)}G^{(t-1)T})_{ij}} F_{ik}^{(t)}$;
4: Test for convergence;
5: **if** Some convergence condition is satisfied **then**
6: $F = F^{(t)}$;
7: $G = G^{(t)}$;
8: **Break**
9: **end if**
10: $t = t + 1$;
11: **end while**

Project Gradient Algorithm ([45]). The project gradient descent method is generally designed for bound-constrained optimization problems. In order to use this method, a sufficiently large upper bound U is firstly set for F and (since the upper bound U is sufficiently large, the solutions of the revised mod will be identical with the original one). The objective optimization function selected as the least squares error. The K-L divergence is not suitable becau this divergence is not well-defined on the boundary of the constraints (the lo function is defined for positive reals). The method can then be summarized i Algorithm 3. Note that $(P[\bullet])_{ij} = \begin{cases} \bullet_{ij}, & 0 \leqslant \bullet_{ij} \leqslant U, \\ 0. & \bullet_{ij} < 0, \\ U, & \bullet_{ij} > U. \end{cases}$

Newton Algorithm ([46]). The Newton algorithm is designed for the leas squares error (Indeed, the idea of quasi-Newton method is employed). Basicall it can be summarized in Algorithm 4. Note that D is an appropriate positiv definite gradient scaling matrix, and $[Z_+(X)]_{ij} = \begin{cases} X_{ij}, & (i,j) \notin I_+, \\ 0. & \text{otherwise} \end{cases}$ and I_+ will be given in the algorithm. The details are omitted due to space limitation.

The Newton algorithm and the Quasi-Newton algorithm presented below have utilized the second order information of the model (Hessian matrix), hence one can expect that they have better numerical performance than the multiplicative update rules and the projected gradient descent though they should be more time-consuming.

Quasi-Newton Method ([47]). The Quasi-Newton algorithm is designed fo the $\alpha-$divergence. As we have discussed above, this divergence is a general case several useful objective optimization functions including the K-L divergence. Bu note that the least squares error is not included. The proposed Quasi-Newto algorithm is summarized in Algorithm 5. Note that $H_J^{(F)}$ and $H_J^{(G)}$ are th Hessian matrices of F and G, and $\nabla_F J$ and $\nabla_G J$ are the gradients of F and G

Active Set Algorithm ([48]). The active set algorithm is designed for th least squares error. The basic idea is to decompose the original optimizatio problem $\min\limits_{F \geqslant 0, G \geqslant 0} \|X - FG^T\|_F^2$ into several separate subproblems, then solv them independently using the standard active set method and finally merg the solutions obtained. In other words, firstly, fixing F, decompose the proble $\min\limits_{F \geqslant 0, G \geqslant 0} \|X - FG^T\|_F^2$ into the following series of subproblems: $\min\limits_{G_{i,:} \geqslant 0} \|X_{:,i} - FG_{i,:}^T\|_F^2$, $i = 1, 2, \cdots, m$, then solve them independently and finally update G. Then fixing G, update F similarly.

Hereto, we have reviewed several newly developed algorithms, most of which are nonlinear-programming-originated but are specially designed for NMF model. Note that the technical details are omitted here due to space limitation. One can get more information from the corresponding references.

Algorithm 3. Nonnegative Matrix Factorization (Least Squares Error, Projected Gradient Method)

Input: $F^{(0)}, G^{(0)}, t = 1$.
Output: F, G.
1: **while** 1 **do**
2: $F^{(old)} = F^{(t-1)}$;
3: **while** 1 **do**
4: Compute the gradient matrix $\nabla_F J(X, F^{(old)} G^{(t-1)T})$;
5: Compute the step length α;
6: Update $F^{(old)}$:
$F^{(new)} = P[F^{(old)} - \alpha \nabla_F J(X, F^{(old)} G^{(t-1)T})]$;
7: $F^{(old)} = F^{(new)}$;
8: Test for convergence;
9: **if** Some convergence condition is satisfied **then**
10: $F^{(t)} = F^{(old)}$;
11: **Break**
12: **end if**
13: **end while**
14: $G^{(old)} = G^{(t-1)}$;
15: **while** 1 **do**
16: Compute the gradient matrix $\nabla_G J(X, F^{(t)} G^{(old)T})$;
17: Compute the step length α;
18: Update $G^{(old)}$:
$G^{(new)} = P[G^{(old)} - \alpha \nabla_G J(X, F^{(t)} G^{(old)T})]$;
19: $G^{(old)} = G^{(new)}$;
20: Test for convergence;
21: **if** Some convergence condition is satisfied **then**
22: $G^{(t)} = G^{(old)}$;
23: **Break**
24: **end if**
25: **end while**
26: **if** Some stopping criteria are met **then**
27: $F = F^{(t)}$; $G = G^{(t)}$;
28: **Break**
29: **end if**
30: $t = t + 1$;
31: **end while**

Algorithm 4. Nonnegative Matrix Factorization (Least Squares Error, Newton Algorithm)

Input: $F^{(0)}, G^{(0)}, D, t = 1$.
Output: F, G.
1: **while** 1 **do**
2: $F^{(old)} = F^{(t-1)}$;
3: **while** 1 **do**
4: Compute the gradient matrix $\nabla_F J(X, F^{(old)} G^{(t-1)T})$;
5: Compute fixed set $I_+ := \{(i,j) : F_{ij}^{(old)} = 0, [\nabla_F J(X, F^{(old)} G^{(t-1)T})]_{ij} > 0\}$ for $F^{(old)}$;
6: Compute the step length vector α;
7: Update $F^{(old)}$:

$$U = Z_+[\nabla_F J(X, F^{(old)} G^{(t-1)T})]; \quad U = Z_+(DU);$$
$$F^{(new)} = \max(F^{(old)} - U diag(\alpha), 0);$$

8: $F^{(old)} = F^{(new)}$;
9: Update D if necessary;
10: Test for convergence;
11: **if** Some convergence condition is satisfied **then**
12: $F^{(t)} = F^{(old)}$;
13: **Break**
14: **end if**
15: **end while**
16: $G^{(old)} = G^{(t-1)}$;
17: **while** 1 **do**
18: Compute the gradient matrix $\nabla_G J(X, F^{(t)} G^{(old)T})$;
19: Compute fixed set $I_+ := \{(i,j) : G_{ij}^{(old)} = 0, [\nabla_G J(X, F^{(t)} G^{(old)T})]_{ij} > 0\}$ for $G^{(old)}$;
20: Compute the step length vector α;
21: Update $G^{(old)}$:

$$U = Z_+[\nabla_G J(X, F^{(t)} G^{(old)T})]; \quad U = Z_+(DU);$$
$$G^{(new)} = \max(G^{(old)} - U diag(\alpha), 0);$$

22: $G^{(old)} = G^{(new)}$;
23: Update D if necessary;
24: Test for convergence;
25: **if** Some convergence condition is satisfied **then**
26: $G^{(t)} = G^{(old)}$;
27: **Break**
28: **end if**
29: **end while**
30: **if** Some stopping criteria are met **then**
31: $F = F^{(t)}$; $G = G^{(t)}$;
32: **Break**
33: **end if**
34: $t = t + 1$;
35: **end while**

Algorithm 5. Nonnegative Matrix Factorization (α−Divergence, Quasi-Newton Algorithm)

Input: $F^{(0)}, G^{(0)}, t = 1$.
Output: F, G.
1: **while** 1 **do**
2: Update $F^{(t)} := \max(F^{(t-1)} - [H_J^{(F)}]^{-1}\nabla_F J, 0)$;
3: Update $G^{(t)} := \max(G^{(t-1)} - [H_J^{(G)}]^{-1}\nabla_G J, 0)$;
4: Test for convergence;
5: **if** Some convergence condition is satisfied **then**
6: $F = F^{(t)}$;
7: $G = G^{(t)}$;
8: **Break**
9: **end if**
10: $t = t + 1$;
11: **end while**

4 Applications of NMF

Nonnegative Matrix Factorization has been proved to be valuable in many fields of data mining, especially in unsupervised learning. In this part, we will briefly review its applications in image processing, data clustering, semi-supervised clustering, bi-clustering (co-clustering) and financial data mining. Note that we cannot cover all the interesting applications of NMF, but generally speaking, the special point on NMF is its ability to recover the hidden patterns or trends behind the observed data automatically, which makes it suitable for image processing, feature extraction, dimensional reduction and unsupervised learning. The preliminary theoretical analysis concerning this ability will be reviewed in the next section, in other words, the relations between NMF and some other unsupervised learning models will be discussed.

4.1 Image Processing

Though the history of Nonnegative Matrix Factorization was traced back to 1970's, NMF was attracted lots of attention due to the research of Lee & Seung ([1,2]). In their works, the model was applied to image processing successfully. Hence we review the applications of NMF on this aspect firstly.

In image processing, the data can be represented as $n \times m$ nonnegative matrix X, each column of which is an image described by n nonnegative pixel values. Then NMF model can find two factor matrices F and G such that $X \approx FG^T$. F is the so-called basis matrix since each column can be regarded as a part of the whole such as nose, ear or eye, etc. for facial image data. G is the coding matrix and each row is the weights by which the corresponding image can be reconstructed as the linear combination of the columns of F.

In summary, NMF can discover the common basis hidden behind the observations and the way how the images are reconstructed by the basis. Indeed, the psychological and physiological researches have shown evidence for part-based representation in the brain, which is also the foundation of some computational theories ([1]). But further researches have also shown that the standard NMF model does not necessarily give the correct part-of-whole representations ([25,27]), hence many efforts have been done to improve the sparseness of NMF in order to identify more localized features that are building parts for the whole representation (See Sect. 2).

4.2 Clustering

One of the most interesting and successful applications of NMF is to cluster data such as text, image or biology data, i.e. discovering patterns automatically from data. Given a nonnegative $n \times m$ matrix X, each column of which is a sample and described by n features, NMF can be applied to find two factor matrices F and G such that $X \approx FG^T$, where F is $n \times r$ and G is $m \times r$, and r is the cluster number. Columns of F can be regarded as the cluster centroids while G is the cluster membership indicator matrix. In other words, the sample i is of cluster k if G_{ik} is the largest value of the row $G_{i,:}$.

The good performance of NMF in clustering has been validated in several different fields including bioinformatics (tumor sample clustering based on microarray data, [14]), community structure detection of the complex network ([49]) and text clustering ([10,11,12]).

4.3 Semi-supervised Clustering

In many cases, some background information concerning the pairwise relations of some samples are known and we can add them into the clustering model in order to guide the clustering process. The resulting constrained problem is called semi-supervised clustering. Specifically, the following two types of pairwise relations are often considered:

- *Must-link* specifies that two samples should have the same cluster label;
- *Cannot-link* specifies that two samples should not have the same cluster label.

Then, one can establish two nonnegative matrices $W_{\text{reward}} = \{w_{ij} :$ sample i and sample j are in the same class$\}$ and $W_{\text{penalty}} = \{w_{ij} :$ sample i and sample j are not in the same class$\}$ based on the above information, and the similarity matrix $W = X^T X$ of the samples (columns of X are samples) can then be replaced by $W - W_{\text{reward}} + W_{\text{penalty}}$ (note that it is still a symmetric matrix). Finally, NMF is applied:

$$\min_{S \geqslant 0, G \geqslant 0} \|(W - W_{\text{reward}} + W_{\text{penalty}}) - GSG^T\|_F^2,$$

where G is the cluster membership indicator, i.e., sample i is of cluster k if the element G_{ik} is the largest value of the row $G_{i,:}$. Theoretical analysis and practical applications have been contributed by [50]. We summarize the main theoretical results but omit the details here.

Theorem 2. *Orthogonal Semi-Supervised NMF clustering is equivalent to Semi-Supervised Kernel K-means ([51]).*

Theorem 3. *Orthogonal Semi-Supervised NMF clustering is equivalent to Semi-Supervised Spectral clustering with Normalized Cuts ([52]).*

4.4 Bi-clustering (co-clustering)

Bi-clustering was recently introduced by Cheng & Church ([53]) for gene expression data analysis. In practice, many genes are only active in some conditions or classes and remain silent under other cases. Such gene-class structures, which are very important to understand the pathology, can not be discovered using the traditional clustering algorithms. Hence it is very necessary to develop bi-clustering models/algorithms to identify the local structures. Bi-clustering models/algorithms are different from the traditional clustering methodologies which assign the samples into specific classes based on the genes' expression levels across *ALL* the samples, they try to cluster the rows (features) and the columns (samples) of a matrix simultaneously.

In other words, the idea of bi-clustering is to characterize each sample by a subset of genes and to define each gene in a similar way. As a consequence, bi-clustering algorithms can select the groups of genes that show similar expression behaviors in a subset of samples that belong to some specific classes such as some tumor types, thus identify the local structures of the microarray matrix data [53,54]. Binary Matrix Factorization (BMF) has been presented for solving bi-clustering problem: the input binary gene-sample matrix X[4] is decomposed into two binary matrices F and G such that $X \approx FG^T$. The binary matrices F and G can explicitly designate the cluster memberships for genes and samples. Hence BMF offers a framework for simultaneously clustering the genes and samples.

An example is given here[5] to demonstrate the biclustering capability of BMF. Given the original data matrix

$$X = \begin{pmatrix} 0 & 0 & 0 & 0 & 0 & 0 & 1 & 1 \\ 0 & 0 & 0 & 0 & 0 & 1 & 1 & 0 \\ 0 & 1 & 1 & 1 & 0 & 1 & 1 & 1 \\ 1 & 0 & 1 & 1 & 0 & 1 & 1 & 1 \\ 0 & 1 & 0 & 1 & 0 & 0 & 0 & 0 \end{pmatrix}.$$

One can see two biclusters, one in the upper-right corner, and one in lower-left corner. Our BMF model gives

[4] [21] has discussed the details on how to discretize the microarray data into a binary matrix.

[5] Another example is given in the appendix to illustrate the limitations of NMF for discovering bi-clustering structures.

$$F = (F_{:,1}, F_{:,2}) = \begin{pmatrix} 0 & 1 \\ 0 & 1 \\ 1 & 1 \\ 1 & 1 \\ 1 & 0 \end{pmatrix}; \quad G = (G_{:,1}, G_{:,2}) = \begin{pmatrix} 0 & 1 & 1 & 1 & 0 & 0 & 0 & 0 \\ 0 & 0 & 0 & 0 & 0 & 1 & 1 & 1 \end{pmatrix};$$

The two discovered biclusters are recovered in a clean way:

$$FG^T = \begin{pmatrix} 0\,0\,0\,0\,0\,1\,1\,1 \\ 0\,0\,0\,0\,0\,1\,1\,1 \\ 0\,1\,1\,1\,0\,1\,1\,1 \\ 0\,1\,1\,1\,0\,1\,1\,1 \\ 0\,1\,1\,1\,0\,0\,0\,0 \end{pmatrix}.$$

4.5 Financial Data Mining

Underlying Trends in Stock Market: In the stock market, it has been observed that the stock price fluctuations does not behave independently of each other but are mainly dominated by several underlying and unobserved factors. Hence identification the underlying trends from the stock market data is an interesting problem, which can be solved by NMF. Given an $n \times m$ nonnegative matrix X, columns of which are the records of the stock prices during n time points, NMF can be applied to find two nonnegative factors F and G such that $X \approx FG^T$, where columns of F are the underlying components. Note that identifying the common factors that drive the prices is somewhat similar to blind source separation (BSS) in signal processing. Furthermore, G can be used to identify the cluster labels of the stocks (see Sect. 4.2) and the most interesting result is that the stocks of the same sector are not necessarily assigned into the same cluster and vice versa, which is of potential use to guide diversified portfolio, in other words, investors should diversify their money into not only different sectors, but also different clusters. More details can be found in [55].

Discriminant Features Extraction in Financial Distress Data: Building appropriate financial distress prediction model based on the extracted discriminative features is more and more important under the background of financial crisis. In [56] it has presented a new prediction model which is indeed a combination of K-means, NMF and Support Vector Machine (SVM). The basic idea is to train a SVM classifier in the reduced dimensional space which is spanned by the discriminative features extracted by NMF, the algorithm of which is initialized by K-means. The details can be found in [56].

5 Relations with Other Relevant Models

Indeed, the last ten years have witnessed the boom of Nonnegative Matrix Factorization in many fields including bioinformatics, images processing, text mining, physics, multimedia, etc. But it is still not very clear that why the model works. Researches on the relations between NMF and other unsupervised learning models such as K-means and Probabilistic Latent Semantic Indexing try to give us a preliminary interpretation of this question. The basic results of this part are: i) the model of soft K-means can be rewritten as symmetric-NMF model. Hence K-means and NMF are equivalent, which justifies the ability of NMF for data clustering. But this does not mean that K-means and NMF will generate identical cluster results since they employ different algorithms; ii) Probabilistic Latent Semantic Indexing (PLSI) and NMF optimize the same objective function (K-L divergence), but PLSI has additional constraints. The algorithms of the two models can generate equivalent solutions, but they are different in essence.

5.1 Relations between NMF and K-means

In [17] it has been shown that the model of K-means can be written in a special form of NMF with orthogonal constraints, in which the objective function is the least squares error and the objective matrix W is the similarity matrix of the original samples and symmetric. This result is important and interesting because it gives a solid foundation for NMF used for data clustering.

K-means is one of the most famous and traditional methods for clustering analysis. It aims to partition m samples into $K-$clusters. The motivation is very intuitive: the samples that are close to each other should share the same cluster indicators. Hence K-means algorithm alternatively gives the cluster index of each sample by the nearest cluster center and gives the cluster center by the centroid of its members. The major drawback of K-means is that it is very sensitive to the initializations and prone to local minima. Mathematically, K-means can be formulated as minimizing a sum of squares cost function: $\min J_K = \sum_{k=1}^{K} \sum_{i \in C_k} \|x_i - m_k\|^2$, where $x_i, i = 1, 2, \cdots m$ are the data samples and $X = (x_1, x_2, \cdots, x_m)$ is the data matrix, $m_k = \sum_{i \in C_k} x_i / n_k$ is the centroid of cluster C_k with n_k samples. This optimization problem can be equivalently solved by a special type of nonnegative matrix factorization $W = HH^T$, where $W = X^T X$, with orthogonal constraint $H^T H = I$, i.e., nonnegative matrix factorization is equivalent to soft K-means (i.e., $H^T H = I$ is relaxed).

Theorem 4. $\min \|W - HH^T\|^2$, *where* $W = X^T X$, *is equivalent to soft K-means.*

Proof. See Appendix.

The model equivalence of K-means and NMF has established the theoretical foundation of NMF used for data clustering. Though NMF has been applied for clustering successfully, there is still a lack of theoretical analysis until this equivalent result is proved. But one should be noted that it does not mean that NMF and K-means generate identical results. The algorithms that used to solve

NMF and K-means are quite different. NMF uses gradient descent method while K-means uses coordinate descent method ([57]). A general conclusion is that NMF almost always outperforms K-means. Maybe this is due to the flexibility of NMF which has more parameters to be decided. In fact, K-means always wants to find the ellipsoidal-shaped clusters while NMF does not. When the data distribution is far from an ellipsoidal-shaped clustering, which is often the case for real data, NMF may have advantages ([22]). In summary, though NMF is equivalent to K-means, it often generates a different and better result.

Moreover, it has been proved that the solution of soft K-means can also be given by Principal Component Analysis (PCA), which builts closer relationships between PCA and NMF ([58]) . A systematic numerical comparison and analysis of K-means, PCA and NMF is of interesting, but is beyond the scope of this chapter.

5.2 Relations between NMF and PLSI

Probabilistic Latent Semantic Indexing (PLSI) is one of the state-of-the-art unsupervised learning models in data mining, and has been widely used in many applications such as text clustering, information retrieval and collaborative filtering. In this section, relations between NMF and PLSI, including the differences of their models and the differences of their algorithms will be given. In summary, NMF and PLSI optimize the same objective function; but their algorithms are different due to the additional constraints in PLSI.

Probabilistic Latent Semantic Indexing (PLSI, [59]) is a probabilistic model stemmed from Latent Semantic Analysis (LSA, [60]). Compared to LSA, PLSI has a more solid theoretical foundation in statistics and thus is a more principled approach for analyzing text, discovering latent topics and information retrieval, etc. ([59,61,62]). PLSI is a kind of topic model and, given a joint probabilistic matrix X (i.e., $\sum_{i,j} X_{ij} = 1.$), aims to get three nonnegative matrices C, diagonal S and H such that CSH^T is the approximation of X. The parameters in PLSI model are trained by the Expectation Maximization (EM) algorithm which iteratively increases the objective likelihood function until some convergence condition is satisfied and, at each step, PLSI maintains the column normalization property of C, S and H ($\sum_i C_{ik} = 1, \sum_k S_{kk} = 1, \sum_j H_{jk} = 1$).

For simplifying explanation, we take the document analysis task as an example. Given a document collection $X_{n \times m}$ of m documents and a vocabulary of n words, where each element X_{ij} indicates whether a word w_i occurs in document d_j, the learning task in PLSI is to find three matrices C,H and S, such that X is approximated by CSH^T, where C_{ik} is the probability of $P(w_i|z_k)$[6], H_{jk} is the probability of $P(d_j|z_k)$ and S is diagonal matrix with diagonal element $S_{kk} = P(z_k)$.

To learn the PLSI model, we can consider maximizing the log-likelihood of the PLSI model $L = \sum_{i,j} n(i,j) log P(w_i, d_j)$, where $n(i,j)$ is the co-occurrence

[6] z_k means the kth latent topic.

number of word i and document j, and $P(w_i, d_j) = \sum_k P(w_i|z_k)P(z_k)P(d_j|z_k) = \sum_k C_{ik}S_{kk}H_{jk}$. Here we normalize X to satisfy $\sum_{i,j} X_{ij} = 1$, and the log-likelihood function can then be rewritten as:

$$L = \sum_{i,j} X_{ij} \log P(w_i, d_j). \tag{7}$$

The parameters C, S and H are then iteratively got by Expectation-Maximization (EM) algorithm. The EM algorithm begins with some initial values of C, H, S and iteratively updates them according to the following formulas:

$$C_{ik} := \frac{\sum\limits_{j} X_{ij} P_{ij}^k}{\sum\limits_{i,j} X_{ij} P_{ij}^k}; \quad S_{kk} := \sum_{i,j} X_{ij} P_{ij}^k; \quad H_{jk} := \frac{\sum\limits_{i} X_{ij} P_{ij}^k}{\sum\limits_{i,j} X_{ij} P_{ij}^k}. \tag{8}$$

where P_{ij}^k is the probability of

$$P(z_k|w_i, d_j) = \frac{S_{kk}C_{ik}H_{jk}}{\sum_k S_{kk}C_{ik}H_{jk}}. \tag{9}$$

By combining (8) and (9), one can get:

$$C_{ik} := \frac{\sum\limits_{j} X_{ij} \frac{S_{kk}C_{ik}H_{jk}}{\sum\limits_{k} S_{kk}C_{ik}H_{jk}}}{\sum\limits_{i,j} X_{ij} \frac{S_{kk}C_{ik}H_{jk}}{\sum\limits_{k} S_{kk}C_{ik}H_{jk}}} \quad H_{jk} := \frac{\sum\limits_{i} X_{ij} \frac{S_{kk}C_{ik}H_{jk}}{\sum\limits_{k} S_{kk}C_{ik}H_{jk}}}{\sum\limits_{i,j} X_{ij} \frac{S_{kk}C_{ik}H_{jk}}{\sum\limits_{k} S_{kk}C_{ik}H_{jk}}} \quad S_{kk} := S_{kk} \frac{\sum\limits_{ij} X_{ij}C_{ik}H_{jk}}{\sum\limits_{k} S_{kk}C_{ik}H_{jk}}$$

$$= C_{ik} \frac{(\frac{X.}{CSH^T})H)_{ik}}{(C^T \frac{X.}{CSH^T} H)_{kk}}; \qquad = H_{jk} \frac{(\frac{X.}{CSH^T})^T C)_{jk}}{(C^T \frac{X.}{CSH^T} H)_{kk}}; \qquad = S_{kk}(C^T \frac{X.}{CSH^T} H)_{kk}. \tag{10}$$

The algorithm of PLSI is summarized in Algorithm 6:

Consequently, we will review the relations between NMF and PLSI. The basic conclusions are: 1) maximizing the objective likelihood function in PLSI is equivalent to minimizing the K-L divergence in NMF. Hence NMF and PLSI optimize the same objective function, i.e., K-L divergence ([18]); 2) their solutions are equivalent because of the fixed row sum and fixed column sum property of NMF with K-L divergence; 3) Their algorithms are different because of the additional constraints in PLSI.

To begin with, we give the following lemma:

Lemma 1 (fixed row and column sums property, [18,63]). *In NMF, under the update rules:*

$$F_{ik} := \frac{F_{ik}}{\sum_j G_{jk}} \sum_j \frac{X_{ij}}{(FG^T)_{ij}} G_{jk};$$
$$G_{jk} := \frac{G_{jk}}{\sum_i F_{ik}} \sum_i \frac{X_{ij}}{(FG^T)_{ij}} F_{ik},$$

Algorithm 6. Probabilistic Latent Semantic Indexing

Input: $C^0, S^0, H^0, t = 1$.
Output: C, S, H.
1: **while** 1 **do**
2: Update $C_{ik}^{(t)} := C_{ik}^{(t-1)} \frac{(\frac{X.}{C^{(t-1)}S^{(t-1)}H^{(t-1)T}})H^{(t-1)})_{ik}}{(C^{(t-1)T}\frac{X.}{C^{(t-1)}S^{(t-1)}H^{(t-1)T}}H^{(t-1)})_{kk}}$;
3: Update $S_{kk}^{(t)} := S_{kk}^{(t-1)}(C^{(t)T}\frac{X.}{C^{(t)}S^{(t-1)}H^{(t-1)T}}H^{(t-1)})_{kk}$;
4: Update $H_{jk}^{(t)} := H_{jk}^{(t-1)} \frac{(\frac{X.}{C^{(t)}S^{(t)}H^{(t-1)T}})^T C^{(t)})_{jk}}{(C^{(t-1)T}\frac{X.}{C^{(t)}S^{(t)}H^{(t-1)T}}H^{(t-1)})_{kk}}$;
5: Test for convergence.
6: **if** Some convergence condition is satisfied **then**
7: $C = C^{(t)}$;
8: $S = S^{(t)}$;
9: $H = H^{(t)}$;
10: **Break**
11: **end if**
12: $t = t + 1$;
13: **end while**

we have, at convergence:

$$\sum_{i=1}^{n}(FG^T)_{ij} = \sum_{i=1}^{n} X_{ij}; \quad \sum_{j=1}^{m}(FG^T)_{ij} = \sum_{j=1}^{m} X_{ij}.$$

Proof. See Appendix.

Now we proceed to prove the model equivalence between NMF and PLSI.

Theorem 5. *NMF and PLSI optimize the same objective function.*

Proof. See Appendix.

Theorem 6. *([18,19]) Any local maximum likelihood solution (C, S, H) of PLSI is a solution of NMF with K-L divergence and vice versa.*

Proof. This is obviously true by letting $F = C$ and $G = HS$ (or $F = CS$ and $G = H$) at convergence.

The conclusion that any local minimum solution (F, G) of NMF is a solution of PLSI can be proved similarly by normalizing F and G at convergence. □

From above analysis, one can see that NMF and PLSI optimize the same objective function, and the solution (F, G) of NMF and the solution (C, S, H) of PLSI are equivalent. Furthermore, we observe that at convergence, $FG^T = CSH^T$.

Consequently we will show that the algorithms of NMF and PLSI are different. To show this, we will firstly study the normalization of NMF. In other words, to compare the differences between NMF and PLSI more explicitly, we column normalize F and G at each step in NMF.

Obviously, in Algorithm 2, it holds that $F^{(t)}G^{(t-1)T} = (F^{(t)}A)(G^{(t-1)}B)^T$ for any two matrices A and B as long as $AB^T = I$ and $F^{(t)}A \geqslant 0$, $G^{(t-1)}B \geqslant 0$. If we select special A and B such that A is diagonal with $A_{kk} = \sum_i F_{ik}$ and $B = A^{-1}$, then $(F^{(t)}A)$ is column normalization of $F^{(t)}$. Similarly, we can get the column normalization of $G^{(t)}$. Based on these observations, we can revise the standard NMF algorithm as follows: after line 2 in Algorithm 2, we firstly column normalize $F^{(t)}$, and then replace $G^{(t-1)}$ by $(G^{(t-1)}B)^T$, consequently update $G^{(t-1)}$, then normalize $G^{(t)}$ and so on. Thus we get the normalization version of NMF algorithm:

Consequently, we give a conclusion on normalization of NMF. This conclusion can help us understand the algorithm differences between PLSI and NMF more clearly.

Theorem 7. *For NMF, at the $t-th$ iteration, given the triple factors $C^{(t-1)}$, diagonal matrix $S^{(t-1)}$ and $H^{(t-1)}$, which satisfy $\sum_i C_{ik}^{(t-1)} = 1, \sum_k S_{kk}^{(t-1)} = 1$ and $\sum_j H_{jk}^{(t-1)} = 1$, as initializations such that $F^{(t-1)} = C^{(t-1)}S^{(t-1)}$ and $G^{(t-1)} = H^{(t-1)}$ or $F^{(t-1)} = C^{(t-1)}$ and $G^{(t-1)} = H^{(t-1)}S^{(t-1)}$, the result $F^{(t)}$ can be equivalently formulated as*

$$C_{ik}^{(t)} := C_{ik}^{(t-1)} \frac{(\frac{X.}{C^{(t-1)}S^{(t-1)}H^{(t-1)T}} H^{(t-1)})_{ik}}{(C^{(t-1)T}\frac{X.}{C^{(t-1)}S^{(t-1)}H^{(t-1)T}} H^{(t-1)})_{kk}}, \tag{11}$$

$$S_{kk}^{(t)} := S_{kk}^{(t-1)}(C^{(t-1)T}\frac{X.}{C^{(t-1)}S^{(t-1)}H^{(t-1)T}} H^{(t-1)})_{kk} \tag{12}$$

such that

$$F^{(t)} = C^{(t)}S^{(t)}. \tag{13}$$

The proof is omitted due to space limitation.

From above theorem, we can see that $C^{(t)}$ is column normalization of $F^{(t)}$, and the update rule of C is given. In corollary 1, we give an interesting property of $S^{(t)}$.

Corollary 1. *For NMF, at the $t-th$ iteration, $\sum\limits_i C_{ik}^{(t)} = 1$ and $\sum\limits_k S_{kk}^{(t)} = 1$.*

For G in NMF, we have similar result.

Corollary 2. *For NMF, at the $t-th$ iteration, given the triple factors $C^{(t-1)}$, diagonal matrix $S^{(t-1)}$ and $H^{(t-1)}$, which satisfy $\sum_i C_{ik}^{(t-1)} = 1, \sum_k S_{kk}^{(t-1)} = 1$ and $\sum_j H_{jk}^{(t-1)} = 1$, as initializations such that $F^{(t-1)} = C^{(t-1)}S^{(t-1)}$ and $G^{(t-1)} = H^{(t-1)}$ or $F^{(t-1)} = C^{(t-1)}$ and $G^{(t-1)} = H^{(t-1)}S^{(t-1)}$, the result $G^{(t)}$ can be equivalently formulated as*

$$H_{jk}^{(t)} := H_{jk}^{(t-1)} \frac{\left(\left(\frac{X.}{C^{(t-1)}S^{(t-1)}H^{(t-1)T}}\right)^T C^{(t-1)}\right)_{jk}}{\left(C^{(t-1)T}\frac{X.}{C^{(t-1)}S^{(t-1)}H^{(t-1)T}}H^{(t-1)}\right)_{kk}},$$

$$S_{kk}^{(t)} := S_{kk}^{(t-1)}\left(C^{(t-1)T}\frac{X.}{C^{(t-1)}S^{(t-1)}H^{(t-1)^T}}H^{(t-1)}\right)_{kk}$$

such that $G^{(t)} = H^{(t)}S^{(t)}$.

Based on the above discussions, we can revise Algorithm 2 to Algorithm 7.

Algorithm 7. Nonnegative Matrix Factorization*

Input: $C^{(0)}, S^{(0)}, H^{(0)}, t = 1$.
Output: C, S, H.
1: **while** 1 **do**
2: Update $C_{ik}^{(t)} := C_{ik}^{(t-1)} \frac{\left(\frac{X.}{C^{(t-1)}S^{(t-1)}H^{(t-1)T}}H^{(t-1)}\right)_{ik}}{\left(C^{(t-1)T}\frac{X.}{C^{(t-1)}S^{(t-1)}H^{(t-1)T}}H^{(t-1)}\right)_{kk}}$;
3: Update $S_{kk}^{(t)} := S_{kk}^{(t-1)}\left(C^{(t-1)T}\frac{X.}{C^{(t-1)}S^{(t-1)}H^{(t-1)^T}}H^{(t-1)}\right)_{kk}$;
4: Update $H_{jk}^{(t)} := H_{jk}^{(t-1)} \frac{\left(\left(\frac{X.}{C^{(t)}S^{(t)}H^{(t-1)T}}\right)^T C^{(t)}\right)_{jk}}{\left(C^{(t)T}\frac{X.}{C^{(t)}S^{(t)}H^{(t-1)T}}H^{(t-1)}\right)_{kk}}$;
5: Update $S_{kk}^{(t)} := S_{kk}^{(t)}\left(C^{(t)T}\frac{X.}{C^{(t)}S^{(t)}H^{(t-1)^T}}H^{(t-1)}\right)_{kk}$;
6: Test for convergence.
7: **if** Some convergence condition is satisfied **then**
8: $C = C^{(t)}$;
9: $S = S^{(t)}$;
10: $H = H^{(t)}$;
11: **Break**
12: **end if**
13: $t = t + 1$;
14: **end while**

Note that the normalization version of NMF will converge to a different local optimum from the standard NMF. But the revised version has a close relation with the standard one: any local optimum of Algorithm 7 is also a solution of Algorithm 2, and vice versa.

Theorem 8. *Any local optimum of Algorithm 7 is a solution of Algorithm 2.*

Proof. This is obviously true by joining line 2 and line 3, line 4 and line 5 in Algorithm 7.

After studying normalization of NMF carefully, we can now have a better insight into the algorithm differences between PLSI and NMF.

The following conclusions give the relations of C (in PLSI) and F (in NMF), H (in PLSI) and G (in NMF).

Theorem 9. *For PLSI and NMF, at the $t-th$ iteration, given the triple factors $C^{(t-1)}, S^{(t-1)}$ and $H^{(t-1)}$ as initializations of PLSI and $F^{(t-1)}, G^{(t-1)}$ as initializations of NMF such that $C^{(t-1)}S^{(t-1)} = F^{(t-1)}$ and $H^{(t-1)} = G^{(t-1)}$ or $C^{(t-1)} = F^{(t-1)}$ and $H^{(t-1)}S^{(t-1)} = G^{(t-1)}$ (i.e., $C^{(t-1)}S^{(t-1)}H^{(t-1)T} = F^{(t-1)}G^{(t-1)T}$), the update rules of C and F have the following relations: except for additional normalization, the update rule of C is identical with that of F in NMF, i.e., $C^{(t)} = F^{(t)}D_F^{-1}$, where D_F is diagonal matrix and the diagonal element $(D_F)_{kk} = \sum\limits_i F_{ik}^{(t)}$.*

Proof. The result is obviously true from (10), (11) , (12) and (13).

Corollary 3. *For PLSI and NMF, at the $t-th$ iteration, given the triple factors $C^{(t-1)}, S^{(t-1)}$ and $H^{(t-1)}$ as initializations of PLSI and $F^{(t-1)}, G^{(t-1)}$ as initializations of NMF such that $C^{(t-1)}S^{(t-1)} = F^{(t-1)}$ and $H^{(t-1)} = G^{(t-1)}$ or $C^{(t-1)} = F^{(t-1)}$ and $H^{(t-1)}S^{(t-1)} = G^{(t-1)}$ (i.e., $C^{(t-1)}S^{(t-1)}H^{(t-1)T} = F^{(t-1)}G^{(t-1)T}$), the update rules of H and G have the following relations: except for additional normalization, the update rule of H is identical with that of G in NMF, i.e., $H^{(t)} = G^{(t)}D_G^{-1}$, where D_G is diagonal matrix and the diagonal element $(D_F)_{kk} = \sum\limits_j G_{jk}^{(t)}$.*

Hence, NMF with normalization at each iteration has close relationship with PLSI. But this does not mean that PLSI can be replaced by NMF by normalizing F and G at each step, which can be observed from Algorithm 6 and Algorithm 7.

The key reason is that PLSI imposes normalization conditions on the factors explicitly. In [18] it has been shown that PLSI and NMF optimize the same objective function, hence PLSI can be seen as NMF-based model with additional normalization constraints ($\sum_i C_{ik} = 1, \sum_j H_{jk} = 1, \sum_k S_{kk} = 1$). The derivation process of PLSI update rules of C and H can be separated into two steps. Take the update rule of C while fixing S and H for example: firstly one gets the un-normalized C by gradient descent (identical with NMF), and then normalizes C to satisfy the constraint $\sum_i C_{ik} = 1$. The update rule of H is got in a similar way. The update rule of S can be got even more simply, just by gradient descent, and the normalization constraints will be satisfied automatically. In detail, at the $t-$th iteration, firstly, the derivative of the cost function $J(X, CSH^T)$ with respect to S while fixing C and H is:

$$\frac{\partial}{\partial S_{kk}} J = -\sum_{ij} \frac{X_{ij} C_{ia} H_{ja}}{\sum_k S_{kk} C_{ik} H_{jk}} + \sum_{ij} C_{ia} H_{ja}$$
$$= -\sum_{ij} \frac{X_{ij} C_{ia} H_{ja}}{\sum_k S_{kk} C_{ik} H_{jk}} + 1.$$

Let the step size $\eta_{kk} = S_{kk}$, then the update rule of S is:

$$S_{kk} = S_{kk} + \eta_{kk} (\sum_{ij} \frac{X_{ij} C_{ia} H_{ja}}{\sum_k S_{kk} C_{ik} H_{jk}} - 1)$$
$$= S_{kk} (C^T \frac{X}{CSH^T} H)_{kk}.$$

Theorem 6 has shown that any local optimal solution of PLSI is also a solution of NMF with K-L divergence, and vice versa, and Theorem 8 has shown similar results between normalized NMF and standard NMF. These results mean that given the same initializations, PLSI, NMF and normalized NMF will give equivalent solutions. Furthermore, we observe that their solution values are always identical:

$$CSH^{T7} = FG^{T8} = F^* G^{*T9}. \tag{14}$$

Indeed, this phenomenon is very common in NMF. Roughly speaking, the standard NMF algorithm can be expressed like this: `update` F, then `update` G and so on. Now we revise it to: $\underbrace{\texttt{update } F, \texttt{update } F, \cdots, \texttt{update } F}_{\texttt{m times}}$, then $\underbrace{\texttt{update } G, \texttt{update } G, \cdots, \texttt{update } G}_{\texttt{n times}}$, and so on. Choosing different m and n, we can get infinitely many solutions even if given the same initializations. But these solutions are all having the same solution values.

Note that since PLSI has to update S at each iteration, it needs more running time than NMF.

6 Conclusions and Future Works

This chapter presents an overview of the major directions for research on Nonnegative Matrix Factorization, including the models, objective functions and algorithms, and the applications, as well as its relations with other models. We highlights the following conclusions: 1) Compared with Principal Component Analysis, NMF is more interpretable due to its nonnegative constraints; 2) NMF is very flexible. There are several choices of objective functions and algorithms to accommodate a variety of applications; 3) NMF has linked K-means and PLSI,

[7] Results by PLSI.
[8] Results by NMF.
[9] Results by normalized NMF.

the two state-of-the-art unsupervised learning models, under the same framework; 4) NMF has a wide variety of applications and often has better numerical performance when compared with the other models/algorithms.

Finally, we list several open problems that are related to this chapter:

- there is still lack of systematic comparisons of the concordances and differences among the sparse variants of NMF. Note that generally speaking, the penalty that uses 1-norm should give more sparse results when compared with 2-norm since 2-norm often gives values that are very small rather than zeros, but 2-norm penalty is easier to calculate ([64,5]);
- what are the relationships among the objective divergence functions, the algorithms and the applications? There is still lack of systematic analysis;
- why (14) holds? In other words, since they converge to different local solutions, why the solution values are always identical?
- how to tackle very large scale dataset in real applications? Distributed NMF([65]) seems an interesting direction.

Acknowledgement. The author is very appreciated the valuable comments of Dr. Jie Tang (Department of Computer Science and Technology, Tsinghua University, P.R.China) and Dr. Yong Wang (Academy of Mathematics and Systems Science, Chinese Academy of Sciences, P.R.China). This work is supported by the Foundation of Academic Discipline Program at Central University of Finance and Economics, P.R.China.

Appendix

Proof of Theorem 1:

First of all, rewrite $F = (F_{:,1}, F_{:,2}, \cdots, F_{:,r}), G = (G_{:,1}, G_{:,2}, \cdots, G_{:,r})$. Let

$$\begin{aligned} D_F &= diag(\max(F_{:,1}), \max(F_{:,2}), \cdots, \max(F_{:,r})), \\ D_G &= diag(\max(G_{:,1}), \max(G_{:,2}), \cdots, \max(G_{:,r})), \end{aligned}$$

where $\max(\bullet)$ is the largest element of column $\bullet$.

Note

$$D_F = D_F^{1/2} D_F^{1/2}, \qquad D_G = D_G^{1/2} D_G^{1/2}.$$

$$D_F^{-1} = D_F^{-1/2} D_F^{-1/2}, \qquad D_G^{-1} = D_G^{-1/2} D_G^{-1/2}.$$

We obtain

$$\begin{aligned} X = FG^T &= (FD_F^{-1})(D_F D_G)(GD_G^{-1})^T \\ &= (FD_F^{-1/2} D_G^{1/2})(GD_G^{-1/2} D_F^{1/2})^T. \end{aligned}$$

Construct D as $D = D_G^{-1/2} D_F^{1/2}$, then

$$F^* = F D_F^{-1/2} D_G^{1/2}, \qquad G^* = G D_G^{-1/2} D_F^{1/2}.$$

Thus (4) is proved.

Furthermore,

$$\begin{aligned}(F D_F^{-1/2} D_G^{1/2})_{ij} &= F_{ij} \cdot \sqrt{\frac{\max(G_{:,j})}{\max(F_{:,j})}} \\ &= \frac{F_{ij}}{\max(F_{:,j})} \cdot \sqrt{\max(F_{:,j}) \max(G_{:,j})}.\end{aligned}$$

Without loss of generality, assuming that

$$\max(F_{:,j}) = F_{tj}, \qquad \max(G_{:,j}) = G_{lj},$$

then we have

$$\begin{aligned}\max(F_{:,j}) \cdot \max(G_{:,j}) &\le F_{t1} G_{1l}^T + \cdots F_{tj} G_{jl}^T + \cdots + F_{tr} G_{rl}^T \\ &= \sum_k F_{tk} G_{kl}^T = X_{tl} \le M.\end{aligned}$$

So $0 \le F_{ij}^* \le \sqrt{M}$ and $0 \le G_{ij}^* \le \sqrt{M}$.
If X is symmetric and $F = G^T$,

$$G_{ij}^* = G_{ij} \cdot \sqrt{\frac{\max(G_{:,i})}{\max(G_{:,i})}} = G_{ij},$$

which implies $G^* = G$. □

Proof of Theorem 4:

Firstly, J_K can be rewritten as:

$$\begin{aligned}J_K &= \sum_{k=1}^{K} \sum_{i \in C_k} \|x_i - m_k\|^2 \\ &= c_2 - \sum_{k=1}^{K} \frac{1}{n_k} \sum_{i,j \in C_k} x_i^T x_j,\end{aligned}$$

where $c_2 = \sum_i \|x_i\|^2$. The clustering result can be represented by K nonnegative indicator vectors:

$$H = (h_1, h_2, \cdots, h_K), \quad h_k^T h_l = \delta_{kl} = \begin{cases} 1 & k = l \\ 0 & k \ne l \end{cases}$$

where $h_k = (0, \cdots, 0, \underbrace{1, \cdots, 1}_{n_k}, 0, \cdots, 0)^T / n_k^{1/2}$.

Now J_K becomes: $J_K = Tr(X^TX) - Tr(H^TX^TXH)$, where $Tr(\bullet)$ is the trace of matrix $\bullet$. Thus $\min J_K$ becomes

$$\max_{H^TH=I, H\geqslant 0} Tr(H^TWH), \tag{15}$$

where $W = X^TX$.

But $-2Tr(H^TWH) = \|W\|^2 - 2Tr(H^TWH) + \|H^TH\|^2 = \|W - H^TH\|^2$, hence,

$$\begin{aligned} H &= \arg \min_{H^TH=I, H\geqslant 0} -2Tr(H^TWH) \\ &= \arg \min_{H^TH=I, H\geqslant 0} \|W - H^TH\|^2. \end{aligned}$$

Relaxing the orthogonal constraint $H^TH = I$ completes the proof. □

Proof of Lemma 1:

At convergence, one has:

$$G_{jk} = \frac{G_{jk}}{\sum_i F_{ik}} \sum_i \frac{X_{ij}F_{ik}}{(FG^T)_{ij}}.$$

Hence

$$\begin{aligned} \sum_{i'} (FG^T)_{i'j} &= \sum_{i',k} F_{i'k}G_{jk} \\ &= \sum_{i',k} F_{i'k} \frac{G_{jk}}{\sum_i F_{ik}} \sum_i \frac{X_{ij}F_{ik}}{(FG^T)_{ij}} \\ &= \sum_k G_{jk} \sum_i \frac{X_{ij}F_{ik}}{(FG^T)_{ij}} \\ &= \sum_{i=1}^m X_{ij}. \end{aligned}$$

The other equality can be proven similarly. □

Proof of Theorem 5:

Firstly, we note that maximizing (7) can be rewritten as:

$$\min -\sum_{i=1}^m \sum_{j=1}^n X_{ij} \log P(w_i, d_j),$$

which is equivalent to

$$\min \sum_{i=1}^m \sum_{j=1}^n -X_{ij} \log P(w_i, d_j) + \sum_{i=1}^m \sum_{j=1}^n (X_{ij} \log X_{ij} - X_{ij} + (FG^T)_{ij}),$$

or

$$\min \sum_{i=1}^{m} \sum_{j=1}^{n} (X_{ij} \log \frac{X_{ij}}{P(w_i, d_j)} - X_{ij} + (FG^T)_{ij}),$$

since $\sum_{i=1}^{m} \sum_{j=1}^{n} X_{ij} \log X_{ij}$ is a constant and $\sum\limits_{i=1}^{m} \sum\limits_{j=1}^{n} (-X_{ij} + (FG^T)_{ij})$ cancels out at convergence by Lemma 1. Hence, by Theorem 6, PLSI and NMF optimize the same objective function. □

An Example to Illustrate the Limitations of NMF for Discovering Bi-clustering Structures

In fact, several papers [14,15] have discussed about the bi-clustering aspect of NMF. But the key difficulty is that one can not identify the binary relationship of genes and samples exactly since the resulting matrices F and G are not binary. Here we give an example to illustrate the limitations of NMF for discovering bi-clustering structures. Given the original data matrix

$$X = \begin{pmatrix} 0.8 & 0.8 & 0.8 & 0.64 & 0.64 & 0.64 \\ 0.76 & 0.76 & 0.76 & 0.68 & 0.68 & 1.68 \\ 0.64 & 0.64 & 0.64 & 0.80 & 0.80 & 0.80 \\ 0.68 & 0.68 & 0.68 & 0.76 & 0.76 & 0.76 \\ 0.64 & 0.64 & 0.64 & 0.80 & 0.80 & 0.80 \end{pmatrix}.$$

Each row of X is a feature and each column of X is a sample.

We get the factor matrices F and G as follows:

$$F = \begin{pmatrix} 0.80 & 0.40 \\ 0.70 & 0.50 \\ 0.40 & 0.80 \\ 0.50 & 0.70 \\ 0.40 & 0.80 \end{pmatrix}; \ G^T = \begin{pmatrix} 0.8 & 0.8 & 0.8 & 0.4 & 0.4 & 0.4 \\ 0.4 & 0.4 & 0.4 & 0.8 & 0.8 & 0.8 \end{pmatrix}.$$

One can easily observe the clustering structures of the columns from G, but when identifying the bi-clustering structures, he(or she) has difficulties to identify an appropriate threshold to select which features should be involved in bi-clustering structures. From this small example we can see that standard NMF has limitations to discover bi-clustering structures explicitly.

References

1. Lee, D.D., Seung, H.S.: Learning the parts of objects by non-negative matrix factorization. Nature 401(6755), 788–791 (1999)
2. Lee, D.D., Seung, H.S.: Algorithms for non-negative matrix factorization. In: Annual Conference on Neural Information Processing Systems, pp. 556–562 (2000)
3. Paatero, P., Tapper, U.: Positive matrix factorization: A non-negative factor model with optimal utilization of error estimates of data values. Environmetrics 5(2), 111–126 (1994)
4. Jolliffe, I.T.: Principal Component Analysis, 2nd edn. Springer, Heidelberg (2002)
5. Hastie, T., Tibshirani, R., Friedman, J.: The Elements of Statistical Learning: Data Mining, Inference, and Prediction, 2nd edn., corr. 3rd printing edn. Springer Series in Statistics. Springer, Heidelberg (2009)
6. Tropp, J.A.: Literature survey: Non-negative matrix factorization. University of Texas at Austin, Austin, TX (2003) (unpublished document)
7. Xie, Y.L., Hopke, P., Paatero, P.: Positive matrix factorization applied to a curve resolution problem. Journal of Chemometrics 12(6), 357–364 (1999)
8. Li, S.Z., Hou, X.W., Zhang, H.J., Cheng, Q.S.: Learning spatially localized, parts-based representation. In: Proceedings of the 2001 IEEE Computer Society Conference on Computer Vision and Pattern Recognition, vol. 1, pp. I-207– I-212 (2001)
9. Cooper, M., Foote, J.: Summarizing video using non-negative similarity matrix factorization. In: IEEE Workshop on Multimedia Signal Processing, pp. 25–28 (2002)
10. Pauca, V.P., Shahnaz, F., Berry, M.W., Plemmons, R.J.: Text mining using non-negative matrix factorizations. In: Proceedings of the Fourth SIAM International Conference on Data Mining (2004)
11. Shahnaz, F., Berry, M.W., Pauca, P.R.J.: Document clustering using nonnegative matrix factorization. Information Processing & Management 42(2), 373–386 (2006)
12. Xu, W., Liu, X., Gong, Y.: Document clustering based on non-negative matrix factorization. In: SIGIR 2003: Proceedings of the 26th Annual International ACM SIGIR Conference on Research and Development in Informaion Retrieval, pp. 267–273. ACM Press, New York (2003)
13. Nielsen, F.A., Balslev, D., Hansen, L.K.: Mining the posterior cingulate: Segregation between memory and pain components. NeuroImage 27(3), 520–532 (2005)
14. Brunet, J.P., Tamayo, P., Golub, T.R., Mesirov, J.P.: Metagenes and molecular pattern discovery using matrix factorization. Proc. Natl. Acad. Sci. USA 101(12), 4164–4169 (2004)
15. Pascual-Montano, A., Carazo, J.M., Kochi, K., Lehmann, D., Pascual-Marqui, R.D.: Nonsmooth nonnegative matrix factorization (nsNMF). IEEE transactions on Pattern Analysis and Machine Intelligence 28(3), 403–415 (2006)
16. Devarajan, K.: Nonnegative matrix factorization: An analytical and interpretive tool in computational biology. PLoS Comput. 4(7), e1000029 (2008)
17. Ding, C., He, X., Simon, H.D.: On the equivalence of nonnegative matrix factorization and spectral clustering. In: SIAM Data Mining Conf. (2005)
18. Ding, C., Li, T., Peng, W.: On the equivalence between non-negative matrix factorization and probabilistic latent semantic indexing. Comput. Stat. Data Anal. 52(8), 3913–3927 (2008)
19. Gaussier, E., Goutte, C.: Relation between PLSA and NMF and implications. In: SIGIR 2005: Proceedings of the 28th Annual International ACM SIGIR Conference on Research and Development in Information Retrieval, pp. 601–602. ACM, New York (2005)

20. Zhang, Z.Y., Li, T., Ding, C., Zhang, X.S.: Binary matrix factorization with applications. In: IEEE International Conference on Data Mining, pp. 391–400 (2007)
21. Zhang, Z.Y., Li, T., Ding, C., Ren, X.W., Zhang, X.S.: Binary matrix factorization for analyzing gene expression data. Data Min. Knowl. Discov. 20(1), 28–52 (2010)
22. Ding, C.H.Q., Li, T., Jordan, M.I.: Convex and semi-nonnegative matrix factorizations. IEEE Trans. Pattern Anal. Mach. Intell. 32(1), 45–55 (2010)
23. Ding, C., Li, T., Peng, W., Park, H.: Orthogonal nonnegative matrix tfactorizations for clustering. In: KDD 2006: Proceedings of the 12th ACM SIGKDD International Conference on Knowledge Discovery and Data mining, pp. 126–135. ACM, New York (2006)
24. Li, T., Ding, C.: The relationships among various nonnegative matrix factorization methods for clustering. In: ICDM 2006: Proceedings of the Sixth International Conference on Data Mining, pp. 362–371. IEEE Computer Society, Washington, DC, USA (2006)
25. Li, S.Z., Hou, X.W., Zhang, H.J., Cheng, Q.S.: Learning spatially localized, parts-based representation. In: Proceedings of the 2001 IEEE Computer Society Conference on Computer Vision and Pattern Recognition, CVPR 2001, vol. 1 (2001)
26. Feng, T., Li, S., Shum, H.Y., Zhang, H.: Local non-negative matrix factorization as a visual representation. In: International Conference on Development and Learning (2002)
27. Hoyer, P.O.: Non-negative matrix factorization with sparseness constraints. Journal of Machine Learning Research 5, 1457–1469 (2004)
28. Hoyer, P.O.: Non-negative sparse coding. In: Proceedings of the, 12th IEEE Workshop on Neural Networks for Signal Processing, pp. 557–565 (2002)
29. Liu, W., Zheng, N., Lu, X.: Non-negative matrix factorization for visual coding. In: Proc. IEEE Int. Conf. on Acoustics, Speech and Signal Processing, ICASSP 2003 (2003)
30. Gao, Y., Church, G.: Improving molecular cancer class discovery through sparse non-negative matrix factorization. Bioinformatics 21(21), 3970–3975 (2005)
31. Pauca, V.P., Piper, J., Plemmons, R.J.: Nonnegative matrix factorization for spectral data analysis. Linear Algebra and its Applications 416(1), 29–47 (2006)
32. Hoyer, P.O.: Non-negative matrix factorization with sparseness constraints. J. Mach. Learn. Res. 5, 1457–1469 (2004)
33. Kim, H., Park, H.: Sparse non-negative matrix factorizations via alternating nonnegativity- constrained least squares for microarray data analysis. Bioinformatics 23(12), 1495–1502 (2007)
34. Mahoney, M.W., Drineas, P.: CUR matrix decompositions for improved data analysis. Proc. Natl. Acad. Sci. USA 106(3), 697–702 (2009)
35. Cichocki, A., Zdunek, R., Amari, S.: Csiszár's divergences for non-negative matrix factorization: Family of new algorithms. In: Proc. Int'l Conf. Independent Component Analysis and Blind Signal Separation, pp. 32–39 (2006)
36. Cichocki, A., Lee, H., Kim, Y.D., Choi, S.: Non-negative matrix factorization with -divergence. Pattern Recogn. Lett. 29(9), 1433–1440 (2008)
37. Cichocki, A., Amari, S.-i., Zdunek, R., Kompass, R., Hori, G., He, Z.: Extended SMART Algorithms for Non-negative Matrix Factorization. In: Rutkowski, L., Tadeusiewicz, R., Zadeh, L.A., Żurada, J.M. (eds.) ICAISC 2006. LNCS (LNAI), vol. 4029, pp. 548–562. Springer, Heidelberg (2006)
38. Liu, W., Yuan, K., Ye, D.: On alpha-divergence based nonnegative matrix factorization for clustering cancer gene expression data. Artif. Intell. Med. 44(1), 1–5 (2008)

39. Cichocki, A., Zdunek, R., Choi, S., Plemmons, R., Amari, S.: Nonnegative tensor factorization using alpha and beta divergencies. In: Proc. IEEE International Conference on Acoustics, Speech, and Signal Processing (ICASSP 2007), pp. 1393–1396 (2007)
40. Dhillon, I.S., Sra, S.: Generalized nonnegative matrix approximations with bregman divergences. In: Proc. Advances in Neural Information Proc. Systems (NIPS), pp. 283–290 (2005)
41. Kompass, R.: A generalized divergence measure for nonnegative matrix factorization. Neural Comput. 19(3), 780–791 (2007)
42. Cichocki, A., Zdunek, R., Phan, A.H., Amari, S.-i.: Nonnegative Matrix and Tensor Factorizations: Applications to Exploratory Multi-way Data Analysis and Blind Source Separation. A John Wiley and Sons, Ltd, Publication, Chichester (2009)
43. Févotte, C., Bertin, N., Durrieu, J.L.: Nonnegative matrix factorization with the itakura-saito divergence: With application to music analysis. Neural Comput. 21(3), 793–830 (2009)
44. Gonzalez, E.F., Zhang, Y.: Accelerating the lee-seung algorithm for nonnegative matrix factorization. Technical Report (2005)
45. Lin, C.J.: Projected gradient methods for nonnegative matrix factorization. Neural Comput. 19(10), 2756–2779 (2007)
46. Kim, D., Sra, S., Dhillon, I.S.: Fast newton-type methods for the least squares nonnegative matrix approximation problem. In: Proceedings of SIAM Conference on Data Mining, pp. 343–354 (2007)
47. Zdunek, R., Cichocki, A.: Non-negative Matrix Factorization with Quasi-Newton Optimization. In: Rutkowski, L., Tadeusiewicz, R., Zadeh, L.A., Żurada, J.M. (eds.) ICAISC 2006. LNCS (LNAI), vol. 4029, pp. 870–879. Springer, Heidelberg (2006)
48. Kim, H., Park, H.: Nonnegative matrix factorization based on alternating nonnegativity constrained least squares and active set method. SIAM J. Matrix Anal. Appl. 30(2), 713–730 (2008)
49. Long, B., Wu, X., Zhang, Z., Yu, P.S.: Community learning by graph approximation. In: Proceedings of the 2007 Seventh IEEE International Conference on Data Mining, ICDM 2007, pp. 232–241 (2007)
50. Chen, Y., Rege, M., Dong, M., Hua, J.: Incorporating user provided constraints into document clustering. In: Proceedings of the 2007 Seventh IEEE International Conference on Data Mining, ICDM 2007, pp. 103–112 (2007)
51. Kulis, B., Basu, S., Dhillon, I., Mooney, R.: Semi-supervised graph clustering: a kernel approach. In: ICML 2005: Proceedings of the 22nd International Conference on Machine Learning, pp. 457–464. ACM, New York (2005)
52. Ji, X., Xu, W.: Document clustering with prior knowledge. In: SIGIR 2006: Proceedings of the 29th Annual International ACM SIGIR Conference on Research and Development in Information retrieval, pp. 405–412. ACM, New York (2006)
53. Cheng, Y., Church, G.M.: Biclustering of expression data. In: Proceedings of the Eighth International Conference on Intelligent Systems for Molecular Biology, pp. 93–103. AAAI Press, Menlo Park (2000)
54. Prelić, A., Bleuler, S., Zimmermann, P., Wille, A., Bühlmann, P., Gruissem, W., Hennig, L., Thiele, L., Zitzler, E.: A systematic comparison and evaluation of biclustering methods for gene expression data. Bioinformatics 22(9), 1122–1129 (2006)
55. Drakakis, K., Rickard, S., de Frein, R., Cichocki, A.: Analysis of financial data using non-negative matrix factorization. International Mathematical Forum 3(38), 1853–1870 (2008)

56. Ribeiro, B., Silva, C., Vieira, A., Neves, J.: Extracting Discriminative Features Using Non-negative Matrix Factorization in Financial Distress Data. In: Kolehmainen, M., Toivanen, P., Beliczynski, B. (eds.) ICANNGA 2009. LNCS, vol. 5495, pp. 537–547. Springer, Heidelberg (2009)
57. Zha, H., He, X., Ding, C., Simon, H.: Spectral relaxation for k-means clustering. In: Proc. Advances in Neural Information Proc. Systems (NIPS), pp. 1057–1064 (2001)
58. Ding, C., He, X.: K-means clustering via principal component analysis. In: Proceedings of the twenty-first international conference on Machine learning (ICML 2004), pp. 225–232 (2004)
59. Hofmann, T.: Probabilistic latent semantic indexing. In: SIGIR 1999: Proceedings of the 22nd Annual International ACM SIGIR Conference on Research and Development in Information Retrieval, pp. 50–57. ACM Press, New York (1999)
60. Deerwester, S.C., Dumais, S.T., Landauer, T.K., Furnas, G.W., Harshman, R.A.: Indexing by latent semantic analysis. Journal of the American Society of Information Science 41(6), 391–407 (1990)
61. Wu, X., Yan, J., Liu, N., Yan, S., Chen, Y., Chen, Z.: Probabilistic latent semantic user segmentation for behavioral targeted advertising. In: ADKDD 2009: Proceedings of the Third International Workshop on Data Mining and Audience Intelligence for Advertising, pp. 10–17. ACM, New York (2009)
62. Cohn, D., Hofmann, T.: The missing link - a probabilistic model of document content and hypertext connectivity. In: Proc. Advances in Neural Information Proc. Systems, NIPS (2001)
63. Ho, N.D., Dooren, P.V.: Non-negative matrix factorization with fixed row and column sums. Linear Algebra and its Applications 429, 1020–1025 (2008)
64. Tibshirani, R.: Regression shrinkage and selection via the lasso. Journal of the Royal Statistical Society, Series B 58, 267–288 (1996)
65. Liu, C., Yang, H.: c., Fan, J., He, L.W.,Wang, Y.M.: Distributed nonnegative matrix factorization for web-scale dyadic data analysis on mapreduce. In: Proceedings of the 19th International Conference on World wide web (WWW 2010), pp. 681–690 (2010)

Chapter 7
Visual Data Mining and Discovery with Binarized Vectors

Boris Kovalerchuk[1], Florian Delizy[1], Logan Riggs[1], and Evgenii Vityaev[2]

[1] Dept. of Computer Science, Central Washington University, Ellensburg, WA, 9896-7520, USA
[2] Institute of Mathematics, Russian Academy of Sciences, Novosibirsk, 630090, Russia

Abstract. The emerging field of Visual Analytics combines several fields where Data Mining and Visualization play leading roles. The fundamental departure of visual analytics from other approaches is in extensive use of visual analytical tools to discover patterns not only to visualize pattern that have been discovered by traditional data mining methods. High complexity data mining tasks often require employing a multi-level top-down approach, where first at the top levels a qualitative analysis of the complex situation is conducted and top-level patterns are discovered. This paper presents the concept of Monotone Boolean Function Visual Analytics (MBFVA) for such top level pattern discovery. This approach employs binarization and monotonization of quantitative attributes to get a top level data representation. The top level discoveries form a foundation for next more detailed data mining levels where patterns are refined. The approach is illustrated with application to the medical, law enforcement and security domains. The medical application is concerned with discovering breast cancer diagnostic rules (i) interactively with a radiologist, (ii) analytically with data mining algorithms, and (iii) visually. The coordinated visualization of these rules opens an opportunity to coordinate the multi-source rules, and to come up with rules that are meaningful for the expert in the field, and are confirmed with the database. Often experts and data mining algorithms operate at the very different and incomparable levels of detail and produce incomparable patterns. The proposed MBFVA approach allows solving this problem. This paper shows how to represent and visualize binary multivariate data in 2-D and 3-D. This representation preserves the structural relations that exist in multivariate data. It creates a new opportunity to guide the visual discovery of unknown patterns in the data. In particular, the structural representation allows us to convert a complex border between the patterns in multidimensional space into visual 2-D and 3-D forms. This decreases the information overload on the user. The visualization shows not only the border between classes, but also shows a location of the case of interest relative to the border between the patterns. A user does not need to see the thousands of previous cases that have been used to build a border between the patterns. If the abnormal case is deeply inside in the abnormal area, far away from the border between "normal" and "abnormal" classes, then this shows that

D.E. Holmes, L.C. Jain (Eds.): Data Mining: Found. & Intell. Paradigms, ISRL 24, pp. 135–156.
springerlink.com

this case is very abnormal and needs immediate attention. The paper concludes with the outline of the scaling of the algorithm for the large data sets and expanding the approach for non-monotone data.

Keywords: Data Mining, Visual discovery, Monotone chains, Multi-level Data Mining, Monotone Boolean Function, Visual Analytics.

1 Introduction

Visual data mining (VDM) assists a user in detecting interesting knowledge, and in gaining a deep visual understanding of the data in combination with advanced visualization [Beilken & Spenke, 1999; Keim et al., 2002; Schulz, et al, 2006; Badjio, Pouletm 2005; Zhao et al, 2005, Lim, 2009, 2010; Oliveira, Levkowitz, 2003, Pak, Bergeron, 1997; Wong et al, 1999,]. *Visualizing the border* between classes is one of the especially important aspects of visual data mining. The well-separated classes that are visually far away from each other with simple border between classes match our intuitive concept of the patterns. This simple separation serves as an important support for the idea that the data mining result is robust and not accidental. Moreover, for many situations, a user can easily catch a border visually, but its analytical form can be quite complex and difficult to discover. This visual simple border for a human may not be a simple mathematically.

VDM methods have shown benefits in many areas. However, available methods do not address the specifics of data, with little variability in the traditional visual representation of different objects such as parallel coordinates. VDM is an especially challenging task when data richness should be preserved without the excessive aggregation that often happens with simple and intuitive presentation graphics such as bar charts [Keim, Hao, et al., 2002]. Another challenge is that often such data lack the natural 3-D space and time dimensions [Groth, 1998] and instead require the visualization of an abstract feature.

We begin with an analysis of the currently available methods of data visualization. Glyphs can visualize *nine attributes* (three positions x, y, and z; three size dimensions; color; opacity; and shape). Texture can add more dimensions. Shapes of the glyphs are studied in [Shaw, et al., 1999], where it was concluded that with large super-ellipses, about 22 separate shapes can be distinguished on the average. An overview of multivariate glyphs is presented in [Ward, 2002].

In this paper, we show that the placement based on the use of the *data structure* is a promising approach to visualize a border between classes for multidimensional data. We call this the **GPDS** approach (**Glyph Placement on a Data Structure**). It is important to note that in this approach, some attributes are *implicitly* encoded in the data structure while others are *explicitly* encoded in the glyph or icon. Thus, if the structure carries ten attributes and a glyph/icon carries nine attributes, nineteen attributes are encoded. Below to illustrate the use of the data structure concept, we consider simple 2-D icons as *bars* of different colors. Adding texture, motion and other icon characteristics can increase dimensions of the data visualized.

Alternative techniques such as Generalized Spiral and Pixel Bar Chart are developed in [Keim, Hao, et al., 2002]. These techniques work with large data sets without overlapping, but only with a few attributes, (these range from a single attribute to perhaps four to six attributes).

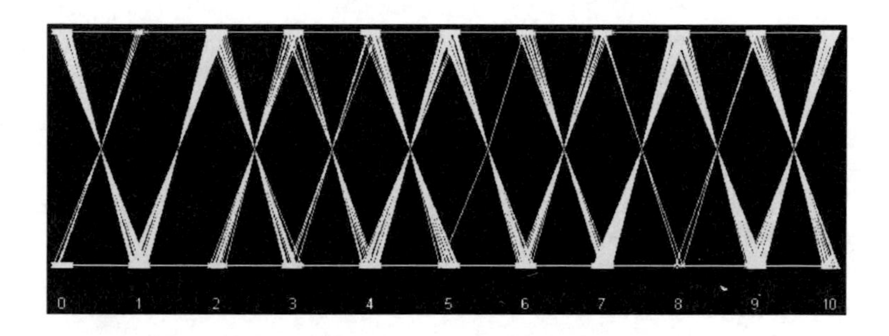

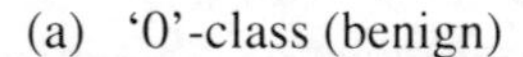
(a) '0'-class (benign)

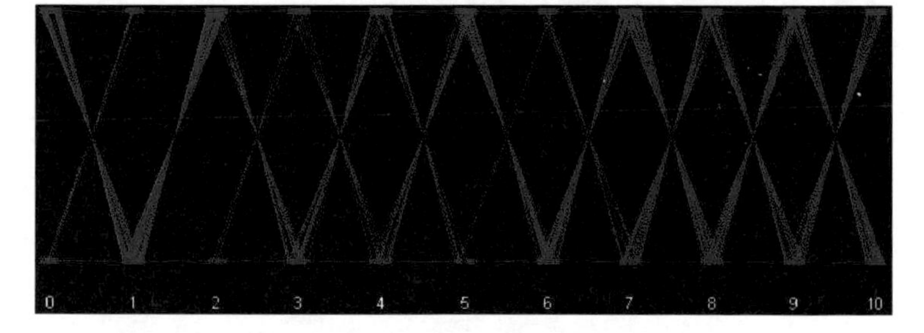

(b) '1'-class (malignant)

Fig. 1. Breast cancer data in parallel coordinates

The parallel coordinate visualization [Inselberg, Dimsdale, 1990] can show ten or more attributes in 2-D, but suffers from record overlap and thus is limited to tasks with well-distinguished cluster records. In parallel coordinates, each vertical axis corresponds to a data attribute (x_i) and a line connecting points on each parallel coordinate corresponds to a record. Figure 1 (a)-(c) depicts about a hundred breast cancer cases (each of them is an 11-dimensional Boolean vector in Boolean space E^{11}). Classes '0' and '1' look practically the same as Figures 1 (a) and (b) show. Thus, parallel coordinates were are not able to discover visually the pattern that would separate classes 0' and '1' (benign and malignant) in these dataset. In this paper, we will show that the proposed GPDS method is able to do this.

Parallel coordinates belong to a class of methods that explicitly visualize *every* attribute x_i of an n-dimensional vector $(x_1, x_2, \ldots, x_n)$ and place the vector using *all* attributes x_i but each attribute is placed on its own parallel coordinate *independently* of the placing other attributes of this vector and other vectors. This is one of the major reasons of occlusion and overlap of visualized data. The GPDS approach constructs a data structure and can place objects using *attribute relations*.

2 Method for Visualizing Data

Below **we** describe Monotone Boolean Function Visual Analytics (**MBFVA**) method and its implementation called **VDATMIN** that exploit Glyph Placement on a Data Structure in combination with Monotone Boolean Functions approach. As was discussed above many data mining problems can be encoded using Boolean vectors, where each record is a set of binary values {0; 1} and each record belongs to one of two classes (categories) that are also encoded as 0 and 1. For instance, a patient can be represented as a Boolean vector of symptoms along with an indication of the diagnostic class (e.g., benign or malignant tumor) [Kovalerchuk, Vityaev, Ruiz, 2001, Kovalerchuk et al, 1996]. For Boolean vectors, our VDM method relies on **monotone structural relations** between them in the n-dimensional binary cube, E^n based on the theory of monotone Boolean functions.

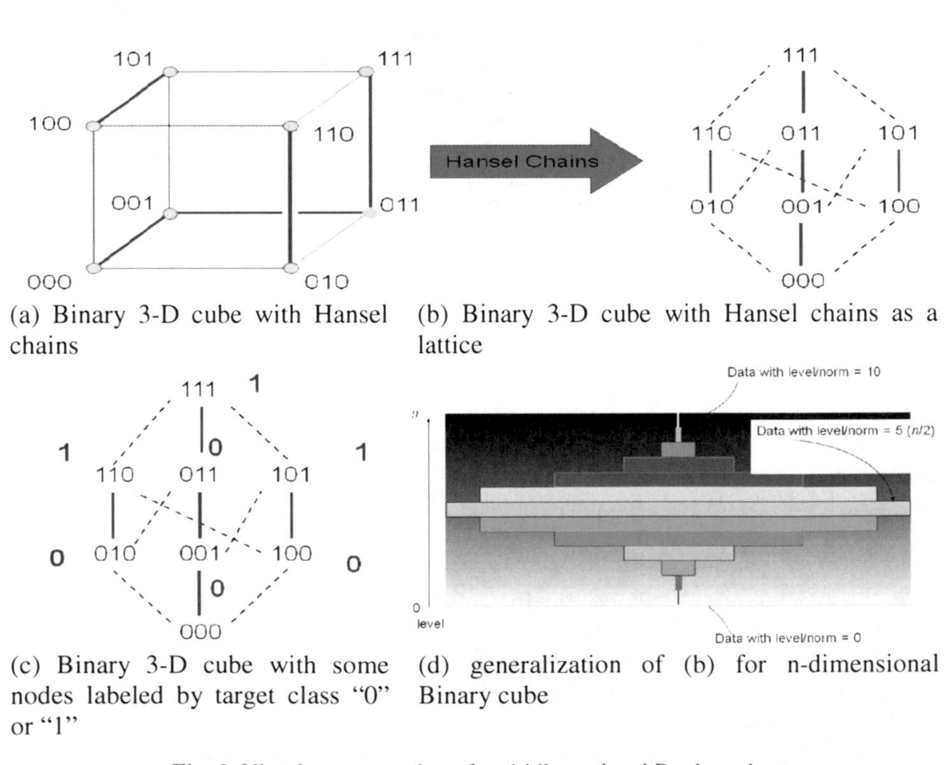

(a) Binary 3-D cube with Hansel chains

(b) Binary 3-D cube with Hansel chains as a lattice

(c) Binary 3-D cube with some nodes labeled by target class “0” or “1”

(d) generalization of (b) for n-dimensional Binary cube

Fig. 2. Visual representation of multidimensional Boolean data

Figure 2(a) illustrates the concept of monotonicity in 3-D Boolean cube, where red lines show three monotone chains (known as Hansel chains [Kovalerchuk et al, 1996; Hansel, 1966]):

chain 1: (000), (001), (011), (111),
chain 2: (100), (101),
chain 3: (011), (110).

In each Hansel chain, each next vector is greater than a preceding vector. In the next vector, exactly one attribute is greater than in the preceding vector. Together these Hansel chains cover the whole 3-D Boolean cube and none of vectors is repeated (chains do not overlap). There is a general recursive process [Kovalerchuk et al, 1996; Hansel, 1966] to construct Hansel chains for a Boolean cube, E^n of any dimension n without overlap of chains.

Figure 2 (b) shows the same Boolean cube as a lattice with Hansel chains drawn in parallel with the largest vector (111) on the top and the smallest vector (000) on the bottom. Figure 2(c) shows the same binary 3-D cube with some nodes labeled by target class "0" or "1". In this way, training and testing data can be shown. Figure 2(d) presents a generalization of the lattice visualization shown in Figure 29b) for n-dimensional Binary cube. This visualization is used for the user interface in the VDATMIN system.

The concept of the monotone Boolean function from discrete mathematics [Korshunov, 2003, Keller, Pilpel, 2009] is defined below. Let $E^n=\{0,1\}^n$ be a binary *n*- dimensional cube then vector $\mathbf{y}=(y_1,y_2,\ldots,y_n)$ is no greater than vector $\mathbf{x}=(x_1,x_2,\ldots,x_n)$ from E^n if for every i $x_i \geq y_i$, i.e.,

$$\mathbf{x} \geq \mathbf{y} \Leftrightarrow \forall i \; x_i \geq y_i$$

In other words, vectors **x** and **y** are ordered. In general relation ≥ for Boolean vectors in E^n is a *partial order* that makes E^n a *lattice* with a max element (1,1,…,1) and min element (0,0,…,0).

Boolean function f: $E^n \rightarrow E$ is called a *monotone Boolean function* if

$$\forall \; \mathbf{x} \geq \mathbf{y} \Rightarrow f(\mathbf{x}) \geq f(\mathbf{y}).$$

Figure 3 demonstrates the user interface of visual data mining system VDATMIN. Figure 3(a) shows all 2^{12}=4096 nodes of n-dimensional binary cube E^n for n=12. Each node (12-dimemtional Boolean vector) is represented as a blue bar. The bar that represents the vector **x** containing all zeros is located in the lowest layer in the middle of the picture. The bar representing the vector **x** that contains all "1" ($|x|=12$) is located at the top of the picture in the middle. All other bars are located in between.

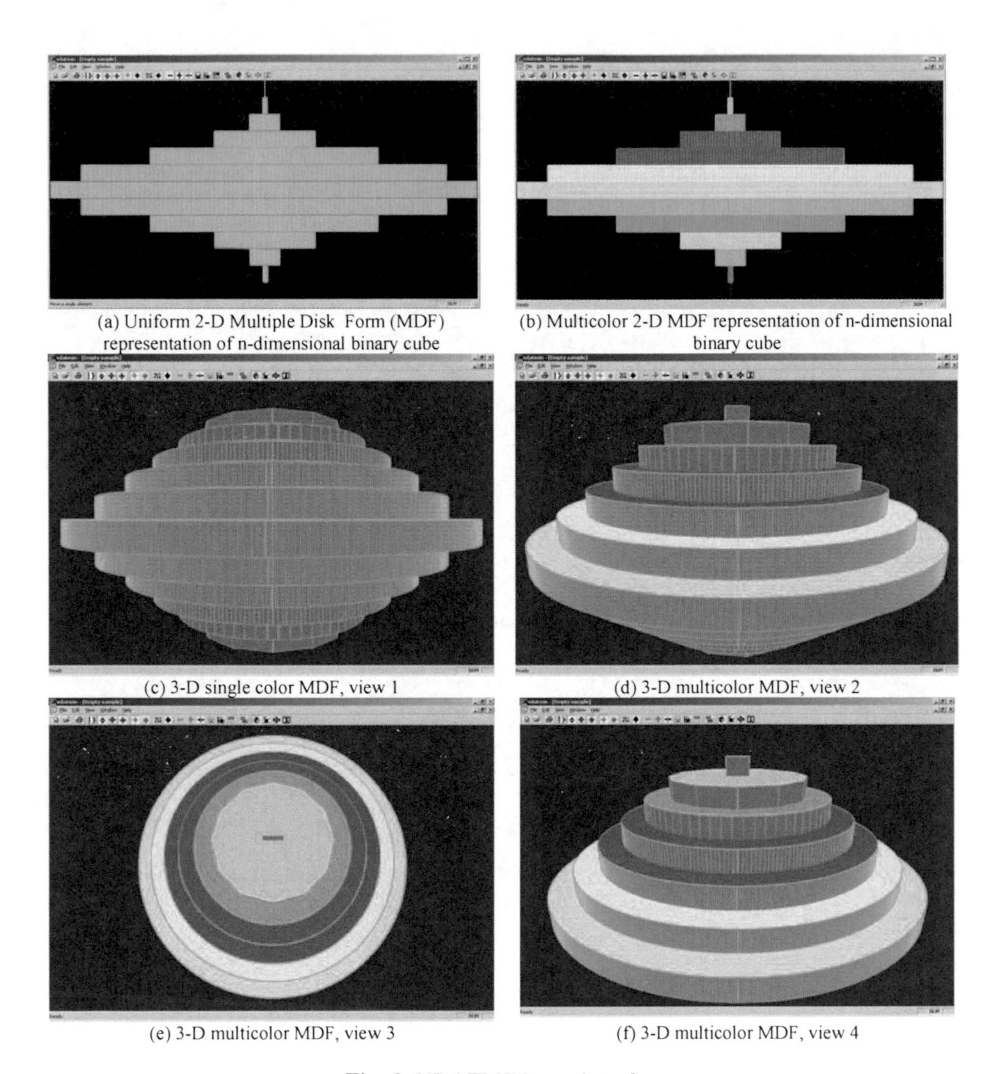

(a) Uniform 2-D Multiple Disk Form (MDF) representation of n-dimensional binary cube

(b) Multicolor 2-D MDF representation of n-dimensional binary cube

(c) 3-D single color MDF, view 1

(d) 3-D multicolor MDF, view 2

(e) 3-D multicolor MDF, view 3

(f) 3-D multicolor MDF, view 4

Fig. 3. VDATMIN user interface

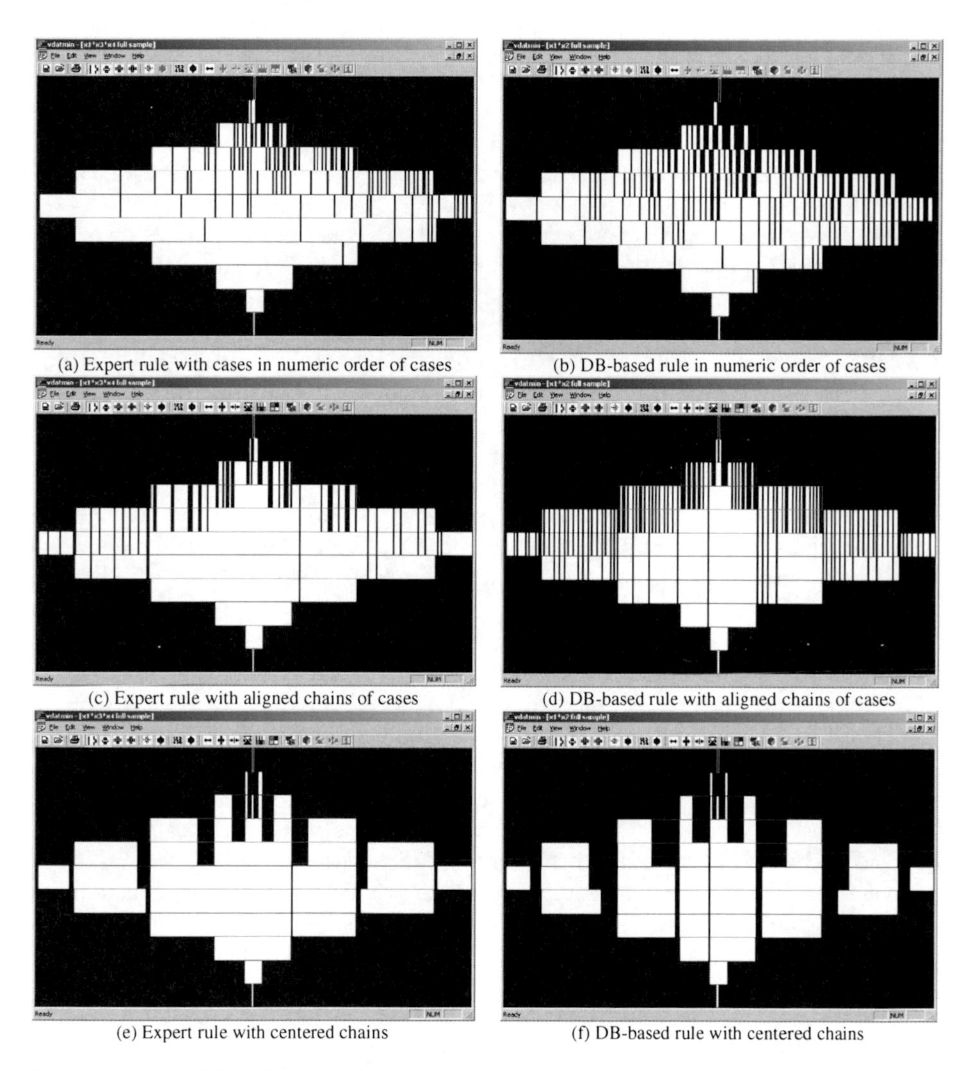

(a) Expert rule with cases in numeric order of cases

(b) DB-based rule in numeric order of cases

(c) Expert rule with aligned chains of cases

(d) DB-based rule with aligned chains of cases

(e) Expert rule with centered chains

(f) DB-based rule with centered chains

Fig. 4. (a),(c),(e) Visualization of the expert cancer rule in 10-D feature space, (b), (d),(f) visualization of the closest cancer rule extracted from the data base 10-D feature space

The bar layer next from the bottom contains all 12 vectors that have norm |**x**|=1. All vectors on the layers above it have norms from 2 to 12, respectively. The largest number or vectors is in the middle level (norm |**x**|=6) for n=12. Therefore, that middle layer is the longest one. In 3-D, each layer is represented as a disk as shown in Figure 3 (c)-(f). This visual data representation is called *Multiple Disk Form* (**MDF**). It shows all 4096 12-D vectors without any overlap.

The MDF visualization is applied in Figure 4 to visualize cancer rules discovered by using relational data mining and by "expert" mining [Kovalerchuk, Vityaev, Ruiz, 2001]. The rule generated by the expert radiologist is shown in Figure 4 (a),(c),(e) and the cancer rule extracted from the database by a relational data mining algorithm MMDR [Kovalerchuk, Vityaev, 2000] is shown in Figure 4 (b), (d),(f). Each rule is described by showing all cases where it is true, as black bars and as white bars where it is false. In other words, each Boolean vector **x** (case, patient, element) is represented in MDF as a *black bar* if the target value for **x** is equal to 1 (cancer), *f*(**x**)=1, and it is a *white bar* if *f*(*x*)=0 (benign).

The VDATMIN also allows using other bar colors to indicate the status of the vector. For instance, Figure 3(b) shows each layer of vectors in different color. This system can indicate another status of the vector (case) which shows whether it is derived from target values (e.g., cancer, benign) of other cases using the monotonicity hypothesis. The vector **y** is rendered as a *light grey bar* if its target value *f*(**y**)=0 is *derived* from the target value for the vector **x**, such that $\mathbf{y} \leq \mathbf{x}$ and *f*(**x**)=0. Alternatively, the vector **y** is rendered as a *dark grey bar* if **y≥x** and *f*(**x**)=1. In this case *f*(**y**)=1. Vector **y** is called an *expanded vector*. The idea is that if the monotonicity hypothesis holds, then the value of *f*(**y**) can be derived by expanding the value *f*(**x**) as shown above. In other words, for white **x**, vector **y** is rendered as a light gray bar, which shows its similarity to **x** in the target variable value (e.g., cancer), and its status as derived from x is not directly observed. Similarly the dark gray color is used for vector **y** with the target value derived from *f*(**x**)=1. While grey scale metaphor with black and white extremes is a common one, sometimes it is better visually to use the darkness scale with other colors. Specifically VDATMIN uses the scale of blue color as well.

Figure 5 explains the visualization used in Figure 4 (b),(d),(f) related to aligning chains of vectors. Say we have a set of Boolean vectors:

(0000 0000 100) < (0000 1000 100) < (0001 1000 100) < (0001 1010 100) <
(0001 1010 110) < (0001 1011 110)

with a lexicographical order. This means that every coordinate in the previous vector is less than or equal to the same coordinate in the next vector. In Figure 5(a) all vectors are ordered in each layer independently from vectors on other layers. It is done by using their binary numeric value, while in Figure 5(b) it is done in accordance with their lexicographical order. They form a straight line of bars starting from the smallest one. This makes the visualization much clearer and simpler.

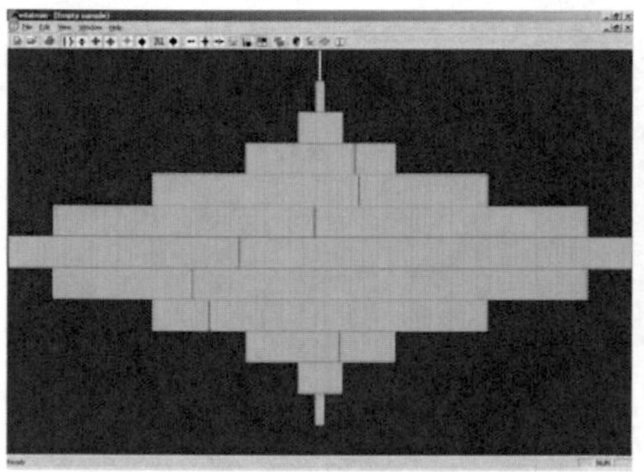

(a) Monotone increasing vectors rendered in the numeric order

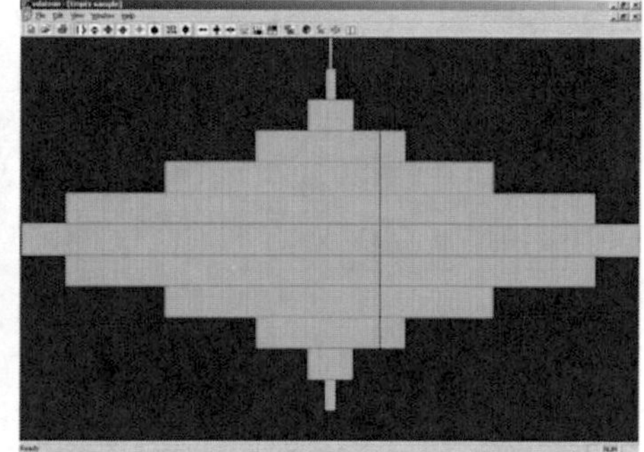

(b) The same elements aligned as a vertical chain

Fig. 5. Alternative visualizations of increasing vectors

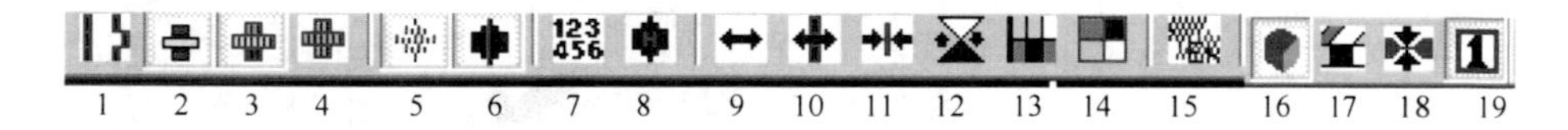

Fig. 6. Details of the user interface to support viewing monotone chains of elements. (1) Align Chains vertically, (2) Show Layer Borders, (, (3) Show Element Borders, (4) Show Element Borders in one color, (5) Show Bush Up (elements that are greater than a selected element) , (6) Highlight a chain, (7) Sort elements using their numerical values (natural order), (8) Align Chains (sort the data using the Hansel chains algorithm), (9) Move an element by dragging, (10) Move a chain by dragging, (11) Automatically center Hansel chains, (12) Expand Elements, (13) Show Monotonicity Violations, (14) Change expanded to real elements, (15) Expand Monotonicity, (16) Show 3D view, (17) Show 3D plot view, (18) Show 3D compressed view, (19) show initial position of disk.

Figure 6 shows the details of the user interface. Button 12 "Expand Elements" toggles the ability to click on a 2D element and expands down the chain if the element is white and expands up the chain if the element is black. Button 13 "Show Monotonicity Violations" will show violations as red elements. Button 14 "Change expanded to real elements" toggles the ability to click on an element and change it from expanded status (dark gray or light gray) to real (black or white). Button (16) "Show 3D view" toggles between 2D and 3D view. Button (16) "Show 3D plot view" is a 3D view that draws on the tops and bottoms of disks. Button (17) "Show 3D compressed view" is a view that compresses the data based on it being close to other data. Button (18) "Show the initial position of the disk" draws a red box around the 1st element in each layer. In the 3D a user has abilities to change the view of the MDF by controlling the camera that include rotating left - right, moving left-right, up-down, and zooming in and out.

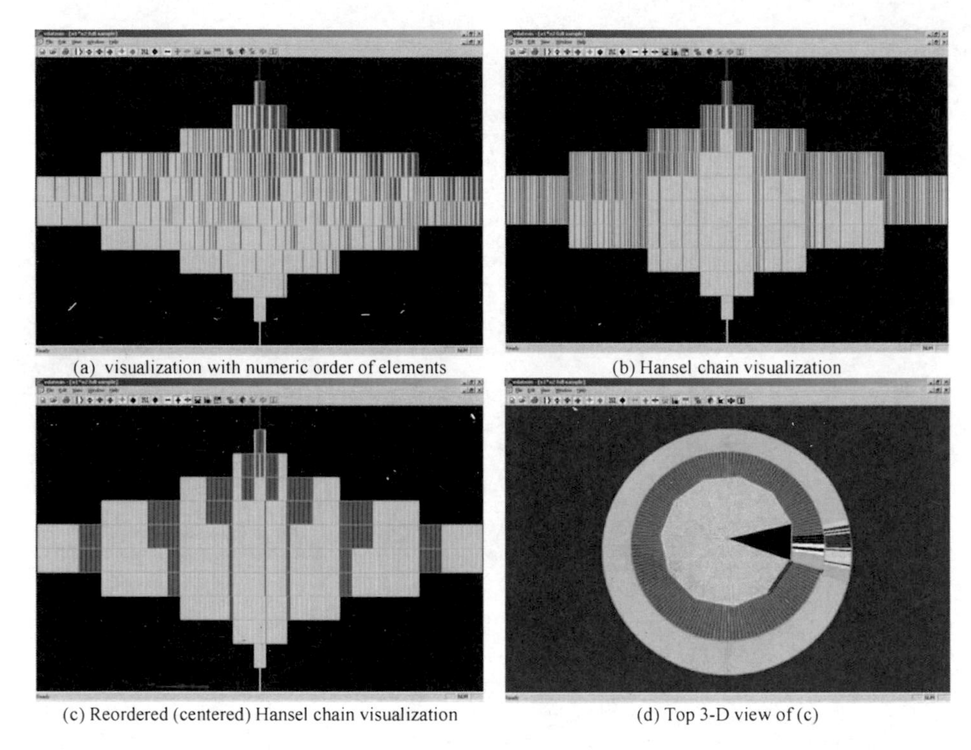
(a) visualization with numeric order of elements
(b) Hansel chain visualization
(c) Reordered (centered) Hansel chain visualization
(d) Top 3-D view of (c)

Fig. 7. The visualization of the Boolean rule y= x_1&x_2 in 11-dimensional space

Figure 7 shows the visualization of the Boolean rule $f(\mathbf{x}) = x_1\&x_2$ in 11-dimensional space, e.g. if in $x=(x_1,x_2,x_3,\ldots,x_{11})$ we have $x_1=x_2=1$, $x_i=0$, i= 3,4,...,11 then $f(\mathbf{x})=1$. In Figure 7, all vectors that have $f(\mathbf{x})=1$ are black bars in and all vectors that have $f(\mathbf{x})=0$ are white bars. There is no vector **x** with $f(\mathbf{x})$ expanded by monotonicity because all values of the target are given explicitly by the rule $f(\mathbf{x}) = x_1\&x_2$. This is the case when we have a complete rule. However, this is not the case in data-driven data mining where training data represent only a fraction of all vectors **x** in E^n. The first black bar (on the third layer from the bottom) represents the vector **x** with $x_1=x_2=1$, $x_i=0$, i= 3,4,...,11. All other vectors on the same layer with norm $|\mathbf{x}|=2$ are white because they cannot have $x_1=x_2=1$. The next layer ($|\mathbf{x}|=3$) contains 9 vectors and respectively 9 black bars.

In Figure 7(a), all vectors are ordered in each layer in accordance with their binary value (e.g., vector (000...111) is numerically smaller than (111...000)), where it is assumed that x_1 represents a lowest bit and x_{11} represents the highest bit. This our vector with $x_1=x_2=1$, $x_i=0$, i= 3,4,...,11 is shown on the right end of the layer with $|\mathbf{x}|=2$.

Figure 7(b) shows a border between two classes of $f(\mathbf{x})$ values 0 and 1 much better than (a) representation. It is based on monotone chains of elements of E^n called Hansel chains [Hansel, 1966]. Mathematical details how these layers are built are given in [Kovalerchuk, Delizy, 2005, Kovalerchuk, et al., 1996].

To be able to visualize data of the larger dimension we use grouping of Hansel chains and visualize groups of similar chains as a single chain. Thus, less area is needed to show the same data. The user has abilities to enter data to be visualized in two ways: (1) as formulas such as any disjunctive normal form (e.g., $x_1\&x_2 \vee x_3\&x_4\&x_5$) or as actual vectors in n-D. In the first case, the program parses the logical formulas.

3 Visualization for Breast Cancer Diagnistics

We already presented in Figure 4 MDF visualization of one of the expert cancer rule and the cancer rule extracted from the database by the data mining algorithm. Below we expand this analysis and show it in Figure 8.

A more complete **cancer rule** produced by the "expert mining" process that involves 11 features is as follows:

$$f(\mathbf{x}) = x_5x_{10} \vee x_4x_{10} \vee x_6x_7x_8x_{10} \vee x_5x_9x_{11} \vee x_4x_9x_{11} \vee x_6x_7x_8x_9x_{11} \vee x_5x_3 \vee x_4x_3 \vee x_6x_7x_8x_3 \vee x_2x_3 \vee x_1 \quad (2)$$

This formula is from [Kovalerchuk, Vityaev Ruiz, 2001] converted to the disjunctive normal form with the renaming variables to be able to feed VDATMIN directly. Figure 8 shows this rule with all three MDF visualization options.

Expert rules for the **biopsy** also have been developed in by using the expert mining technique based on Monotone Boolean Functions approach in [Kovalerchuk, Vityaev, Ruiz, 2001]. It is shown below again in a modified notation to be able to feed VDATMIN:

$$f(\mathbf{x}) = x_5x_{10} \vee x_4x_{10} \vee x_6x_7x_8x_{10} \vee x_5x_9x_{11} \vee x_4x_9x_{11} \vee x_6x_7x_8x_9x_{11} \vee x_5x_3 \vee x_4x_3 \vee x_6x_7x_8x_3 \vee x_2x_3 \vee x_1 \quad (3)$$

Figure 8 shows the advantages of chain-based MDF visualization relative to visualization that does not exploit monotone chains. The chain-based border between classes is much clearer. This advantage gives an immediate benefit: visual comparison of rules for biopsy and cancer. It also helps to identify the level of consistency of cancer and biopsy rules provided by the expert. It is expected that a biopsy rules should be less stringent than a cancer rules. For instance if the presence of $x_2\&x_3$ is a cancer indicator but only presence of x_3 can be sufficient to recommend biopsy test. In visual terms it means that the border of the biopsy class should be lower or at the same as cancer class for them to be consistent. This is exactly the case as Figure 8 (c) and (f) show. The black areas in the ovals in Figure 8 (f) for biopsy are lower than the same areas for cancer in Figure 8 (f). Figure 8 (j) shows highly overlapped parallel coordinate visualization of the same data (yellow - benign, red – malignant). The same classes are shown separately in Figure 1 (c). It shows advantages of VDATMIN relative to parallel coordinates for Boolean data. Figure 8(k) shows types of source X-ray mammography images used to derive Boolean vectors.

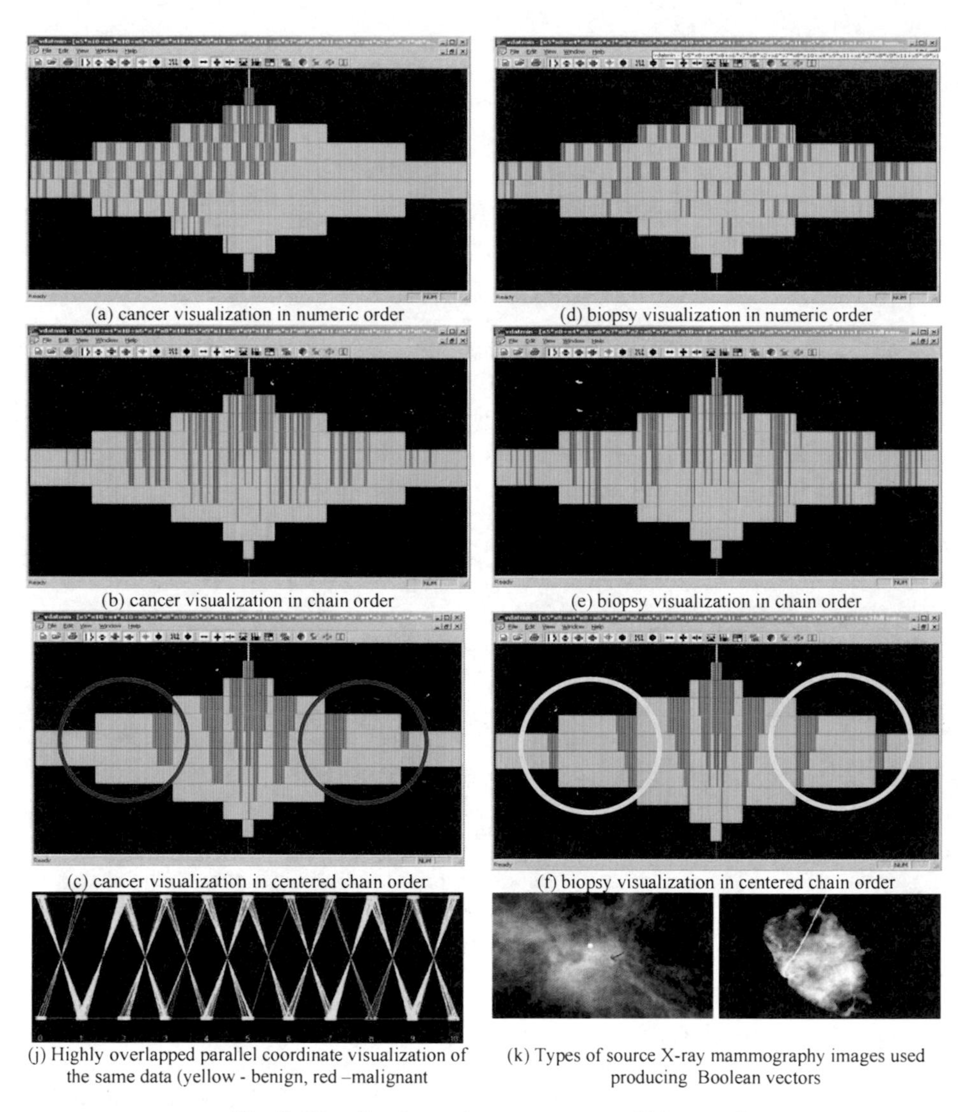

(a) cancer visualization in numeric order
(d) biopsy visualization in numeric order
(b) cancer visualization in chain order
(e) biopsy visualization in chain order
(c) cancer visualization in centered chain order
(f) biopsy visualization in centered chain order
(j) Highly overlapped parallel coordinate visualization of the same data (yellow - benign, red –malignant
(k) Types of source X-ray mammography images used producing Boolean vectors

Fig. 8. Visualizations of expert cancer and biopsy rules

4 General Concept of Using MDF in Data Mining

Figure 9 illustrates the general concept of simultaneous coordinated visualization of multiple components of the analytics: original available training data, rules extracted from these data by using data mining, rules extracted from the expert. Often the data and rules are in two categories: “final” and “warning”. In many applications, final rules produce a “final” decision, e.g., cancer, crime, security breach, but “warning” rules produce warnings about possible final state, e.g., biopsy positive, crime warning, and security alert. There are must be consistency between final and warning rules from data mining and expert mining. The VDATMIN allows capturing discrepancies and consistency visually as Figure 9 shows on the illustrative examples for “final” and “warning” rules. Comparison of Figure 9(a) and 9(b) shows discrepancy between “final” data mining rules and monotonically expanded data. In the cancer example, this may lead to both missed cancer cases and benign cases diagnosed as malignant. In the center of (b) we see that the border of the monotone expansion is below than the border in (a). This means that some cancer case would be diagnosed as benign. In contrast, on the sides for both (a), (b) we see an opposite picture, which may lead to benign cases diagnosed as malignant. Similar interpretation will take place for crimes and security examples. Figure 9(c) and 9(d) show full consistency of expert ‘final” and “warning” rules with each other. All “final” rules are nested in the “warning” rules. Both these rules also much more consistent with data (c) than pure data mining rules (a) as visual comparison shows in a very compact way in Figure 9.

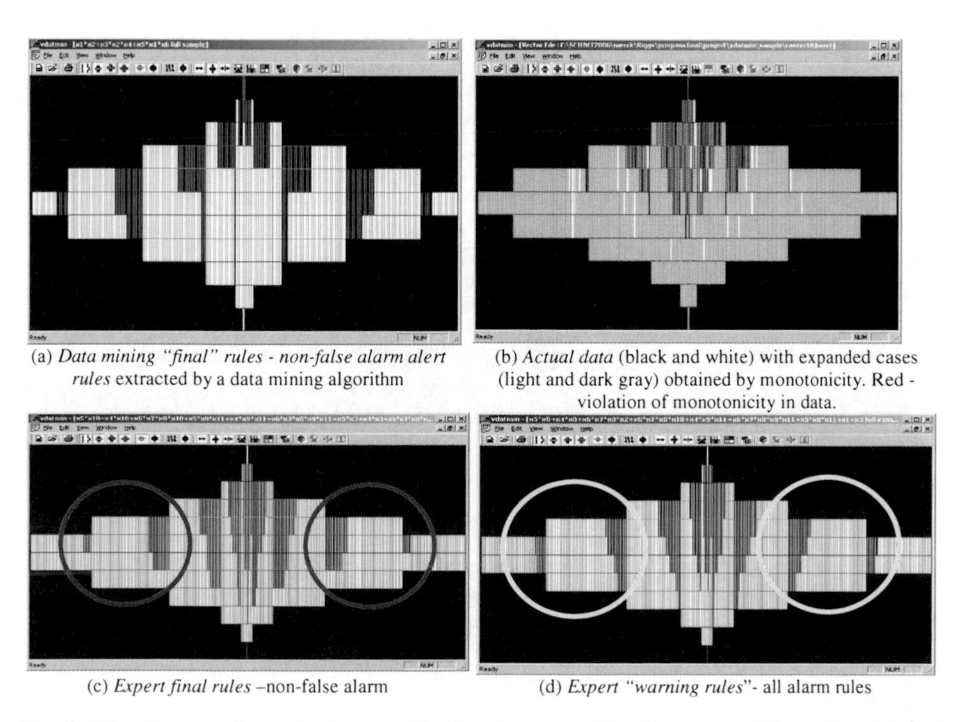

(a) *Data mining “final” rules - non-false alarm alert rules* extracted by a data mining algorithm

(b) *Actual data* (black and white) with expanded cases (light and dark gray) obtained by monotonicity. Red - violation of monotonicity in data.

(c) *Expert final rules* –non-false alarm

(d) *Expert “warning rules”*- all alarm rules

Fig. 9. Visual comparison of rules provided by the expert (a), (b), extracted from data (c) and “visual rule” (d)

5 Scaling Algorithms

5.1 Algorithm with Data-Based Chains

Our goal is to represent the MDF on a single screen with possibly some scrolling. The major factor that is limiting the visualization is the number of Hansel chains that can be visualized as vertical lines. We use two approaches:

(A1) grouping chains with similar height of the border to a cluster,
(A2) constructing chains from only vectors available in the database.

The steps of the algorithm to construct these chains are described below and illustrated in Figures 10 and 11:

Step 1: Order all vectors according their Hamming norm.

Step 2: Loop: for each vector $\mathbf{v}_i$ starting from the first one find all nodes that are greater than this node, $\mathbf{v}_i < \mathbf{v}_j$. This will create a matrix M={m_{ij}}, where m_{ij}=1 if $\mathbf{v}_i < \mathbf{v}_j$ else $m_{ij}= \infty$. We can record only m_{ij}=1. Typically, this is a sparse matrix. This matrix can be interpreted as an incidence matrix of the graph G (directed acyclic graph, DAG), where 1 means that there is direct link between nodes with length 1 and $m_{ij}= \infty$ means the absence of the link and infinite length. Thus this step builds DAG, where arrow between nodes show the direction form smaller Boolean vector to the larger one.

Step 3: Find a longest directed path P in G using M. Call this path chain 1.

Step 4. Move C_1 to the center of MDF

Step 5: Remove all nodes of P from G and find a longest directed path in G with removed P. This path produces chain C_2. Locate C_2 vertically: one vector above another one in MDF.

Step 6: Repeat step 4 until every node of G will belong to some path. Steps 3-5 will produce k chains {C_i} that do not overlap and cover all nodes of G.

Step 7: Compute distances D_{HC} (C_i, C_j) between all chains C_i.

Step 8: Move all other chains in accordance with their distance to C_1 in MDF. The chains with the shorter distance will be the closer to C_1.

Step 9: Assign color to vectors on each chain: black for f(x)=1 and white for f(x)=0.

Step 10: This step contains tree components: expanding chains to have vectors with equal Hamming norms on both chains; equalizing expanded vectors in color with given vectors to see the pattern of the border better, and hiding the empty part of the MDF form.

Consider an example of 200 given vectors in the E^{100}. What is the space needed to visualize them in MDF form? In the best case scenario we would have just two vertical chains that will contains all 200 vectors. Say the longest chain will have 101 vectors and the second chain will contain remaining 99 vectors. This is due to the fact that in100-D the longest chain contains 101 vectors. In the worst case, we would need to visualize 200 chains, if each vector forms its own chain when 200 vectors are incomparable. Similarly, for a much larger set of 10^6 vectors we would need to visualize at least about 10^4 chains ($10^6/101$). For a screen with 2000 pixels, it will result in scrolling the screen 5 times to observe these 10^4 chains in MDF completely for 100-D space and 10^6 vectors. The combining of the scrolling with clustering of chains where each cluster will have about 5 chains per cluster allows to compress all 10^6 vectors in 100-D space into a single screen in the complete multiple disk form (MDF).

On step 7, a user can switch between different distances. To describe distance used we define necessary concepts. Let L(C) be the lower unit of the chain C (the vector $\mathbf{z}$ on the chain with the smallest norm such that $f(\mathbf{z})=1$) Next let $E(C_1,C_2)$ be the smallest element $\mathbf{z}$ of the chain C_2 with f(x)=1 that was obtained by monotone expansion of element $L(C_1)$. This means that is knowing the value $f(L(C_1))=1$ we can expand this value to $\mathbf{z}=E(C_1,C_2)$. Thus, this value $f(\mathbf{z})=1$ cannot be expanded by monotonicity to elements of chain C_2 that are below $E(C_1,C_2)$.

The Hamming distance D between lower units of two chains, $L(C_i)$ and L(Cj), D(L(Ci),L(Cj)) creates a smooth border, but it does not capture the monotone similarity between chains. The Hamming distance combined with Monotone Expansion, called *HME measure* captures both properties. In HME chain C_2 is placed closer to chain C_1 than chain C_3, if the smallest expanded element of C_2 from C_1, $E(C_1,C_2)$, is closer (in Hamming distance D) to $L(C_1)$, which is $D(E(C_1,C_2)) < D(E(C_1,C_3))$. HME is infinite if chain C_2 has no such expanded elements.

5.2 Algorithm with Pixel Chains

This algorithm modifies steps 8-10 from the previous algorithm. To visualize E^{100} it uses a window of 101x100 pixels. The x coordinate is the Hamming-based distance/measure from the longest chain to the current chain H. The y coordinate is the norm (height) of the *lower unit* on the chain H. In E^{100}, this size of the window follows from the fact that the largest Hamming distance is 100 and the longest chain has 101 vectors. See Figure 12. In general for E^n the window is $(n+1)\times n$. Thus a single screen has enough space for E^n with n=1000. This window is called a *Chain Pixel Space* (CPS). Chains are placed in CPS, where each pixel is empty or contains one or more chains. A user can change the visualization by switching the measures used in x (e.g., switching Hamming distance and HME). This visualization is very compact where each pixel can represent hundreds and thousands vectors, but with possible chain overlap. The number of chains overlapped in the pixel is shown by pixel color intensity in 2D or by a bar height when CPS is converted to its 3-D form. The spread of the border is shown in Figure 12(a) in each column. Figure 12(b) shows the lower edge of the border. Similarly, an upper border is visualized.

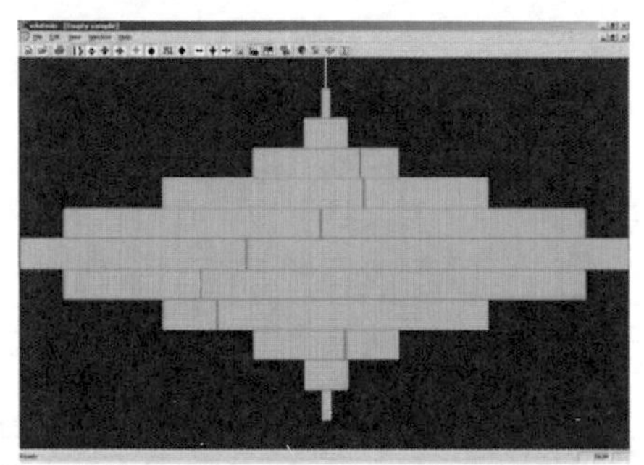

Step 1: Order given vectors according their Hamming norm. Show each vector as a bar in the row of its norm. Vectors with higher norm are on the rows closer to the top.

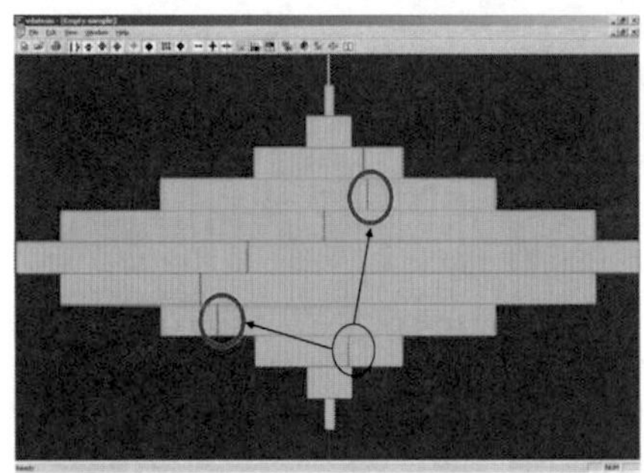

Step 2: Build a graph G of vectors. G has a link from $\mathbf{v}_i$ to $\mathbf{v}_j$. if $\mathbf{v}_i < \mathbf{v}_j$. Vectors in red ovals are greater than the vector in the black oval.

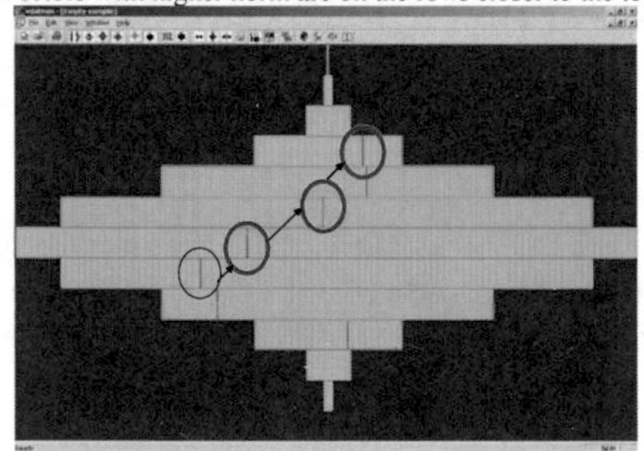

Step 3: Find chain C_1 - a longest directed path in G.

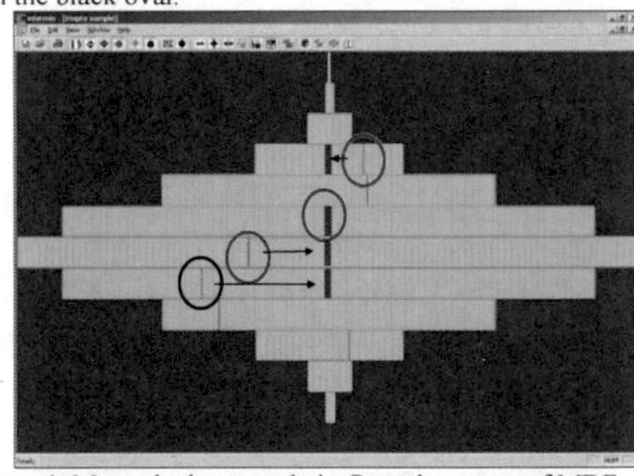

Step 4: Move the longest chain C_1 to the center of MDF

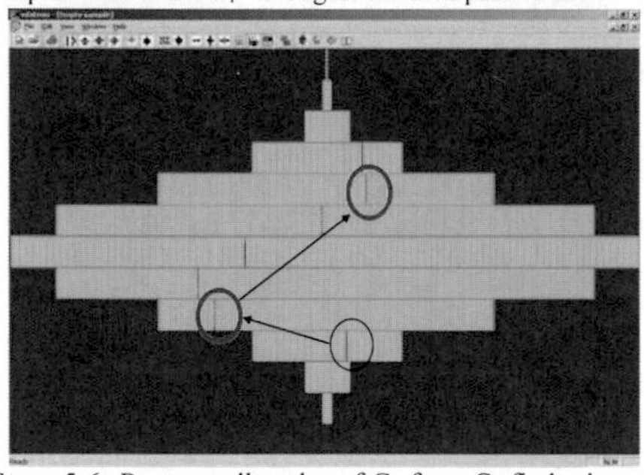

Steps 5-6: Remove all nodes of C_1 from G, find a longest directed path in $G \backslash C_1$. Repeat to get all other chains

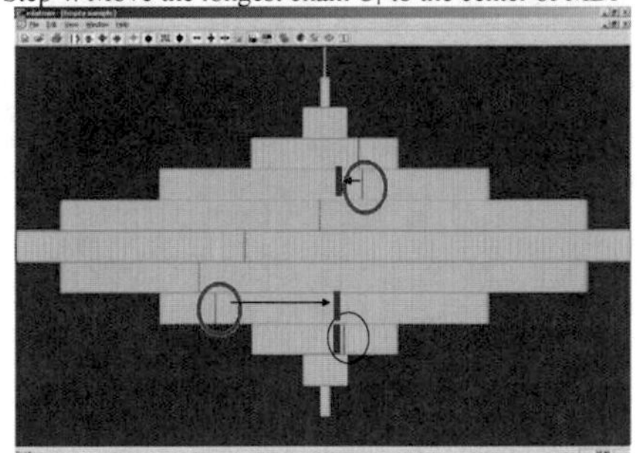

Steps 5-6: Locate chain vertically C_2: one vector above another one in MDF. Repeat this with other chains.

Fig. 10. Illustration of algorithm with data-based chains: part 1

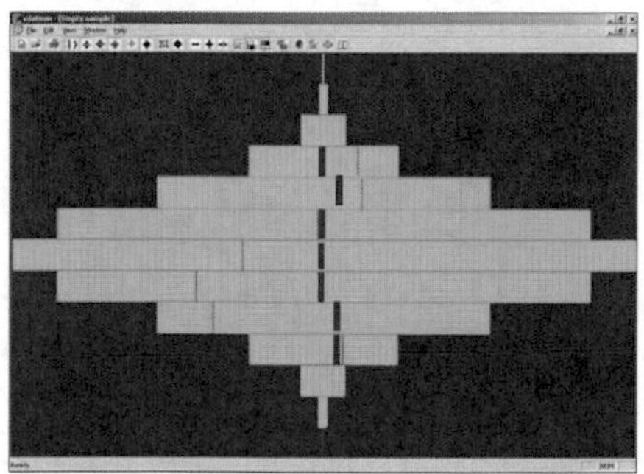

Steps 5-6: Chains C_1 and C_2 located vertically as a result of Steps 5-6.

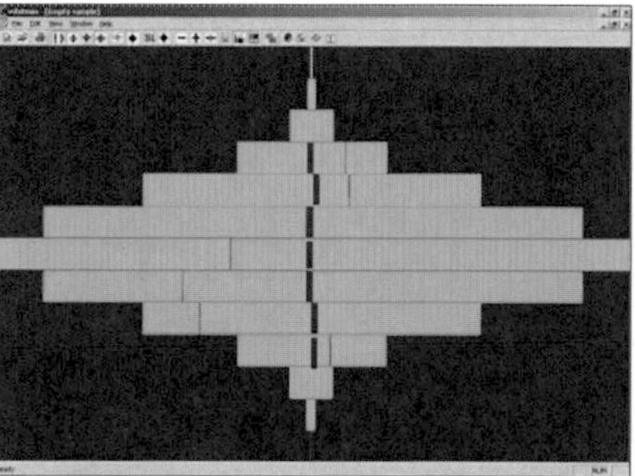

Steps 7-8: Move chains according to their distance to C_1. The chains with the shorter distance are closer to C_1.

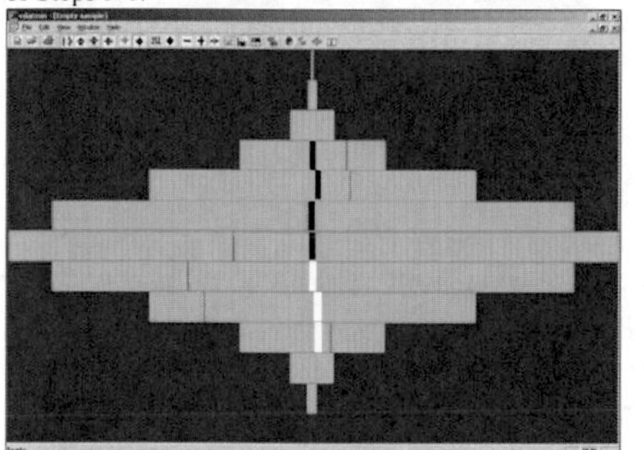

Step 9: Assign colors to vectors on each chain based on target values, black for f(x)=1 and white for f(x)=0.

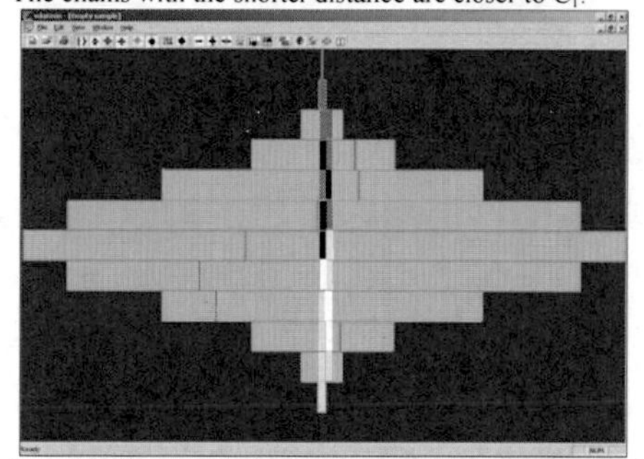

Step 10: Expand chains by monotonicity: f(x)=1 (dark grey), f(x)=0 (light grey), no expansion (yellow).

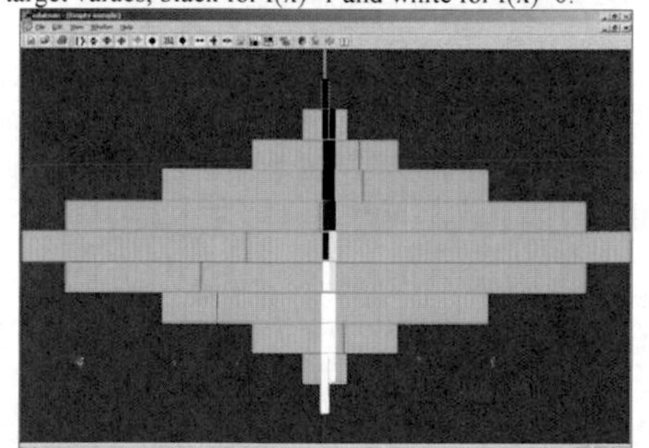

Step 10: Expanded vectors equalized in color with given vectors to see the pattern of the border better.

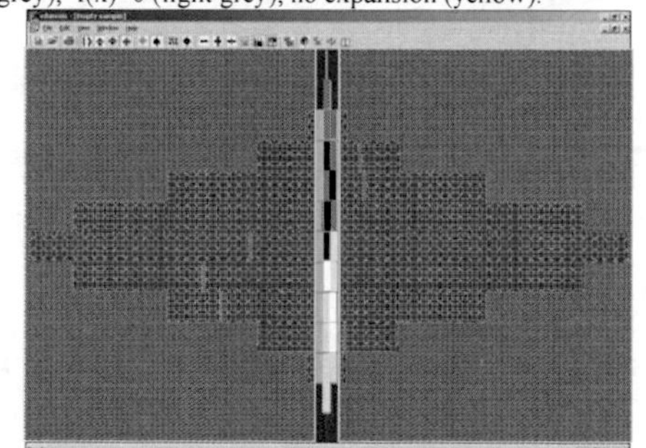

Step 10: Hiding and removing the empty part of the MDF form.

Fig. 11. Illustration of the algorithm with data-based chains: part 2

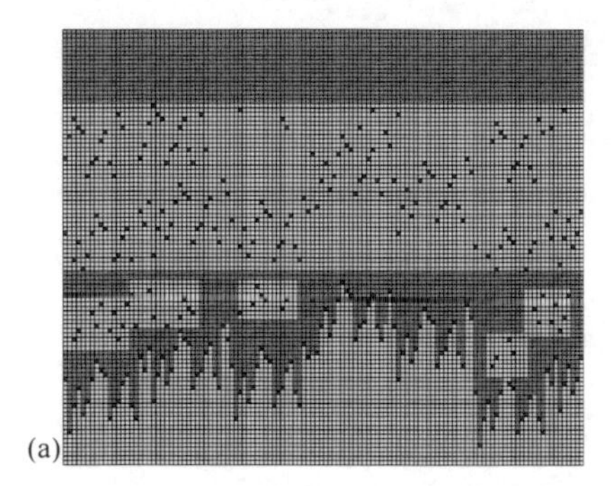

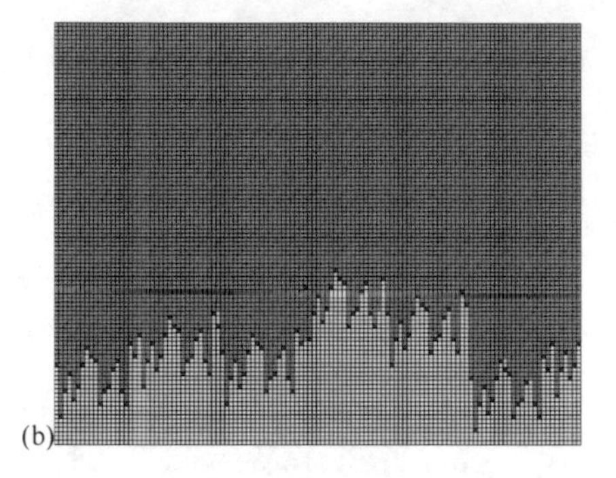

Fig. 12. Pixel-based chain visualization: (a) all chains, (b) lower border between classes

6 Binarization and Monotonization

Above we considered visual data mining with monotone binary data. Below we discuss generalization of this technique for the data that are not binary and not monotone. The simplest way to binarize data is use a threshold with δ-function: δ(x)=1 if x>=T else δ(x)=0. The main reason for binarization is data simplification and getting a qualitative evaluation of the complex situation. Binarization of data is an extreme case of data discretization that is quite common in data mining with multiple techniques developed. Typically, we need to analyze the situation at the different levels of detail. We would prefer first to get a "bird view" of the situation and then 'zoom' to most interesting spots found in the 'bird view". This is not only a question of convenience, but a deep issue of artificial intelligence and brain modeling. In this way humans able to solve tasks that seems computationally intractable. These issues are studied in Dynamic Logic of Phenomena (DLP) [Kovalerchuk, Perlovsky, 2008, 2009].

Example 1: *Crime situation.* Multiple demographic factors contribute to crime level in specific areas. The collected data can be overwhelming, therefore initial qualitative analysis can be done with two target values "growing crime level", and "stable or declining crime level" that can be measured by threshold that the increase in the number of criminal cases is greater than threshold T.

Similarly, we can binarize features that impact the target feature –crime level. For the example 1 it can be: (1) population increase (no significant increase, significant increase); (2) Income (low, high);(3) Tax collected level (low, high), (4) Population percent of age 18-30 (low, high), (5) Mean age (no greater than T, greater than T), (6) Education level as a percent of population with college degree (low- no greater than T, high- greater than T), (7) Unemployment rate (low, high), (8) Law enforcement budget rate (low, high), (9) Crime level in the adjacent neighborhoods, (10) High school dropout level (low, high).

Thus, we can get 10-dimensional Boolean vectors of these exogenous attributes with low encoded as 0 and high as 1. Each available training vector is labeled by 0 or 1, that represent the crime level (low or high). Each such record will be for an individual neighborhood and a specific time. Such binary data representation allows us to use the visual data mining technique described in this paper to discover a visual predictive rule for prediction crime level (low, high). We will also be able to test monotonicity of the attributes (1)-(10) relative to crime level. The lack of monotonicity may mean that some other impact factors are missing or data are corrupted. For instance, some neighborhoods already implemented the neighborhood watch program. This feature is not included in (1)-(10). Several iteration of adding attributes may be required to reach monotonicity. Thus, the proposed visual data mining approach can serve as a *feature augmenting mechanism* that compliment known feature selection mechanisms, which do not guide how to look at new attributes.

Example 2: *Security situation of the port.* Multiple factors within the port and outside contribute to port security level and the collected data can be overwhelming. Therefore initial qualitative analysis can be done with two target values "growing security threats", and "stable or declining security threats" that can be measured by threshold that the increase in the number of security alerts is greater than threshold T in the area.

Similarly, using thresholds we can binarize features that impact the target feature – security level: (1) Cargo in the area (down or no significant increase, significant increase), (2) Real estate value of the area (low, high), (3) Cargo value in the area (low, high), (4) Average number of people in the area (low, high), (5) Average number of non-port employees in the area (low, high), (6) Number of sensors in the area (low, high), (7) Average time a non-employee in the area per day (low, high), (8) Average time an employee in the area per day (low, high), (9) Average number of security people in the area (low, high), (10) Security budget rate in the area per $ of real estate in the area (low, high), (11) Security budget rate in the area per $ of cargo value in the area (low, high), (12) Incident level in the area (high, low).

In this example, final rules could indicate strong and urgent security measures that require significant extra security resource allocated and warning rules could indicate addition attention to the area with minimal additional resources allocated. As above in Figure 9 VDM allows to compare rules "extracted" from the security expert and with rules obtained by data mining and with the date expanded by monotonicity.

Obviously, it is not clear at the beginning how these attributes are related to the number of alerts generated in the area. Answering this question is a data mining task. To solve this task, we can get 10-dimensional Boolean vectors of these exogenous attributes with low encoded as 0 and high as 1. Each vector marked by the security alert rate (low or high encoded by 0 or 1 as well). Each such record will be for an individual area of the port and a specific time. This data binary representation allows us to use the visual data mining technique described above to discover visual predictive rules for prediction security alert level (low, high). We will also be able to test monotonicity of the attributes (1)-(10) relative to alert level. The lack of monotonicity may mean that some other impact factors are missing or data are corrupted. For instance, some port area already implemented the employee security training program, internal alert analysis, etc. These features are not included in (1)-(10). After several iteration of adding attributes, we can reach monotonicity. Thus, similar to the previous example, VDATMIN will serve here as a *feature augmenting mechanism* that compliment known feature selection mechanisms.

7 Monotonization

The algorithm below describes main steps of a monotonization process for the tasks where monotonicity is violated:

Step 1: Find a specific pair of vectors ($\mathbf{x}$,$\mathbf{y}$) with violation of monotonicity, that is $\mathbf{x} > \mathbf{y}$ but $f(\mathbf{x}) < f(\mathbf{y})$

Step 2: Find attributes of ($\mathbf{x}$,$\mathbf{y}$) that led to violation of monotonicity, $\mathbf{x} > \mathbf{y} \Rightarrow f(\mathbf{x}) < f(\mathbf{y})$.

Step 3: Find a subspace S and sub-vectors $\mathbf{x}_s$ and $\mathbf{y}_s$ in subspace S such that monotonicity holds: $\mathbf{x}_s < \mathbf{y}_s \Rightarrow f(\mathbf{x}) < f(\mathbf{y})$.

Step 4: Get attributes U={u} of the total space W that do not belong to S, W\S = U. These attributes cause the violation of monotonicity, $\mathbf{x} > \mathbf{y} \Rightarrow f(\mathbf{x}) < f(\mathbf{y})$ in space W.

Step 5: Modify attributes U.

Example: If attribute (1) "Population increase" is a source of monotonicity violation, it can be modified to a new attribute (g): *"Growth of crime age population"*. The monotone link between this attribute and crime rate seems a reasonable hypothesis (to be tested) if *all other relevant factors* are the same. Under this assumption, the high growth in the crime age population in the area A may lead to a higher crime rate (Cr) than in area B with low growth of this category of the population. In contrast, if areas A and B have different other relevant factors, $F_A \neq F_B$' this may not be the case. Thus, we may have a very specific *restricted type of monotonicity* with the same other relevant factors:

$$[\ (F_A = F_B)\ \&\ g(A) \geq g(B)\ ] \Rightarrow Cr(A) \geq Cr(B), \qquad (1)$$

We will call it *OF-conditional monotonicity* because it holds only under condition that Other Factors (OF) are the same. Mathematically it means that $|\mathbf{a}| = |\mathbf{b}|+1$, that is Boolean vector $\mathbf{a}$ is obtained from Boolean vector $\mathbf{b}$ by changing one of its zero values to one. This is exactly how Hansel chains are built. In other words, this is a *one step up single-attribute monotonicity* because all other attributes of vectors $\mathbf{a}$ and $\mathbf{b}$ are the same.

Step 6: Test monotonicity of modified attributes. In the example above, it means testing (1) on the available data.

Step 7: If Step 6 test succeeded, we can use a modified attribute g instead of the original attribute in the `MBFVA` algorithm. If Step 6 test failed on monotonicity or OF-conditional monotonicity then go to step 8.

Step 8: Decide between two options (i) return to step 5 and make another modification of attributes and (ii) add a new attribute, that is go to step 9.

Note: The failed test result on step 6 can be a very useful result in spite being negative. It indicates that we may miss other relevant factors. Area A can be in the region with historically low crime due to a type population (low migration, high church influence, etc). Thus, even negative test of monotonicity is helpful as a guidance to search new relevant attributes and improving data mining output.

Step 9: Add new attribute. In the example after adding migration level and church influence to $F_A = F_B$ we may generate a new OF-conditional monotonicity hypothesis for (1) and go to step 6 again.

Step 10. Continue looping steps 5-9 until monotonicity produced for all attributes in the original space W or time limit reached.

8 Conclusion

Monotone Boolean Function Visual Analytics (MBFVA) method allows the discovering of rules that are meaningful for the subject matter expert (SME) and are confirmed with the database. The efficiency of the method is illustrated with discovering breast cancer diagnostic rules that are produced by (i) Subject Metter Expert, (ii) the analytical data mining algorithm, and (iii) the visual means from data. The proposed coordinated visualization of these rules is a way to produce high quality rules. Multivariate binary data are visualized in 2-D and 3-D without occlusion. It preserves structural relations in multivariate data. As a result, the complex border between classes in a multidimensional space is converted into visual 2-D and 3-D forms. This decreases the user information overload. To expand the applicability of the described approach, this paper presented an outline of the scaling algorithm for large datasets where each chain of multidimensional vectors is compressed into a single pixel. The detailed development of this algorithm is a topic of future research.

References

[1] Beilken, C., Spenke, M.: Visual interactive data mining with InfoZoom-the Medical Data Set. In: 3rd European Conf. on Principles and Practice of Knowledge Discovery in Databases, PKDD (1999), `http://lisp.vse.cz/pkdd99/Challenge/spenke-m.zip`

[2] Groth, D., Robertson, E.: Architectural support for database visualization. In: Workshop on New Paradigms in Information Visualization and Manipulation, pp. 53–55 (1998)

[3] Hansel, G.: Sur le nombre des functions Bool'eenes monotones de n variables. C.R. Acad. Sci., Paris 262(20), 1088–1090 (1966)

[4] Inselberg, A., Dimsdale, B.: Parallel coordinates: A tool for visualizing multidimensional Geometry. In: Proceedings of IEEE Visualization 1990, pp. 360–375. IEEE Computer Society Press, Los Alamitos (1990)

[5] Keim, D., Hao Ming, C., Dayal, U., Meichun, H.: Pixel bar charts: a visualization technique for very large multiattributes data sets. Information Visualization 1(1), 20–34 (2002)

[6] Keim, D., Müller, W., Schumann, H.: Visual Data Mining. In: EUROGRAPHICS 2002 STAR (2002), `http://www.eg.org/eg/dl/conf/eg2002/stars/s3_visualdatamining_mueller.pdf`

[7] Keim, D.: Information Visualization and Visual Data Mining. IEEE TVCG 7(1), 100–107 (2002)

[8] Keller, N., Pilpel, H.: Linear transformations of monotone functions on the discrete cube. Discrete Mathematics 309(12), 4210–4214 (2009)

[9] Korshunov, A.D.: Monotone Boolean Functions. Russian Math. Surveys 58(5), 929–1001 (2003)

[10] Kovalerchuk, B., Delizy, F.: Visual Data Mining using Monotone Boolean functions. In: Kovalerchuk, B., Schwing, J. (eds.) Visual and Spatial Analysis, pp. 387–406. Springer, Heidelberg (2005)

[11] Kovalerchuk, B., Triantaphyllou, E., Despande, A., Vityaev, E.: Interactive Learning of Monotone Boolean Functions. Information Sciences. Information Sciences 94(1-4), 87–118 (1996)

[12] Kovalerchuk, B., Vityaev, E., Ruiz, J.: Consistent and complete data and "expert" mining in medicine. In: Medical Data Mining and Knowledge Discovery, pp. 238–280. Springer, Heidelberg (2001)

[13] Kovalerchuk, B., Vityaev, E.: Data Mining in Finance: Advances in Relational and Hybrid Methods. Kluwer/Springer, Heidelberg, Dordrecht (2000)

[14] Kovalerchuk, B., Perlovsky, L.: Fusion and Mining Spatial Data in Cyber-physical space with Phenomena Dynamic Logic. In: Proceedings of the 2009 International Joint Conference on Neural Networks, Atlanta, Georgia, USA, pp. 2440–2447 (2009)

[15] Kovalerchuk, B., Perlovsky, L.: Dynamic Logic of Phenomena and Cognition. In: Computational Intelligence: Research Frontiers, pp. 3529–3536. IEEE, Hong Kong (2008)

[16] Lim, S.: Interactive Visual Data Mining of a Large Fire Detector Database. In: International Conference on Information Science and Applications (ICISA), pp. 1–8 (2010), doi:10.1109/ICISA.2010.5480395

[17] Lim, S.: On A Visual Frequent Itemset Mining. In: Proc. of the 4th Int'l Conf. on Digital Information Management (ICDIM 2009), pp. 46–51. IEEE, Los Alamitos (2009)

[18] de Oliveira, M., Levkowitz, H.: From Visual Data Exploration to Visual Data Mining: A Survey. IEEE TVCG 9(3), 378–394 (2003)

[19] Pak, C., Bergeron, R.: 30 Years of Multidimensional Multivariate Visualization. In: Scientific Visualization, pp. 3–33. Society Press (1997)

[20] Shaw, C., Hall, J., Blahut, C., Ebert, D., Roberts, A.: Using shape to visualize multivariate data. In: CIKM 1999 Workshop on New Paradigms in Information Visualization and Manipulation, pp. 17–20. ACM Press, New York (1999)

[21] Ward, M.: A taxonomy of glyph placement strategies for multidimensional data visualization. Information Visualization 1, 194–210 (2002)

[22] Schulz, H., Nocke, T., Schumann, H.: A framework for visual data mining of structures. In: ACM International Conf. Proc Series, vol. 171; Proc. 29th Australasian Computer Science Conf., Hobart, vol. 48, pp. 157–166 (2006)

[23] Badjio, E., Poulet, F.: Dimension Reduction for Visual Data Mining. In: Stochastic Models and Data Analysis, ASMDA-2005 (2002), http://conferences.telecom-bretagne.eu/asmda2005/IMG/pdf/proceedings/266.pdf

[24] Wong, P., Whitney, P., Thomas, j.: Visualizing Association Rules for Text Mining. In: Proc. of the IEEE INFOVIS, pp. 120–123. IEEE, Los Alamitos (1999)

[25] Wong, P.C.: Visual Data Mining. In: IEEE CG&A, pp. 20–21 (September/October 1999)

[26] Zhao, K., Bing, L., Tirpak, T.M., Weimin, X.: A visual data mining framework for convenient identification of useful knowledge. In: Fifth IEEE International Conference on Data Mining, 8 p (2005), doi:10.1109/ICDM.2005.16

Chapter 8
A New Approach and Its Applications for Time Series Analysis and Prediction Based on Moving Average of nth-Order Difference

Yang Lan[1] and Daniel Neagu[2]

[1] Department of Computing, School of Computing, Informatics and Media, University of Bradford, Bradford, BD7 1DP, UK
Y.Lan@bradford.ac.uk

[2] Department of Computing, School of Computing, Informatics and Media, University of Bradford, Bradford, BD7 1DP, UK
D.Neagu@bradford.ac.uk

Abstract. As a typical problem in data mining, Time Series Predictions are widely applied in various domains. The approach focuses on series of observations, with the aim that, using mathematics, statistics and artificial intelligence methods, to analyze, process and make a prediction on the next most probable value based on a number of previous values. We propose an algorithm using the average sum of nth-order difference of series terms with limited range margins, in order to establish a way to predict the next series term based on both, the original data set and a negligible error. The algorithm performances are evaluated using measurement data sets on monthly average Sunspot Number, Earthquakes and Pseudo-Periodical Synthetic Time Series.

1 Introduction

The importance of time for human activities has been emphasized from early times of civilization. Historical data analysis has been related to agriculture (sun and moon cycles, weather) and safety (earthquakes, floods). Nowadays, given technological advances in computational power and memory storage, it becomes a functionality of immediate use for industrial or economical processes.

Time series prediction proposes algorithms for which past data (mainly finite observation sequences of data points related to uniform time intervals) are used to generate models to forecast future data points of the series. It is widely applied in various domains from finance (stock markets) and economy (electricity consumption), meteorology, signal processing to disaster warning (river floods, earthquakes) and solar activity forecasting [2]. The time series analysis was based originally on tools including mathematical modeling [8], time-frequency analysis (Fourier and wavelet transformations) but started using in the last years machine learning methods such as Artificial Neural Networks (ANNs) (time-delay

D.E. Holmes, L.C. Jain (Eds.): Data Mining: Found. & Intell. Paradigms, ISRL 24, pp. 157–182.
springerlink.com

networks [14], recurrent networks [6], Self-Organizing Maps [15]. From a procedural perspective, using computational approaches may first require mathematical analysis to describe and breakdown the initial time series problem into simpler sub-problems for further computational modeling. A well-known approach in time series understanding and prediction is Auto-Regressive Moving Average (ARMA) [1] which comes with the advantage of addressing auto-regressive terms and moving average terms.

A historical main constraint in using mathematical series models for prediction was the fact that the performance of the model is related to the length of data series, but nowadays is not anymore an issue from neither computational nor data storage and processing points of view. However, most machine learning methods face the difficulty of requiring *a priori* knowledge about the problem at hand. On the other hand, results of some traditional methods applied in time series analysis can not satisfy the demand of specific applications. We intend to address these drawbacks for the restricted problem of pseudo-periodical series with limited boundaries by a two-step approach: we propose hereby a new algorithm to approximate the time series terms using the moving average of nth-order difference of already known values and intend to address later the problem of error of approximation by a hybrid model. Therefore future work is proposed to identify as accurately as possible a general approximation by use of a supervised-learning model to forecast a further approximation error if found necessary.

We propose an algorithm for efficient mining of pseudo-periodical time series with direct applications to sunspot number, earthquake and pseudo-periodical synthetic time series prediction, by exploring some interesting properties related to moving average of first-order difference for bounded time series. A further generalization to the use of the sum of nth-order difference to increase forecast performances and a hybrid approach to combine the results of the moving average of nth-order difference of time series with a supervised-learning model of the error of value approximation are also proposed [11]. We study the possibility that pre-processing of time series combined with *a priori* knowledge and hybrid models can increase prediction performances for time series, even for mining noisy data. The results highlight our proposed algorithm's efficiency in mining bounded pseudo-periodical patterns in time series with direct applications in sunspot time series prediction, earthquake time series prediction and pseudo-periodical synthetic time series prediction [12].

The following section introduces the notations and definitions on bounded pseudo-periodical time series. Section 3 describes terms and proofs used in our approach, error approximation with the use of ANNs and our algorithm. Section 4 proposes a way to define the suitable level order n of difference operator and index m for increasing the prediction precision. Case studies on the monthly average of sunspot number time series prediction, earthquake time series prediction and pseudo-periodical synthetic time series prediction are described in sections 5, 6 and 7. Section 8 shows the prediction results comparison between the algorithm we propose, Linear Regression (LR) method and Auto-Regression

Moving Average (ARMA) method. Conclusions, further work and discussions of implementation for the proposed method for a hybrid approach are presented in the last section. The Appendix provides proof to some theoretical results used in Section 3.

2 Definitions Relevant to Time Series Prediction

We will introduce in this section some definitions necessary for the proof of our method and the algorithm proposed in following sections.

Notations:

a_m : *initial data series, $m > 0$ is its index (serial number);*

D_m^n : *n^{th}-order difference, n is the nth-order, m is the serial number;*

E_m^n : *moving average of nth-order difference,*
n is the order of the difference terms, m is the serial number.

Definition 1. ***Time Series*** *represents an ordered sequence of data values related to the same variable, measured typically at successive times, spaced apart in uniform intervals:*

$$A = \{a_1, a_2, a_3, \ldots\} \text{ or } A = \{a_t\},\ t = 1, 2, 3, \ldots \tag{1}$$

where series A is indexed by natural numbers.

Definition 2. ***Time Series Prediction*** *represents the use of a model to predict future events (data points) based on known past events, before they are measured. In other words, given first t measured data points of time series A, the aim of prediction is to develop a model able to advance the value.*

$$a_{t+1} = f(a_1, a_2, a_3, \ldots, a_{t-1}, a_t) \tag{2}$$

Definition 3. ***Pseudo-Periodical Time Series*** *are series of which values repeat over a fixed time interval:*

$$a_t \cong a_{t+d} \cong a_{t+p}, \quad t > 0,\ d > 0,\ p > 0,\ p/d = k > 1, \quad k \in N \tag{3}$$

For real applications time series, there are values showing a pattern of *pseudo-periodical time series*, where values show a repetition over a finite time interval; A consequence for periodical and pseudo-periodical time series is that for a finite d and initial values, the series values are bounded:

$$a_t \in [min(a_1, a_2, \ldots, a_d),\ \ max(a_1, a_2, \ldots, a_d)], \quad d \geq 1 \tag{4}$$

The aim in time series data analysis and prediction is to find a model to provide with a good accuracy a future value of the series. Some research directions indicate as important the immediate future value (see eq.(2)) whereas other problems may indicate a further interval of interest, that it is, the prediction of the following m values of time series:

$$a_m = f(a_1, a_2, \dots a_n), \quad m \in [n+1, n+k], \quad k > 0 \tag{5}$$

We provide below definitions for ARMA model [1] just in terms of highlighting the main track but also our different approach based on the moving average of the nth-order difference.

Definition 4. ***Auto-Regressive Model (ARM)*** *provides a way to express the prediction of the following value in the initial time series by using previous finite number of values affected by white noise and ARM of order q is defined by [1]:*

$$X_t = \sum_{i=1}^{p} a_i X_{t-i} + \varepsilon_t \tag{6}$$

where a_i is the auto-regressive coefficient, X_t is the series under investigation, p is the length of the filter, which is commonly less than the length of the series, and ε_t is a white noise process with zero mean and variance σ^2.

Definition 5. ***Moving Average Model (MAM)*** *of order q is defined as [1]:*

$$X_t = \sum_{i=1}^{q} b_i \varepsilon_{t-i} + \varepsilon_t \tag{7}$$

where b_i is the moving average coefficient, X_t is the series under investigation, q is the length of the filter, which is commonly less than the length of the series, and ε_t represents the error (noise) terms.

Definition 6. ***Auto-Regressive Moving Average (ARMA)*** *model contains infinite (ARM(p)) and finite (MAM(q)) models [1]:*

$$X_t = \sum_{i=1}^{p} a_i X_{t-i} + \sum_{i=1}^{q} b_i \varepsilon_{t-i} + \varepsilon_t \tag{8}$$

Definition 7. ***Linear Regression*** *is a regression method that models the relationship between a dependent variable Y, independent variables X_i, $i = 1, \dots, r$ and a random term ε. The model can be written as:*

$$Y = c_0 + \sum_{i=1}^{r} c_i X_i + \varepsilon \tag{9}$$

where c_0 is the intercept ("constant" term), the c_i are the respective parameters of independent variables and r is the number of parameters to be estimated in the Linear Regression.

Our approach addresses the latter, where the range for the best approximation is also an objective of the algorithm.

3 The Algorithm of Moving Average of nth-order Difference for Bounded Time Series Prediction

Our approach is based on the notion of the difference operator [5] of bounded time series: a nth-order difference array is used to analyze the moving average to predict value(s) for the next period.

Definition 8. ***The Forward Difference Operator*** *for a given functional f with real values a calculates:*

$$\Delta f(a) = f(a+1) - f(a) \tag{10}$$

$\Delta f(a)$ is called first-order difference (or simply difference) of $f(a)$. Following the same principle, the second-order difference is defined:

$$\begin{aligned} \Delta^2 f(a) &= \Delta f(a+1) - \Delta f(a) \\ &= (f(a+2) - f(a+1)) - (f(a+1) - f(a)) \\ &= f(a+2) - 2f(a+1) + f(a) \end{aligned} \tag{11}$$

It's easy to induce that the nth-order difference is defined by:

$$\Delta^n f(a) = \sum_{i=0}^{n} (-1)^{n-i} C_n^i f(a+i) \tag{12}$$

where $C_n^i = \binom{i}{n} = \frac{n!}{i!(n-i)!}$, $0 \le i \le n$ *is the binomial coefficient.*

Definition 9. ***Moving Average*** *is a way of smoothing by averaging n terms of the time series. In mathematics and statistics, moving average is used as a generic smoothing operation or an example of a convolution. A simple moving average is the un-weighted (or weight = 1) mean of previous data points:*

$$SMA_m = \frac{P_1 + P_2 + P_3 + \cdots + P_m}{m} \tag{13}$$

$$\textit{where } m = 1, 2, 3, \cdots$$

Considering the last equation on n, we can find out that the same rule applies for $n+1$: Therefore, based on the induction principle (Peano) eq.(12) is valid for any natural value of n. If $f(a)$, with n a natural number, generates a discrete series a_m, then the previous result can be written (eq.(12))

$$\begin{aligned} \Delta^n f(m) &= \Delta^{n-1} f(m+1) - \Delta^{n-1} f(m) \\ D_m^n &= D_{m+1}^{n-1} - D_m^{n-1} \end{aligned} \tag{14}$$

$$\textit{where } D_m^n \textit{ means } \Delta^n f(m)$$

The proof for eq.(14), a nth-order difference equals the difference of two lower differences ($(n-1)^{th}$-order) is presented in the Appendix.

The nth-order difference is used in the binomial transform of a function, the Newton forward difference equation and the Newton series [5]. These are very useful prediction relationships with the main drawback of difficult numerical evaluation because of rapid grow of the binomial coefficients for large n.

In order to avoid a complex calculus and also to provide a relationship for time series prediction, our idea relates to the fact that applying the difference operator we generate another data series from the initial one, which has the property of pseudo-periodicity [11]. Since the initial series are bounded, the data series generated by the difference operator are also bounded and their average converges to zero.

We provide a proof for this result below, exemplified with the monthly average of Sunspot Number data set case of 600 months values (Fig. 1 - 3).

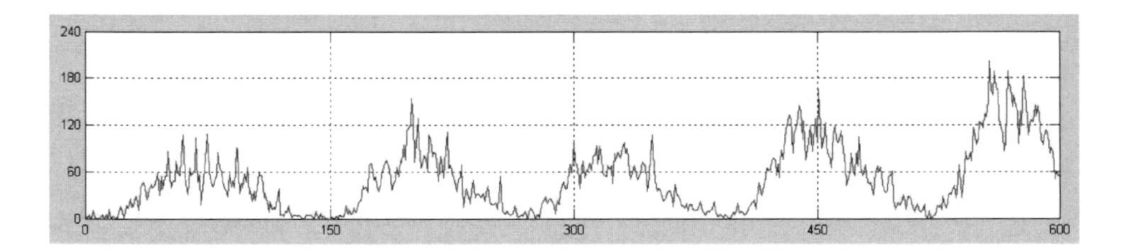

Fig. 1. The Monthly Average Values of Sunspot Number Time Series for 600 Months

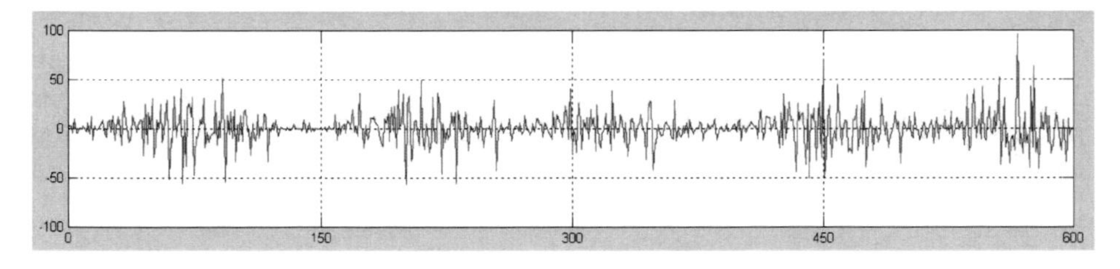

Fig. 2. First-order Difference (D_m^1) of Monthly Average of Sunspot Number Time Series

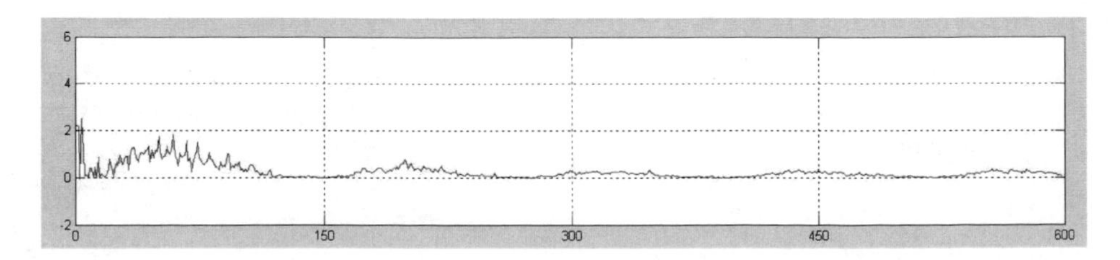

Fig. 3. The Moving Average (E_m^1) of First-order Difference (D_m^1) of Monthly Average of Sunspot Number Time Series

Let D_m^1 represent the first-order difference of initial data set a_m, then:

$$D_m^1 = a_{m+1} - a_m, \quad m \geq 1 \tag{15}$$

as represented in Fig.2.

The first-order difference time series shows a pseudo-periodical bounded shape with amplitude modulated in time. The average of first-order difference time series for initial data set a_m can then be constructed as:

$$E_m^1 = \frac{1}{m}(D_1^1 + D_2^1 + \cdots + D_m^1) = \frac{1}{m}\sum_{i=1}^{m} D_i^1 \tag{16}$$

We calculate below the limit of time series E_m^1 (for an easy calculation we can consider the following)

$$\lim_{m\to\infty} E_m^1 = \lim_{m\to\infty} \frac{1}{m}\sum_{i=1}^{m} D_i^1 \tag{17}$$

And therefore, based on eq.(15) and eq.(17):

$$\begin{aligned}
\lim_{m\to\infty} E_m^1 &= \lim_{m\to\infty} \frac{1}{m}\sum_{i=1}^{m}(a_{i+1} - a_i) \\
&= \lim_{m\to\infty} \frac{1}{m}\big((a_{m+1} - a_m) + (a_m - a_{m-1}) + \cdots + (a_2 - a_1)\big) \\
&= \lim_{m\to\infty} \frac{1}{m}(a_{m+1} - a_1) \\
&= \lim_{m\to\infty} \frac{a_{m+1}}{m} - \lim_{m\to\infty} \frac{a_1}{m}
\end{aligned} \tag{18}$$

For a large m, since a_1 is a limited value, the second term in eq.(18) becomes negligible. Also a_{n+1} is a limited value given the initial constraints on bounded time series we consider of interest and therefore the first term in eq.(18) has a null limit also:

$$\lim_{m\to\infty} E_m^1 = \big(\lim_{m\to\infty} \frac{a_{m+1}}{m} - \lim_{m\to\infty} \frac{a_1}{m}\big) \to 0 \tag{19}$$

Indeed, one can easily see this result is verified for our practical example in Fig.3. Based on the result in eq.(19) as depicted in Fig.3, given a time series $\{a_m\}$, with first-order difference $\{D_m^1\}$, our aim is to determine the value for $\{a_{m+1}\}$ (prediction) based on previous data measurements (and some negligible error). The average for first-order difference (term $n-1$) values is easy to calculate:

$$E_{m-1}^1 = \frac{1}{m-1}(D_1^1 + D_2^1 + \cdots + D_{m-1}^1) \tag{20}$$

Since $E_m^1 \to 0$ for large values of m, then:

$$E_m^1 = E_{m-1}^1 + \varepsilon \tag{21}$$

where $\varepsilon > 0$ is a negligible error for large m. Replacing in eq.(21) E^1_{n-2} from eq.(20):

$$\frac{1}{m}\sum_{i=1}^{m} D^1_i = \frac{1}{m-1}\sum_{i=1}^{m-1} D^1_i + \varepsilon \tag{22}$$

And therefore, from eq.(16)

$$\frac{1}{m}(\sum_{i=1}^{m-1} D^1_i + D^1_m) = \frac{1}{m-1}(\sum_{i=1}^{m-1} D^1_i) + \varepsilon$$

$$D^1_m = m(\frac{1}{m-1}\sum_{i=1}^{m-1} D^1_i + \varepsilon) - \sum_{i=1}^{m-1} D^1_i \tag{23}$$

and because $D^1_m = a_{m+1} - a_m$, we obtain:

$$a_{m+1} = a_m + m(\frac{1}{m-1}\sum_{i=1}^{m-1} D^1_i + \varepsilon) - \sum_{i=1}^{m-1} D^1_i \tag{24}$$

The prediction precision for a_m depends on the nth-order difference D^n_m; in other words, precision of prediction increases in accuracy with the value of m and the order of the difference n. For simplicity, consider the first-order difference of the original bounded pseudo-periodical time series from eq.(24):

$$\begin{aligned} a_{m+1} &= a_m + \frac{m}{m-1}\sum_{i=1}^{m-1} D^1_i + m\varepsilon - \sum_{i=1}^{m-1} D^1_i \\ &= a_m + \frac{1}{m-1}\sum_{i=1}^{m-1} D^1_i + m\varepsilon \end{aligned} \tag{25}$$

and replacing the difference D as from eq.(15):

$$\begin{aligned} a_{m+1} &= a_m + \frac{1}{m-1}(a_m - a_1) + m\varepsilon \\ &= \frac{1}{m-1}(ma_m - a_1) + m\varepsilon \end{aligned} \tag{26}$$

Eq.(26), obtained by considering the average series of first-order difference, suggests a practical way to approximate the prediction a_{m+1} based on previous values a_m and a_1. For large numbers, although the error value is negligible (see eq.(19) and (21) and Fig.3) the accuracy of prediction may still be affected.

At the same time, the moving average E^n_m can be expressed in terms of nth-order difference as:

$$E^n_m = \frac{1}{m}(D^{n-1}_{m+1} - D^{n-1}_1) \tag{27}$$

This is proven by mathematical induction:

$$E_m^n = \frac{1}{m}\sum_{k=1}^{m} D_k^n = \frac{1}{m}(D_{m+1}^{n-1} - D_1^{n-1}) \tag{28}$$

When $n = 1$ *and* $n = 2$*:*

$$\begin{aligned} E_m^1 &= \frac{1}{m}\sum_{k=1}^{m} D_k^1 \\ &= \frac{1}{m}\big((a_{m+1} - a_m) + (a_m - a_{m-1}) + \cdots + (a_3 - a_2) + (a_2 - a_1)\big) \\ &= \frac{1}{m}(a_{m+1} - a_1) \\ &= \frac{1}{m}(D_{m+1}^0 - D_1^0) \end{aligned} \tag{29}$$

$$\begin{aligned} E_m^2 &= \frac{1}{m}\sum_{k=1}^{m} D_k^2 \\ &= \frac{1}{m}\big((a_{m+2} - 2a_{m+1} + a_m) + (a_{m+1} - 2a_m + a_{m-1}) \\ &\qquad + \cdots + (a_4 - 2a_3 + a_2) + (a_3 - 2a_2 + a_1)\big) \\ &= \frac{1}{m}\big((a_{m+2} - a_{m+1}) - (a_2 - a_1)\big) \\ &= \frac{1}{m}(D_{m+1}^1 - D_1^1) \end{aligned} \tag{30}$$

The statement in eq.(28) is verified for $n = 1$ *and* $n = 2$*.*

We assume the statement is true for n*:*

$$E_m^n = \frac{1}{m}\sum_{k=1}^{m} D_k^n = \frac{1}{m}(D_{m+1}^{n-1} - D_1^{n-1}) \tag{31}$$

Then for $n + 1$*:*

$$\begin{aligned} E_m^{n+1} &= \frac{1}{m}\sum_{k=1}^{m} D_k^{n+1} \\ &= \frac{1}{m}(D_m^{n+1} + D_{m-1}^{n+1} + \cdots + D_2^{n+1} + D_1^{n+1}) \\ &= \frac{1}{m}\big((D_{m+1}^n - D_m^n) + (D_m^n - D_{m-1}^n) + \cdots + (D_3^n - D_2^n) + (D_2^n - D_1^n)\big) \\ &= \frac{1}{m}(D_{m+1}^n - D_1^n) \end{aligned} \tag{32}$$

qed.

So for higher order differences, their moving average series for a large value L, where L is in reality still a large but finite value, is:

$$\lim_{m \to L} E_m^n = \lim_{m \to L} (\frac{1}{m} \sum_{k=1}^{m} D_k^n)$$
$$= \lim_{m \to L} (\frac{1}{m} (D_{m+1}^{n-1} - D_1^{n-1})) \tag{33}$$

Since the nth-order difference D_m^n is bounded, then exists a real limited number C for which $|D_{m+1}^{n-1} - D_1^{n-1}| \leq C$;

As a result,

$$\lim_{m \to L} E_m^n = \lim_{m \to L} (\frac{1}{m} \sum_{k=1}^{m} D_k^n) = \lim_{m \to L} (\frac{1}{m} (D_{m+1}^{n-1} - D_1^{n-1})) \to \frac{C}{L} \tag{34}$$

and the Fig.4 shows a map of the limit of the differences:

$$\lim_{m \to L} E_m^n \to \frac{C}{L} \qquad \text{where } \{m|1 \leq m \leq 100\} \text{ and } \{n|1 \leq n \leq 100\}$$

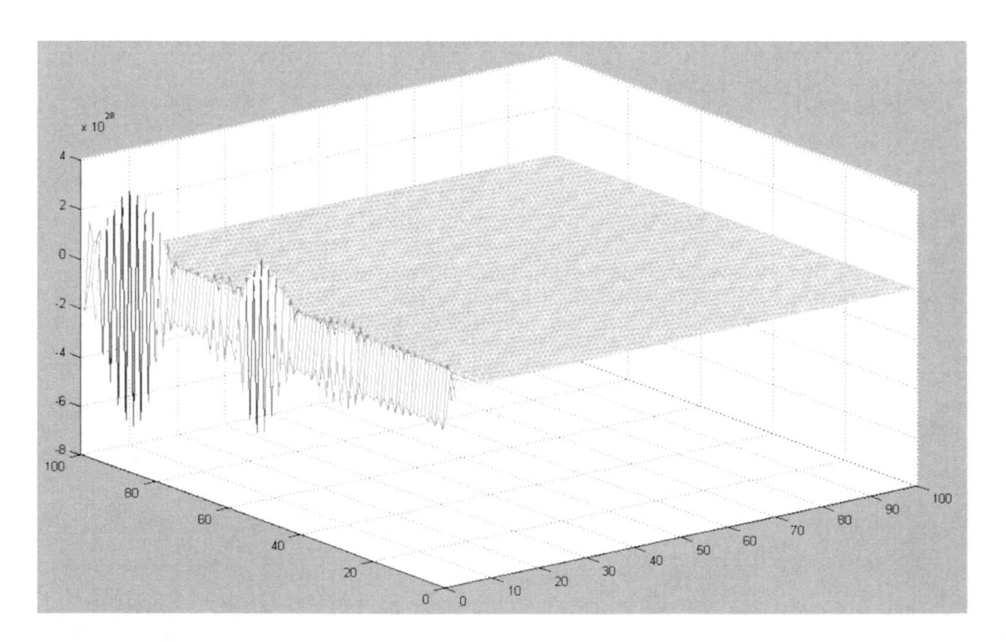

Fig. 4. A Map of Moving Average of nth-order Difference's Limit for Sunspot Number Data Set (X and Y Coordinate Axes Indicate the indexes of Time Intervals; Z Coordinate Axis Denotes the Values of Limit of Moving Average of nth-order Difference for m Data Samples)

The Moving Average of nth-order Difference (MAonDA) algorithm (in pseudo-codes) below implements the results described above for a general time series A (Table 1)

Table 1. An Moving Average of nth-order Difference Algorithm (MAonDA)

```
Input: An Initial Time Series Data;
Method: Moving Average of nth-order Difference Algorithm;
Output: Predicted Time Series Data;
```

```
01. // Input the time series data set;
02. SET A[ ] to READ(An Initial Time Series Data Set)
03. // L records the size of data sequence;
04. SET L to the length of A[ ]
05. // Set maximum difference order level;
06. SET n to value of difference order level
07. // Set the index of difference and it starts from 0;
09. SET counter to 0
10. // Calculate the nth-order difference D[ ] of A[ ]
11. WHILE counter < L-n
12.     SET D[counter] from CALCULATE difference of A[ ]
13. ENDWHILE
14. // Set the index of moving average and it starts from 0;
16. SET counter to 0
17. // Compute the moving average E[ ] of D[ ];
18. FOR each of D[ ]
19.     SET sumTemp to 0
20.     FOR each term of D[0] to D[counter]
21.         SET sumTemp to sum of term of D[0] to D[counter]
22.     ENDFOR
23.     SET E[counter] to divide sumTemp by counter
24.     INCREASE counter
25. ENDFOR
26. // Get the error value by using ANN;
27. GET error from ANN(E[ ])
28. // Give two values Ln and Lm for Finding Function inputs
29. SET Ln and Lm
30. FOR n = 0 to Ln
31.     FOR m = 0 to Lm
32.         SET F[n][m] to COMPUTE Finding Function result
33.     ENDFOR
34. ENDFOR
35. SET Do[n][m] to COMPUTE from A[ ]
36. GET Theta[n][m] to ||F[n][m] - Do[n][m]||
37. GET (m,n) from find(Theta == min(Theta[n][m]))
38. GET the prediction value based on (m,n)
39. OUTPUT(predicted value)
```

4 Finding Suitable Index m and Order Level n for Increasing the Prediction Precision

Now, we have two formulae here:

$$D_m^n = \sum_{i=0}^{n} (-1)^{n-i} C_n^i a_{m+i} = D_{m+1}^{n-1} - D_m^{n-1} \tag{35}$$

$$\sum_{j=1}^{m} D_j^n = D_{m+1}^{n-1} - D_1^{n-1} \tag{36}$$

Based on the above results, we have:

$$E_m^n = \begin{cases} E_{m-1}^n + \varepsilon & \text{if } \varepsilon \neq 0 \\ E_{m-1}^n & \text{if } \varepsilon \cong 0 \end{cases} \tag{37}$$

Then, take eq.(35) and eq.(36) into eq.(37):

$$\begin{aligned} E_m^n &= E_{m-1}^n + \varepsilon \quad \Longleftrightarrow \\ D_{m+1}^{n-1} &= \frac{m}{m-1}\left(D_m^{n-1} + (m-1)\varepsilon\right) - \frac{1}{m-1} D_1^{n-1} \end{aligned} \tag{38}$$

And let $n = n - 1$ in eq.(38) so that:

$$D_{m+1}^n = \frac{m}{m-1}\left(D_m^n + (m-1)\varepsilon\right) + \frac{-1}{m-1} D_1^n \tag{39}$$

Thus, the coefficients can be seen as special "weights" related to two terms of the same order difference level, and they depend on the "start" and the "end" period's values. For greater accuracy (when $\varepsilon \neq 0$), we propose the use of an Artificial Neural Network to approximate the error ε in moving average of nth-order difference algorithm for next period. (see eq.(37)). The moving averages E_m^n, E_{m-1}^n are the inputs of a feed-forward ANN with three layers. The trained network is able to get moving average value E_{m+1}^n for further error approximation (see Fig.5). We used for the 2-inputs, 1-output ANN Back-Propagation training algorithm for 1000 epochs.

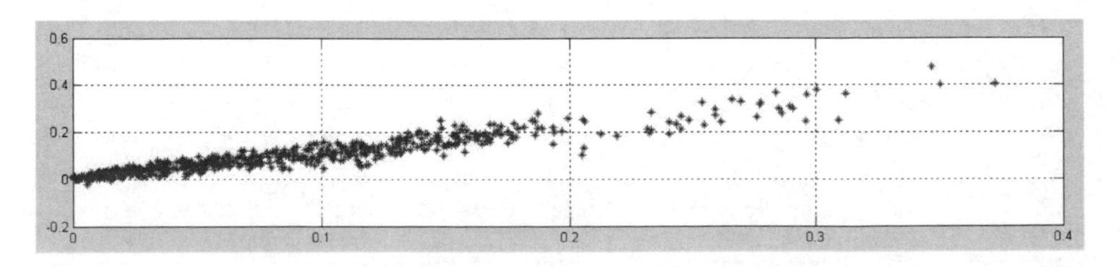

Fig. 5. Analysis and Prediction of Error with Artificial Neural Network

We aim to find a suitable value for m as the prediction of forthcoming value to be well approximated. Since the second "weight" value is negative, and its condition number is so high, eq.(39) is not a "normal" weighted function but Ill-conditioned Function in Short Selling framework [7].

As a result, with $m \to \infty$, its variance increases and the variation of function solution(s) is bigger, therefore the predicted precision may not be good enough. Thus, for $k \in [1, m]$, where m is the length of the initial data series, and the ε is unknown yet, from eq.(39), let:

$$F(k) = \frac{k}{k-1}\left(D_k^n + (k-1)\varepsilon\right) + \frac{-1}{k-1} D_1^n \tag{40}$$

then calculate D_{m+1}^n from the original data set (eq.(12)); next, we suppose Θ represents their Manhattan Distance:

$$\Theta(k) = \|F(k) - D_{k+1}^n\| \tag{41}$$

From the array $\Theta(k)$ we found that, where $\Theta(k_{min}) = \min$, $F(k_{min})$ is the closest value to the real difference D_{m+1}^n. Our aim is to determine the value m for which a_{m+1} is approximated based on the previous data measurements $a_1, a_2, \ldots, a_m$. Fig.6 shows an example of Θ_k^n (when $n = 1$ and $k \in [1, 600]$).

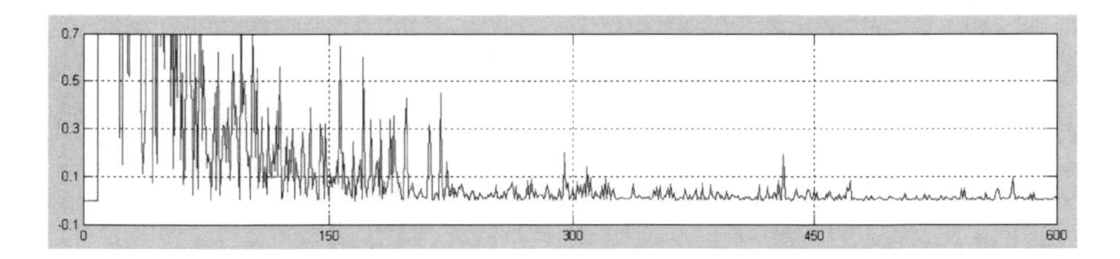

Fig. 6. The values of series: Θ_m^n, when $n = 1, m \in [1, 600]$

According to eq.(41), we may choose a large value of index L_m and order level L_n to locate suitable m and n in:

$$F_{m \times n} = \frac{m}{m-1}\left(D_m^n\right) + \frac{-1}{m-1} D_1^n \tag{42}$$

$$\Theta_{m \times n} = \|F_{m \times n} - D_{m+1}^n\| \quad \text{where } m \in [1, L_m] \text{ and } n \in [1, L_n] \tag{43}$$

in order to identify the area of minimum values.

Fig.7 shows a map of matrix $\Theta_{m \times n}$, where $m \in [1, 500]$ and $n \in [1, 20]$. From eq.(41) we can infer from $\Theta_{m_{min} \times n_{min}} = \min$ to propose the suitable index m_{min} and order level n_{min} for increasing the prediction precision.

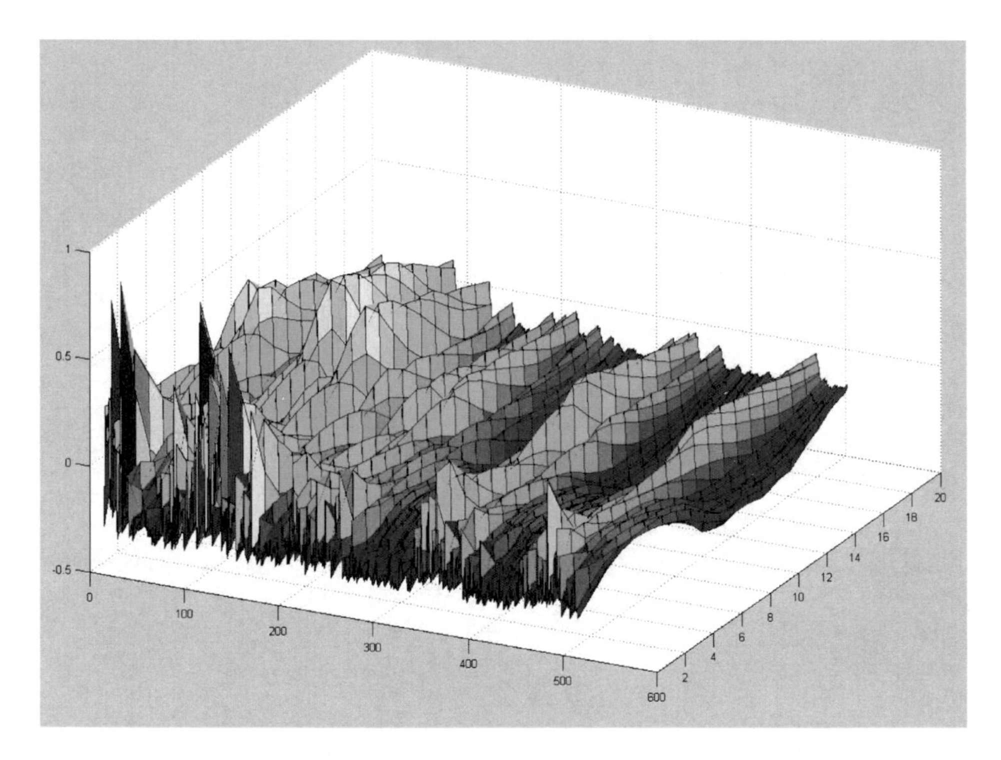

Fig. 7. The Value Map of Matrix: Θ for Sunspot Number Data Set, Where $m \in [1, 500]$ and $n \in [1, 20]$

5 Prediction Results for Sunspot Number Time Series

Early research showing that sunspots have a cycle period start in modern times with George Ellery Hale: he found that the sunspot cycle period is 22 years, because the magnetic polarity of sunspots reverses after 11 years. Rudolf Wolf proposed in 1849 in Zürich to count sunspot numbers by what is nowadays called "Wolfer Number" or "International Sunspot Number" using numeric values related to sunspots' number and size, their geographical location and instrumentation used.

Based on sunspots characterization and observations, Time Series Sunspot Data Set is an ordered data set of sunspot numbers based on observation, which can be treated as a tracking record of solar activities. Of course from the point of view of Definition 3, sunspot data is a pseudo-periodical time series, since there is not a fixed value d, but a series of values with an average of about 22 years (273 month).

The original time series of sunspot number used hereby as a generic data set to describe the application of our algorithm has been generated by the National Geophysical Data Center (NGDC). NGDC provides stewardship, products and services for geophysical data describing the solid earth, marine, and solar-terrestrial environment, as well as earth observations from space [13]. Its data bases currently contain more than 300 digital and analog databases, which include Land, Marine, Satellite, Snow, Ice, Solar-Terrestrial subjects.

NGDC's sunspots databases contain multiform original data from astronomical observatories; the sunspot data sets list various sunspots' attributes in time order, even others solar activities related to sunspots. The time series sunspot data taken as input to the proposed algorithm is based on measurements recorded everyday by observatories through more than 200 years (Fig.8). We used the average sunspot number per month from 1881 A.D to 1981 A.D, and therefore we use a time series data with 1200 data points. Table 2 lists the configuration of data. (Monthly average value reported to Julian date in format YYYY.MM) and Fig.8 depicts these values.

Table 2. An Example of Monthly Average of Sunspot Number Data Set Organization (Time Format: YYYY.MM)

Index	1	2	···	600	601	···	1199	1200
Time	1901.01	1901.02	···	1950.12	1951.01	···	2000.11	2000.12
Value	0.2	2.4	···	54.1	59.9	···	106.8	104.4

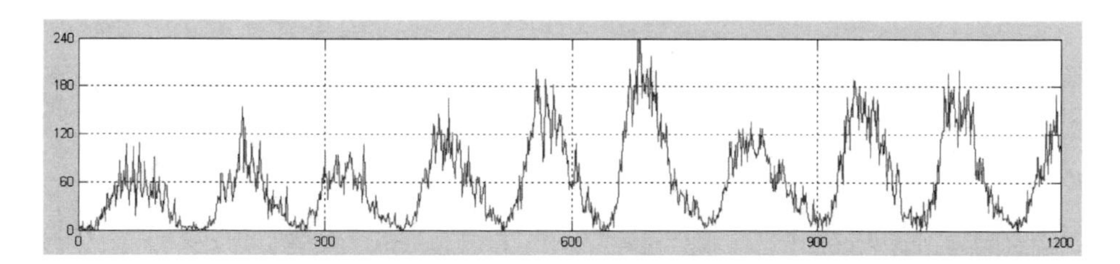

Fig. 8. Monthly Average of Sunspot Number Time Series (X Coordinate Axis Indicates the Index of Time Intervals and Y Coordinate Axis Denotes the Values of Sunspot Number)

The results for the prediction of monthly average of sunspot number [12] are based on values of the fifth-order difference (chose based on the eq.(43)) for the original time series:

$$D_n^5 = a_{n+5} - 5a_{n+4} + 10a_{n+3} - 10a_{n+2} + 5a_{n+1} - a_n \quad (44)$$

which are represented in Fig.9. The average of the difference time series is represented in Fig.10, the prediction of the monthly average of sunspot data generated by our algorithm is given in Fig.11, the prediction of error values using a supervised-trained artificial neural network (ANN) is showed in Fig.12.

We compared the predicted values obtained by running the proposed algorithm MAonDA (for the fifth-order difference) with the original sunspot time

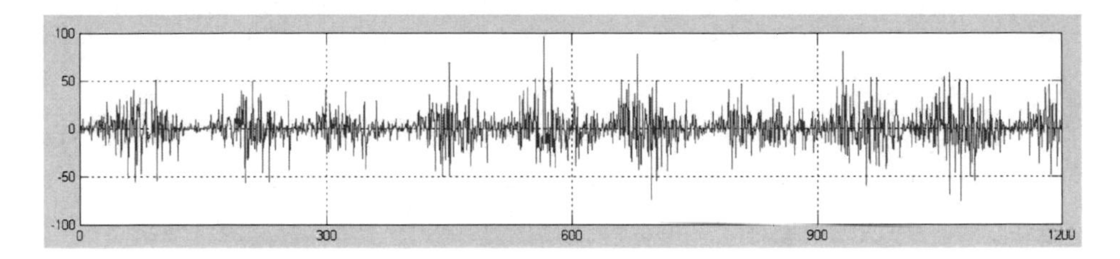

Fig. 9. Fifth-order Difference of Monthly Average of Sunspot Number Time Series

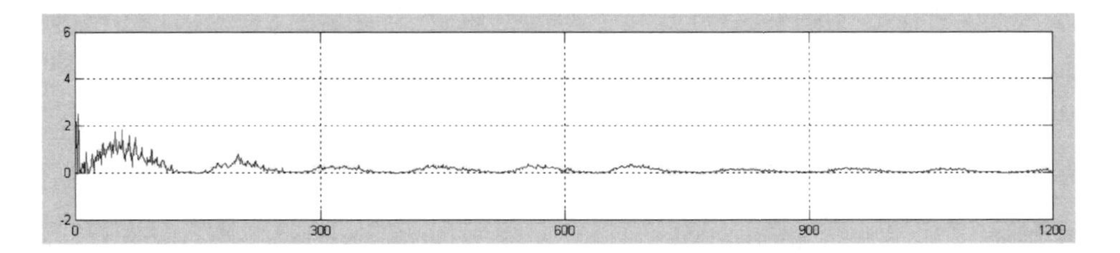

Fig. 10. The Moving Average of Fifth-order Difference of Monthly Average of Sunspot Number Time Series

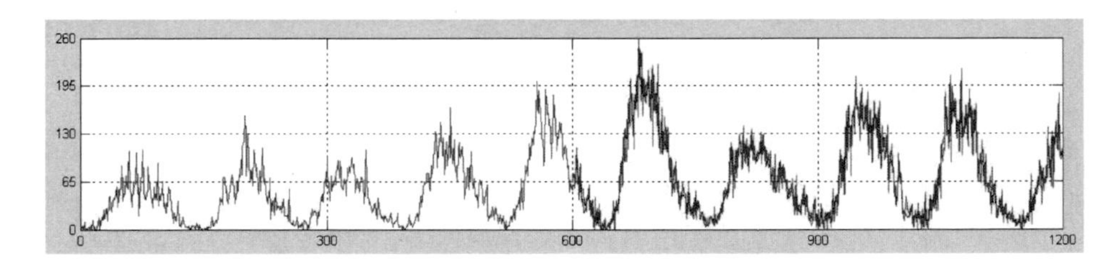

Fig. 11. The Prediction of Values for Monthly Average of Sunspot Number Time Series Based on the Proposed Algorithm

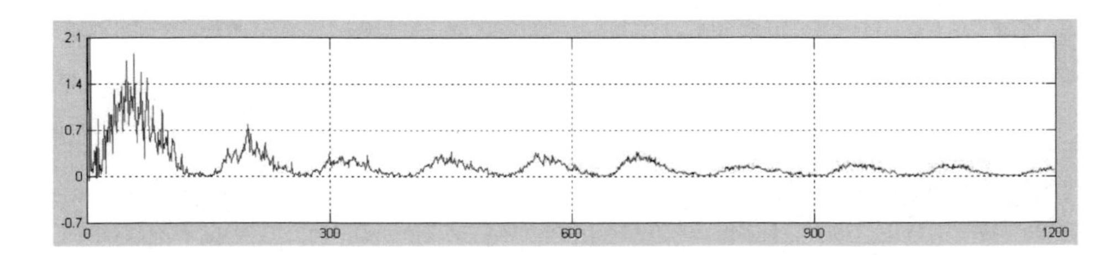

Fig. 12. The Prediction of Error Values Using a Supervised-trained Artificial Neural Network (ANN)

series values and the predictions of a Linear Regression Model (Least-squares Analysis [3] [4]) - the results are depicted in Fig.23. The new algorithm shows a better prediction of time series and suitability to follow closely abnormal trends in the time series, based on tuning parameters m and n (eq.(43)).

6 Prediction Results for Earthquake Time Series

NGDC acquires, processes, and analyzes technical data on earthquake hazards, and disseminates the data in many useable formats. For example, Significant Earthquake Database contains information on more than 5,000 destructive earthquakes from 2150 B.C. to the present; Earthquake Slide Sets NGDC offers fourteen 35-mm slide sets depicting earthquake damage throughout the world; Earthquake Intensity Database contains damage and felt reports for over 22,000 U.S. earthquakes from 1638 to 1985; Worldwide Strong Motion Data Archive contains more than 15,000 digitized and processed accelerograph records over 60 years; The Seismograph Station Bulletins Database contains more than 500,000 microfiche pages from seismograph station bulletins for the years 1900 to 1965. Table 3 shows an example of typical earthquakes time series [13].

Table 3. An Example of Earthquakes Time Series Data Organization

Index	Time	Location	Magnitude	Longitude	Latitude
1	1001.01	China	6.2	34.300	109.000
2	1001.01	Italy	7.0	42.000	13.500
⋮	⋮	⋮	⋮	⋮	⋮
672	1500.01	Hawaii	6.8	19.000	-155.500
⋮	⋮	⋮	⋮	⋮	⋮
1350	2006.08	Argentina	5.6	-33.131	-68.707
1351	2006.08	France	4.3	44.000	6.800

We applied the proposed algorithm (Table 1) for NGDC earthquakes data (see Fig.13) using the fifth-order difference (see Fig.14). Given the pseudo-periodical time series constraint satisfied, the moving average of the fifth-order difference for earthquake time series prediction is around 0 (Fig.15) and therefore our algorithm provides satisfactory results in this case as well.

Figs.13 - 17 show the results for the prediction of earthquakes time series, based on MAonDA algorithm with the fifth-order difference. Fig.13 shows the initial earthquakes time series; Fig.14 represents the values of fifth-order difference earthquakes time series; Fig.15 depicts the moving average of difference earthquakes time series; Fig.16 shows the prediction of earthquakes by using our algorithm and Fig.17 shows the prediction of error values using a supervised-trained artificial neural network (ANN).

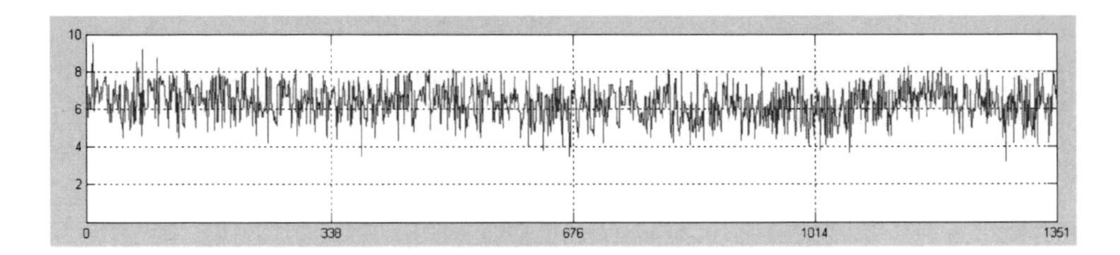

Fig. 13. An Initial Earthquakes Time Series

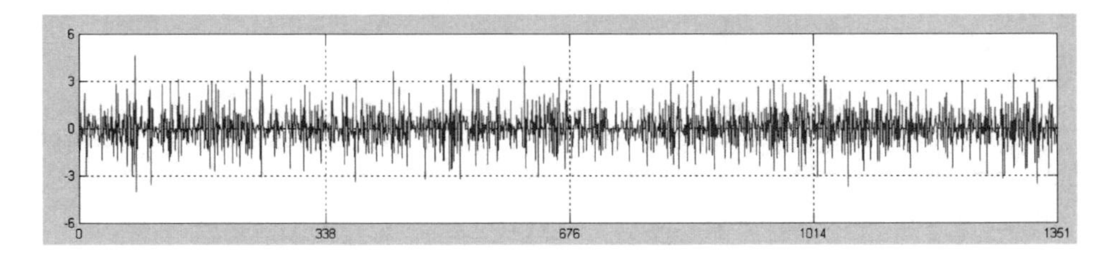

Fig. 14. The Values of Fifth-order Difference of Earthquakes Time Series

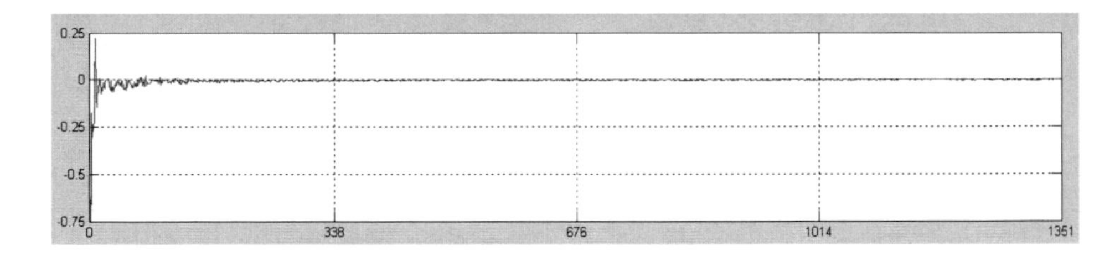

Fig. 15. The moving average of Difference Earthquakes Time Series

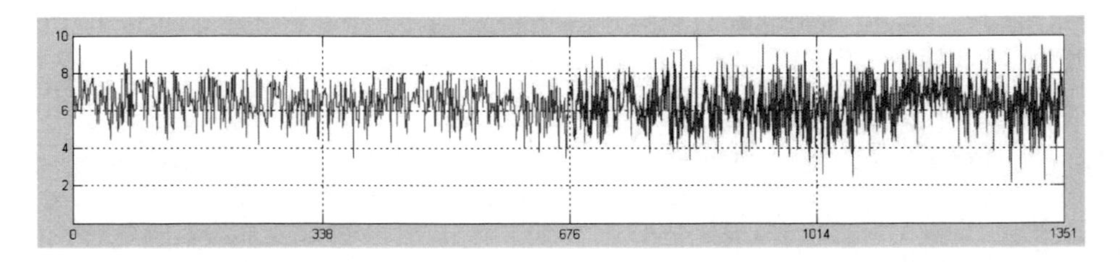

Fig. 16. The Prediction Values of Earthquakes Time Series by the moving average of nth-order Difference Algorithm (MAonDA)

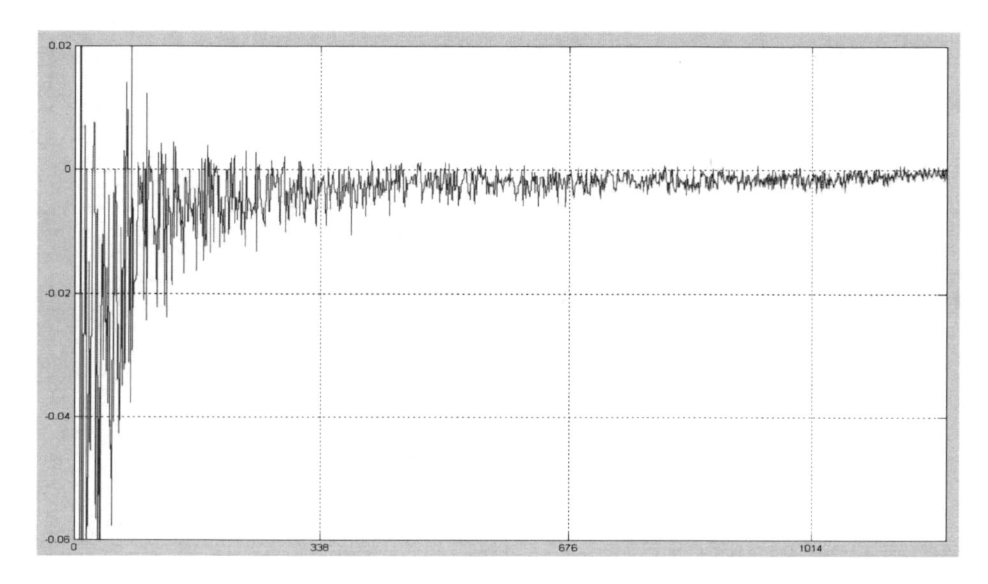

Fig. 17. The Prediction of Error Values Using a Supervised-trained Artificial Neural Network (ANN)

7 Prediction Results for Pseudo-Periodical Synthetic Time Series

The pseudo-periodical synthetic time series data set has been taken from Knowledge Discovery in Databases Archive (KDD Archive), University of California, Irvine [9]. KDD Archive is an online repository of large data sets which encompasses a wide variety of data types, analysis tasks, and application areas. This time series data set is designed for testing indexing schemes in time series databases; The data appears highly periodic, but never exactly repeats itself. This feature is designed to challenge the indexing tasks. This time series data [10] is generated by independent invocations of the function:

$$\overline{y} = \sum_{i=3}^{7} \frac{1}{2^i} \sin(2\pi(2^{2+i} + rand(2^i))\overline{t}), \quad 0 \leq \overline{t} \leq 1 \tag{45}$$

where the function *rand(x)* produces a random integer between *0* and x.

Figs.18 - 20 show the results for the prediction of pseudo-periodical synthetic time series, based on MAonDA algorithm with the fifth-order difference. Fig.18 shows the initial pseudo-periodical synthetic time series; Fig.19 represents the values of fifth-order difference pseudo-periodical synthetic time series; Fig.21 depicts the moving average of difference pseudo-periodical synthetic time series; Fig.22 shows the prediction of pseudo-periodical synthetic time series by using our algorithm and Fig.17 shows the prediction of error values using a supervised-trained artificial neural network (ANN).

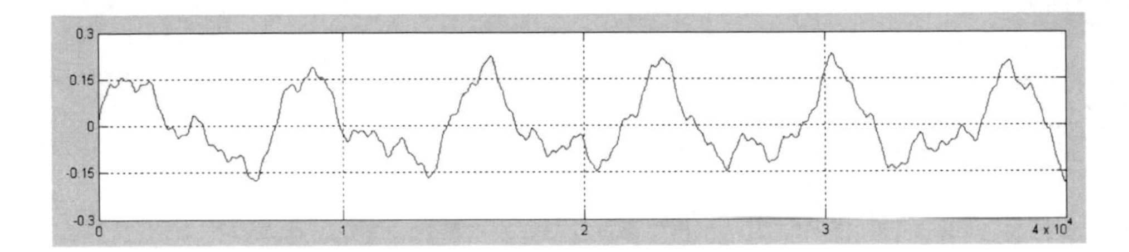

Fig. 18. Fifth-order Difference of Monthly Average of Pseudo-periodical Synthetic Time Series

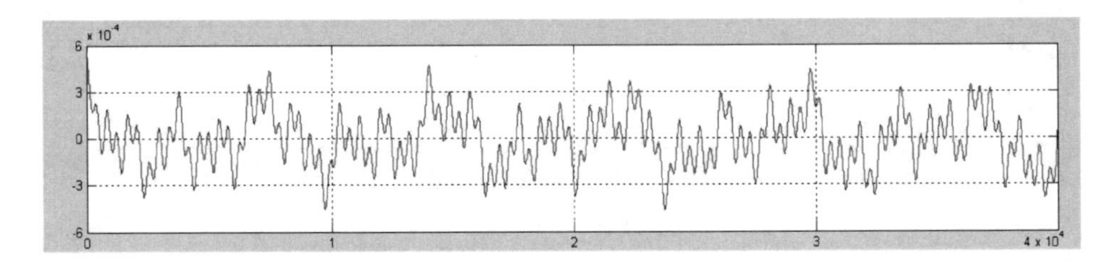

Fig. 19. The Average of Fifth-order Difference of Monthly Average of Pseudo-periodical Synthetic Time Series

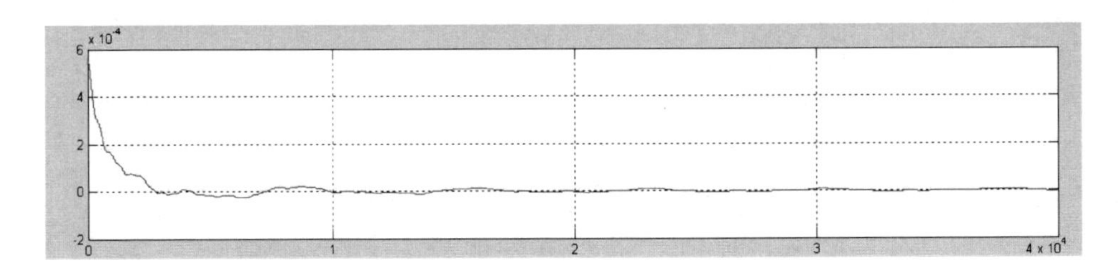

Fig. 20. The Moving Average of Pseudo-periodical Synthetic Time Series

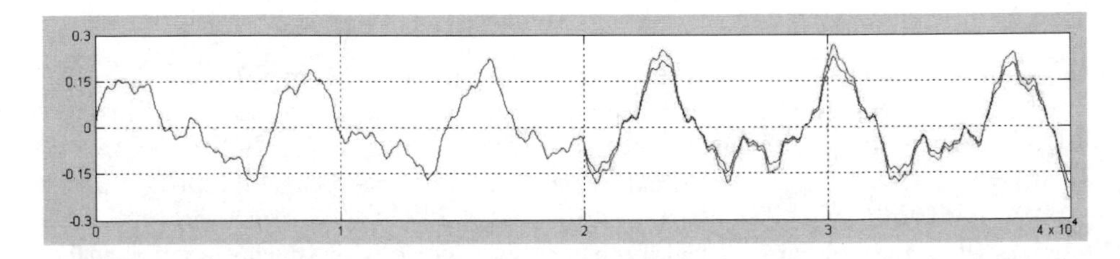

Fig. 21. The Prediction of Values of Pseudo-periodical Synthetic Time Series Based on the Proposed Algorithm

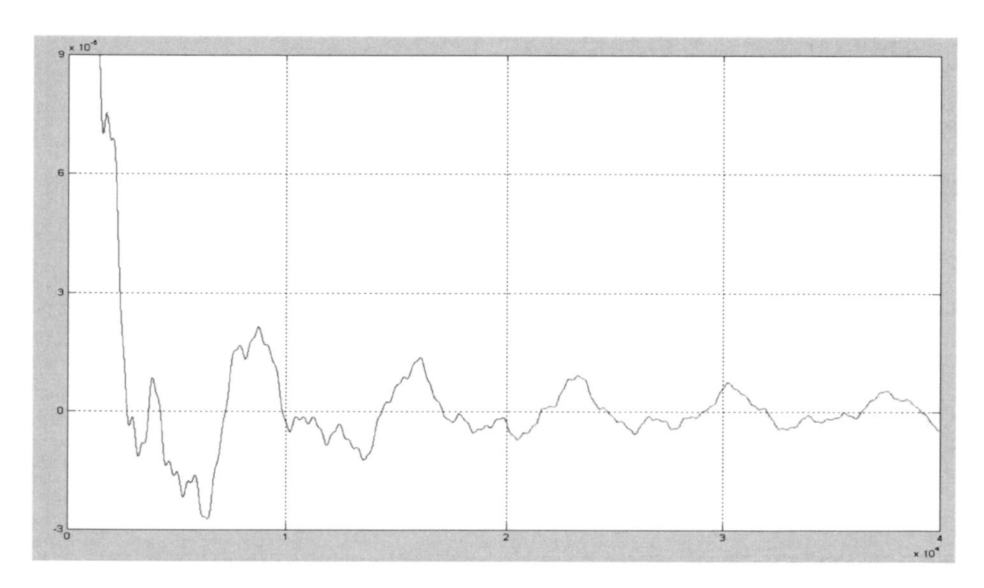

Fig. 22. The Prediction of Error Values Using a Supervised-trained Artificial Neural Network (ANN)

8 Prediction Results Comparison

We also applied the Linear Regression (LR) and Auto-Regression Moving Average (ARMA) algorithm to predict the same sunspot number. In order to check the performance of the algorithms, we used two measures for each prediction method: the Mean Absolute Error (MAE) and Variance-Accounted-For (VAF), to determine how close the predicted values are to the original data sets.

$$E_{MAE} = \frac{1}{N}\sum_{i=1}^{N} \|x_i - \hat{x}_i\| \tag{46}$$

where x_i is prediction value, $\hat{x}_i$ is the original value.

$$E_{VAF} = (1 - \frac{var(y - \hat{y})}{var(y)}) \times 100\% \tag{47}$$

where y is prediction value, $\hat{y}$ is the original value.

Table 4 shows a part of prediction results and also a simplified prediction results comparison for Sunspot Number time series, Earthquakes time series (data sets also from NGDC archive) and Pseudo-periodical Synthetic time series (from KDD archive). As seen in Table 4 and Fig.23, our method provides a better performance for prediction than Linear Regression (LR) and Auto-Regression Moving Average (ARMA), showing lower Mean Absolute Error together with higher Variance-Accounted-For value.

Table 4. Prediction Results Comparison

Sunspot Number Time Series				
Original Values		Prediction Values		
Index	Data	LR	ARMA	MAonDA
600	54.1	55.5154	37.2149	65.7349
601	59.9	65.1697	46.2715	69.3329
⋮	⋮	⋮	⋮	⋮
1191	121.6	5.3972	112.4148	131.4633
1192	124.9	-0.8012	133.6800	146.4852
⋮	⋮	⋮	⋮	⋮
1199	106.8	17.7101	78.7586	97.7593
1200	104.4	22.1878	97.3603	119.1860
E_{MAE}	–	32.2534	20.9931	**15.8002**
E_{VAF}	–	56.70%	70.54%	**81.55%**
Earthquakes Time Series				
Original Values		Prediction Values		
Index	Data	LR	ARMA	MAonDA
600	5.9	7.9146	7.3608	7.0165
601	5.9	6.6744	6.0375	5.9932
⋮	⋮	⋮	⋮	⋮
1000	6.4	2.0708	4.4925	4.0482
1001	6.1	4.1234	7.8364	7.4821
⋮	⋮	⋮	⋮	⋮
1350	7.0	6.0659	6.4603	6.1160
1351	6.0	7.9621	7.5586	7.2143
E_{MAE}	–	2.5863	1.6560	**1.4435**
E_{VAF}	–	59.66%	75.03%	**78.10%**
Pseudo-Periodical Synthetic Time Series				
Original Values		Prediction Values		
Index	Data	LR	ARMA	MAonDA
20000	-0.0497	-0.0893	-0.0611	-0.0419
20001	-0.0500	-0.0905	-0.0615	-0.0422
⋮	⋮	⋮	⋮	⋮
35000	-0.0664	-0.0477	-0.0813	-0.0561
35001	-0.0664	-0.0476	-0.0813	-0.0561
⋮	⋮	⋮	⋮	⋮
39999	-0.1850	-0.02565	-0.2322	-0.1563
40000	-0.1850	-0.02634	-0.2322	-0.1562
E_{MAE}	–	0.1396	0.1148	**0.1048**
E_{VAF}	–	94.98%	96.61%	**97.16%**

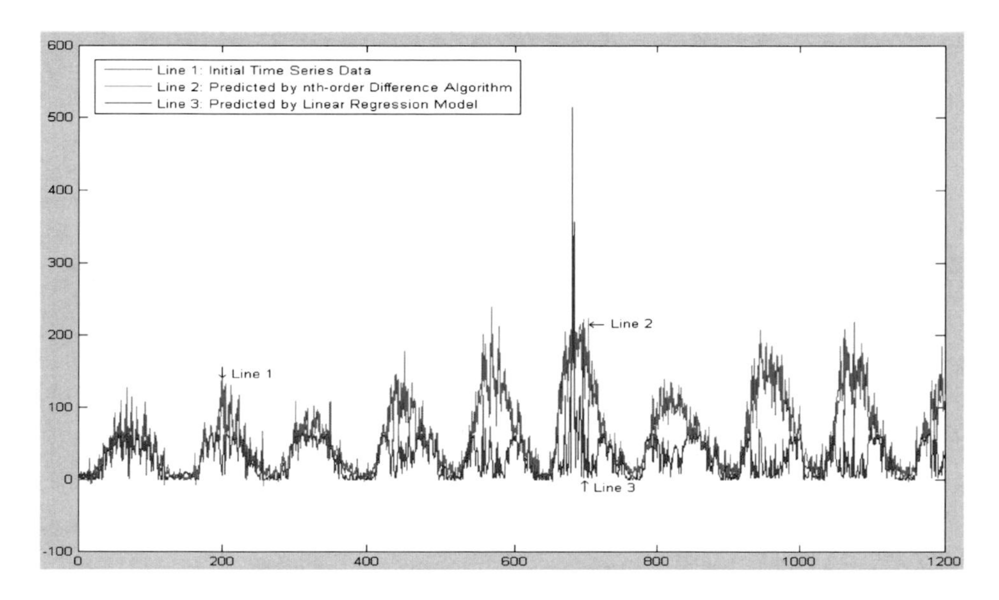

Fig. 23. Prediction Results Compared with Linear Regression Model

9 Conclusions

The moving average of the nth-order difference algorithm proposes a simple approach to reduce the complexity of calculi for prediction in cases of bounded pseudo-periodical time series. We developed an algorithm to predict time series based on a number of previous known values and do not necessarily address the noise but the actual collected values of a time series. The error represents the difference between actual and expected values of moving average. The method also provides a logical development in a transparent way, avoiding the use of Black-box or Grey-box algorithms. We consider further investigating the speed and also the complexity of our solution in comparison with traditional algorithms, such as Auto-Regress Moving Average (ARMA) and also performance issues in comparison with machine learning solutions.

However, this algorithm has the disadvantage of dependency of the (still) error between the average of nth-order difference values at the prediction step, $n+1$ and n. The series average of the nth-order difference algorithm generates therefore a good prediction for the "shape" of the series (including the pseudo-periodicity), but the precision of prediction (amplitude) suffers because of dependence on how many orders (i.e. value of n) difference have been considered, which increases the complexity calculus though and introduces a tuning parameter of the order of difference. A small order of difference reduces the complexity but also the prediction precision, whereas a big order of difference increases the computing effort.

Another direction for further research is the approximation of error in eq.(37) using machine learning techniques, in order to reduce the differences induced by the possibility to obtain a non-zero average of nth-order difference for a period close to the prediction moment (see prediction results differences comparing Fig.8 and Fig.11, Fig.13 and Fig.16, Fig.18 and Fig.21). Provisional encouraging results to approximate the error using a neural network model are depicted in Fig.12, Fig.17 and Fig.22: the connectionist model is trained with the error values for the first 600 cases of Sunspot number time series, the first 675 cases of Earthquakes time series and the first 20000 cases of Pseudo-Periodical Synthetic time series. We propose to study the development of a hybrid model based on the algorithm proposed above by using the average of nth-order difference time series and also a synchronous prediction of the current error given by the trained neural network in an optimized context of a tuned order of the difference.

10 Appendix

The mathematics proof (based on Peano's Induction Axiom) for "a nth-order difference equals the difference of two lower ($(n-1)^t h$-order) differences" (used in eq.(14)):

To Be Proved: $D_m^n = D_{m+1}^{n-1} - D_m^{n-1}$

$$
\begin{aligned}
D_{m+1}^{n-1} &= \sum_{i=0}^{n-1} \frac{(-1)^{(n-1)-i} \cdot (n-1)! \cdot a_{((m+1)+i)}}{i!((n-1)-i)!} \\
&= \frac{(-1)^{(n-1)-0} \cdot (n-1)! \cdot a_{((m+1)+0)}}{0!((n-1)-0)!} \\
&\quad + \frac{(-1)^{(n-1)-1} \cdot (n-1)! \cdot a_{((m+1)+1)}}{1!((n-1)-1)!} \\
&\quad + \cdots\cdots \\
&\quad + \frac{(-1)^{(n-1)-(n-2)} \cdot (n-1)! \cdot a_{((m+1)+(n-2))}}{(n-2)!((n-1)-(n-2))!} \\
&\quad + \frac{(-1)^{(n-1)-(n-1)} \cdot (n-1)! \cdot a_{((m+1)+(n-1))}}{(n-1)!((n-1)-(n-1))!}
\end{aligned}
$$

$$
\begin{aligned}
D_m^{n-1} &= \sum_{i=0}^{n-1} \frac{(-1)^{(n-1)-i} \cdot (n-1)! \cdot a_{(m+i)}}{i!((n-1)-i)!} \\
&= \frac{(-1)^{(n-1)-0} \cdot (n-1)! \cdot a_{(m+0)}}{0!((n-1)-0)!} \\
&\quad + \frac{(-1)^{(n-1)-1} \cdot (n-1)! \cdot a_{(m+1)}}{1!((n-1)-1)!} \\
&\quad + \cdots\cdots
\end{aligned}
$$

$$
\begin{aligned}
&+\frac{(-1)^{(n-1)-(n-2)}\cdot(n-1)!\cdot a_{(m+(n-2))}}{(n-2)!((n-1)-(n-2))!}\\
&+\frac{(-1)^{(n-1)-(n-1)}\cdot(n-1)!\cdot a_{(m+(n-1))}}{(n-1)!((n-1)-(n-1))!}\\
D_{m+1}^{n-1}-D_m^{n-1} &= \sum_{i=0}^{n-1}\frac{(-1)^{(n-1)-i}\cdot(n-1)!\cdot a_{((m+1)+i)}}{i!((n-1)-i)!}\\
&\quad-\sum_{i=0}^{n-1}\frac{(-1)^{(n-1)-i}\cdot(n-1)!\cdot a_{(m+i)}}{i!((n-1)-i)!}\\
&=\frac{(-1)^{(n-1)-(n-1)}\cdot(n-1)!\cdot a_{(m+1)+(n-1)}}{(n-1)!((n-1)-(n-1))!}\\
&\quad+\Big(\frac{(-1)^{(n-1)-(n-2)}\cdot(n-1)!\cdot a_{(m+1)+(n-2)}}{(n-2)!((n-1)-(n-2))!}\\
&\quad-\frac{(-1)^{(n-1)-(n-1)}\cdot(n-1)!\cdot a_{m+(n-1)}}{(n-1)!((n-1)-(n-1))!}\Big)\\
&\quad+\cdots\cdots\\
&\quad+\Big(\frac{(-1)^{(n-1)-0}\cdot(n-1)!\cdot a_{(m+1)+0}}{0!((n-1)-0)!}\\
&\quad-\frac{(-1)^{(n-1)-1}\cdot(n-1)!\cdot a_{m+1}}{1!((n-1)-1)!}\Big)\\
&\quad-\frac{(-1)^{(n-1)-0}\cdot(n-1)!\cdot a_{m+0}}{0!((n-1)-0)!}\\
&=\frac{n}{n}\cdot\frac{(-1)^{n-n}\cdot(n-1)!\cdot a_{m+n}}{0!(n-1)!}\\
&\quad+\Big(\frac{n-1}{n}\cdot\frac{(-1)^{(n-(n-1))}\cdot n!\cdot a_{m+n-1}}{(n-1)!(n-(n-1))!}\\
&\quad-(-1)^{-1}\cdot\frac{1}{n}\cdot\frac{(-1)^{(n-(n-1))}\cdot n!\cdot a_{m+n-1}}{(n-1)!(n-(n-1))!}\Big)\\
&\quad+\cdots\cdots\\
&\quad+\Big(\frac{1}{n}\cdot\frac{(-1)^{(n-1)}\cdot n!\cdot a_{m+1}}{1!(n-1)!}\\
&\quad-(-1)^{-1}\cdot\frac{n-1}{n}\cdot\frac{(-1)^{(n-1)}\cdot n!\cdot a_{m+1}}{1!(n-1)!}\Big)\\
&\quad+\frac{n}{n}\cdot\frac{(-1)^{(n-0)}\cdot(n-1)!\cdot a_{m+0}}{0!((n-1)-0)!}\\
&=\frac{(-1)^{n-n}\cdot n!\cdot a_{m+n}}{n!(n-n)!}+\frac{(-1)^{n-(n-1)}\cdot n!\cdot a_{m+(n-1)}}{(n-1)!(n-(n-1))!}
\end{aligned}
$$

$$
\begin{aligned}
&+\cdots\cdots \\
&+\frac{(-1)^{n-1}\cdot n!\cdot a_{m+1}}{1!(n-1)!}+\frac{(-1)^{n-0}\cdot n!\cdot a_{m+0}}{0!(n-0)!} \\
&=\sum_{i=0}^{n}\frac{(-1)^{n-i}\cdot n!\cdot a_{m+i}}{i!(n-i)!} \\
&=D_m^n
\end{aligned}
$$

References

1. Box, G.E.P., Jenkins, G.M., Reinsel, G.C.: Time Series Analysis: Forecasting and Control. Holden-day San Francisco (1976)
2. Calvo, R.A., Ceccatto, H.A., Piacentini, R.D.: Neural network prediction of solar activity. The Astrophysical Journal 444(2), 916–921 (1995)
3. Cohen, P., Cohen, J., West, S.G., Aiken, L.S.: Applied Multiple Regression/Correlation Analysis for the Behavioral Sciences, 3rd edn. Lawrence Erlbaum, Mahwah (2002)
4. Draper, N.R., Smith, H.: Applied Regression Analysis. John Wiley & Sons Inc., Chichester (1998)
5. Flajolet, P., Sedgewick, R.: Mellin transforms and asymptotics: Finite differences and rice's integrals. Theoretical Computer Science 144(1-2), 101–124 (1995)
6. Giles, C.L., Lawrence, S., Tsoi, A.C.: Noisy time series prediction using recurrent neural networks and grammatical inference. Machine Learning 44(1), 161–183 (2001)
7. Golub, G.H., Loan, C.F.V.: Matrix Computations. Johns Hopkins University Press, Baltimore (1996)
8. Hathaway, D.H., Wilson, R.M., Reichmann, E.J.: The shape of the sunspot cycle. Solar Physics 151(1), 177–190 (1994)
9. KDD: Knowledge discovery in database archive (kdd archive) (2007), `http://kdd.ics.uci.edu/`
10. KDDArchive: Pseudo-periodic synthetic time series (2007), `http://kdd.ics.uci.edu/databases/synthetic/synthetic.html`
11. Lan, Y., Neagu, D.: A New Time Series Prediction Algorithm Based on Moving Average of nth-Order Difference. In: Proceedings of the Sixth International Conference on Machine Learning and Applications, pp. 248–253. IEEE Computer Society, Washington, DC, USA (2007)
12. Lan, Y., Neagu, D.C.: Applications of the Moving Average of nth -Order Difference Algorithm for Time Series Prediction. In: Alhajj, R., Gao, H., Li, X., Li, J., Zaïane, O.R. (eds.) ADMA 2007. LNCS (LNAI), vol. 4632, pp. 264–275. Springer, Heidelberg (2007)
13. NDGC: National geophysical data center (ngdc), `http://www.ngdc.noaa.gov/stp/SOLAR/ftpsunspotregions.html`
14. Saad, E.W., Prokhorov, D.V., Wunsch, D.C.I.: Comparative study of stock trend prediction using time delay, recurrent and probabilistic neural networks. IEEE Transactions on Neural Networks 9(6), 1456–1470 (1998)
15. Simon, G., Lendasse, A., Cottrell, M., Fort, J.C., Verleysen, M.: Time series forecasting: Obtaining long term trends with self-organizing maps. Pattern Recognition Letters 26(12), 1795–1808 (2005)

Chapter 9
Exceptional Model Mining

Arno Knobbe[1], Ad Feelders[2], and Dennis Leman[2]

[1] LIACS, Leiden University, Niels Bohrweg 1,
NL-2333 CA, Leiden, The Netherlands
knobbe@liacs.nl
[2] Utrecht University, P.O. box 80 089,
NL-3508 TB Utrecht, The Netherlands
{ad,dlleman}@cs.uu.nl

Abstract. In most databases, it is possible to identify small partitions of the data where the observed distribution is notably different from that of the database as a whole. In classical subgroup discovery, one considers the distribution of a single nominal attribute, and exceptional subgroups show a surprising increase in the occurrence of one of its values. In this paper, we describe *Exceptional Model Mining* (EMM), a framework that allows for more complicated target concepts. Rather than finding subgroups based on the distribution of a single target attribute, EMM finds subgroups where a model fitted to that subgroup is somehow exceptional. We discuss regression as well as classification models, and define quality measures that determine how exceptional a given model on a subgroup is. Our framework is general enough to be applied to many types of models, even from other paradigms such as association analysis and graphical modeling.

1 Introduction

By and large, subgroup discovery has been concerned with finding regions in the input space where the distribution of a single target variable is substantially different from its distribution in the whole database [3,4]. We propose to extend this idea to targets that are models of some sort, rather than just single variables. Hence, in a very general sense, we want to discover subgroups where a model fitted to the subgroup is substantially different from that same model fitted to the entire database [5].

As an illustrative example, consider the simple linear regression model

$$P_i = a + bS_i + e_i$$

where P is the sales price of a house, S the lot size (measured, say, in square meters), and e the random error term (see Fig. 1 and Section 4 for an actual dataset containing such data). If we think the location of the house might make a difference for the price per square meter, we could consider fitting the same model to the subgroup of houses on a desirable location:

$$P_i = a_D + b_D S_i + e_i,$$

D.E. Holmes, L.C. Jain (Eds.): Data Mining: Found. & Intell. Paradigms, ISRL 24, pp. 183–198.
springerlink.com

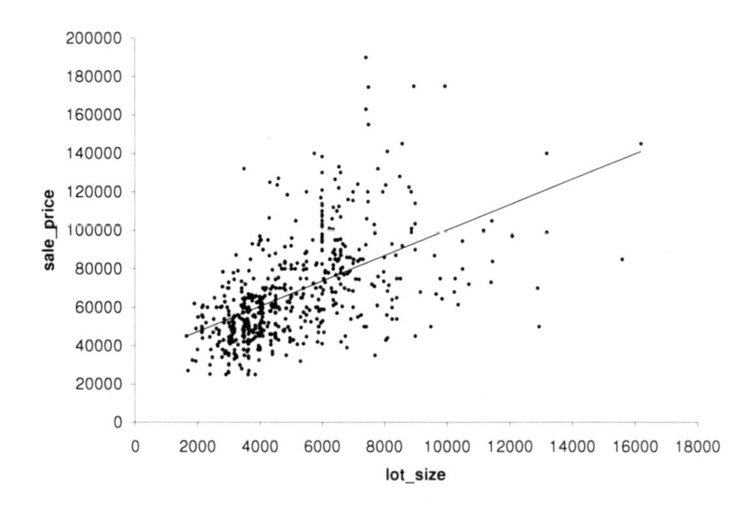

Fig. 1. Scatter plot of *lot_size* and *sales_price* for the housing data

where the subscript D indicates we are only considering houses on a desirable location. To test whether the slope for desirable locations is significantly different, we could perform a statistical test of $H_0 : b = b_D$, or more conveniently, $H_0 : b_D = b_{\bar{D}}$, where $\bar{D}$ denotes the complement of D.

In the above example, we came up ourselves with the idea that houses on a desirable location might have a different slope in the regression model. The main idea presented in this paper is that we can find such groups automatically by using the subgroup discovery framework. Hence, the subgroups are not limited to simple conditions based on a single variable. Their description may involve conjunctions of conditions, and in case of multi-relational data, existential quantification and aggregation as well. In the general case of simple linear regression, we could be looking for subgroups G where the slope b_G in

$$y_i = a_G + b_G x_i + e_i,$$

is substantially different from the slope $b_{\bar{G}}$. The search process only involves the subgroups; the variables y and x are assumed to be determined by the question of the user, that is, they are fixed.

We have stated that the objective is to find subgroups where a model fitted to the subgroup is substantially different from that same model fitted to the entire database. This statement is deliberately general: we can use different types of models in this scheme, and for each type of model we can consider several measures of difference. In this paper we describe a number of model classes and quality measures that can be useful. All these methods have been implemented in the Multi-Relational Data Mining system Safarii [6].

This paper is organized as follows. In Section 2, we introduce some notation that is used throughout the paper, and define the subgroup discovery and exceptional model mining framework. In Section 3, we give examples of three basic types of models for exceptional model mining: correlation, regression and classification. We also propose appropriate quality measures for the types of models discussed. In Section 4, we present the results of exceptional model mining applied to two real-life datasets. Finally, we draw conclusions in Section 5.

2 Exceptional Model Mining

We assume that the database d is a bag of labelled objects $i \in D$, referred to as *individuals*, taken from a domain D. We refer to the size of the database as $N = |d|$. At this point, we do not fix the nature of individuals, be it propositional, relational, or graphical, etc. However, each description of an individual includes a number of attributes $x_1, ..., x_k$ and optionally an output attribute y. These attributes are used in fitting models to subgroups of the data. In regular subgroup discovery, only the y attribute is used, which is typically binary.

We make no assumptions about the syntax of the pattern language, and treat a pattern simply as a function $p : D \to \{0, 1\}$. We will say that a pattern p *covers* an individual i *iff* $p(i) = 1$.

Definition 1 (Subgroup). *A* subgroup *corresponding to a pattern* p *is the set of individuals* $G_p \subseteq d$ *that are covered by* p*:* $G_p = \{i \in d | p(i) = 1\}$.

Definition 2 (Complement). *The* complement *of a subgroup* G_p *is the set of individuals* $\bar{G}_p \subseteq d$ *that are* not *covered by* p*:* $\bar{G}_p = d \backslash G_p$.

When clear from the context, we will omit the p from now on, and simply refer to a subgroup and its complement as G and $\bar{G}$. We use n and $\bar{n}$ to denote the size of G and $\bar{G}$, respectively. In order to judge the quality of candidate patterns in a given database, a *quality measure* needs to be defined. This measure determines for each pattern in a pattern language $\mathcal{P}$ how interesting (exceptional) a model induced on the associated subgroup is.

Definition 3 (Quality Measure). *A* quality measure *for a pattern* p *is a function* $\varphi_d : \mathcal{P} \to \mathbb{R}$ *that computes a unique numeric value for a pattern* p*, given a database* d*.*

Subgroup discovery [3] is a data mining framework aimed at discovering patterns that satisfy a number of user-specified inductive constraints. These constraints typically include an interestingness constraint $\varphi(p) \geq t$, as well as a minimum support threshold $n \geq minsup$ that guarantees the relative frequency of the subgroups in the database. Further constraints may involve properties such as the complexity of the pattern p. In most cases, a subgroup discovery algorithm will traverse a search lattice of candidate patterns in a top-down, general-to-specific fashion. The structure of the lattice is determined by a *refinement operator* $\rho : \mathcal{P} \to 2^{\mathcal{P}}$, a syntactic operation which determines how simple patterns can be extended into more complex ones by atomic additions. In our application (and most others), the refinement operator is assumed to be a *specialisation operator*: $\forall q \in \rho(p) : p \succeq q$ (p is more general than q).

The actual search strategy used to consider candidates is a parameter of the algorithm. We have chosen the *beam search* strategy [14], because it nicely balances the benefits of a greedy method with the implicit parallel search resulting from the beam. Beam search effectively performs a level-wise search that is guided by the quality measure φ. On each level, the best-ranking w patterns are refined to form the candidates for the next level. This means that although the search will be targeted, it is less likely to get stuck in a local optimum, because at each level alternatives are being considered. The search is further bounded by complexity constraints and the *minsup* constraint. The end-result is a ranked list of patterns (subgroups) that satisfy the inductive constraints.

In the case of regular subgroup discovery, with only a single discrete target variable, the quality measure of choice is typically a measure for how different the distribution over the target variable is, compared to that of the whole database (or in fact to that of the complement). As such an unusual distribution is easily produced in small fractions of the database, the deviation is often weighed with the size of the subgroup: a pattern is interesting if it is both exceptional and frequent. Well-known examples of quality measures for binary targets are frequency, confidence, χ^2, and novelty.

The subject of this paper, exceptional model mining (EMM) [5], can now be viewed as an extension of the subgroup discovery framework. The essential difference with standard subgroup discovery is the use of more complex target concepts than the regular single attribute. Our targets are models of some sort, and within each subgroup considered, a model is induced on the attributes $x_1, ..., x_k$, and optionally y. We will define quality measures that capture how exceptional the model within the subgroup is in relation to the model induced on its complement. In the next section, we present a number of model types, and propose one or more quality measures for each. When only the subgroup itself is considered, the quality measures tend to focus on the accuracy of the model, such as the fit of a regression line, or the predictive accuracy of a classifier. If the quality measure captures the difference between the subgroup and its complement, it is typically based on a comparison between more structural properties of the two models, such as the slope of the regression lines, or the make-up of the classifiers (e.g. size, attributes used).

Example 1. Consider again the housing dataset (Fig. 1). Individuals (houses) are described by a number of attributes such as the number of bathrooms or whether the house is located at a desirable location. An example of a pattern (and associated subgroup G) would be:

$$p : nbath \geq 2 \wedge drive = 1$$

which covers 128 houses (about 23% of the data). Its complement (which is often only considered implicitly) is

$$\bar{p} : \neg nbath \geq 2 \vee \neg drive = 1$$

The typical refinement operator will add a single condition on any of the available attributes to the conjunction. In this example, target models are defined over the two attributes $x = lot\_size$ and $y = sales\_price$. Note that these two attributes are therefore not allowed to appear in the subgroup definitions. One possibility is to perform the linear regression of y on x. As a quality measure φ_d, we could consider the absolute difference in slope between the two regression lines fitted to G and $\bar{G}$. In Section 3.2, we propose a more sophisticated quality measure for the difference in slope, that implicitly takes into account the supports n and $\bar{n}$, and thus the significance of the finding.

3 Model Classes

In this section, we discuss simple examples of three classes of models, and suggest quality measures for them. As an example of a model without an output attribute, we consider the correlation between two numeric variables. We discuss linear regression for models with a numeric output attribute, and two simple classifiers for models with discrete output attributes.

3.1 Correlation Models

As an example of a model without an output attribute, we consider two numeric variables x_1 and x_2, and their linear association as measured by the correlation coefficient ρ. We estimate ρ by the sample correlation coefficient r:

$$r = \frac{\sum(x_1^i - \bar{x}_1)(x_2^i - \bar{x}_2)}{\sqrt{\sum(x_1^i - \bar{x}_1)^2 \sum(x_2^i - \bar{x}_2)^2}}$$

where x^i denotes the ith observation on x, and $\bar{x}$ denotes its mean.

Absolute difference between correlations (φ_{abs}). A logical quality measure is to take the absolute difference of the correlation in the subgroup G and its complement $\bar{G}$, that is

$$\varphi_{abs}(p) = |r_G - r_{\bar{G}}|$$

The disadvantage of this measure is that it does not take into account the size of the groups, and hence does not do anything to prevent overfitting. Intuitively, subgroups with higher support should be preferred.

Entropy (φ_{ent}). As an improvement of φ_{abs}, the following quality function weighs the absolute difference between the correlations with the *entropy* of the split between the subgroup and its complement. The entropy captures the information content of such a split, and favours balanced splits (1 bit of information for a 50/50 split) over skewed splits (0 bits for the extreme case of either subgroup or complement being empty). The entropy function $H(p)$ is defined (in this context) as:

$$H(p) = -n/N \lg n/N - \bar{n}/N \lg \bar{n}/N$$

The quality measure φ_{ent} is now defined as:

$$\varphi_{ent}(p) = H(p) \cdot |r_G - r_{\bar{G}}|$$

Significance of Correlation Difference (φ_{scd}). A more statistically oriented approach to prevent overfitting is to perform a hypothesis test on the difference between the correlation in the subgroup and its complement. Let ρ_p and $\rho_{\bar{p}}$ denote the population coefficients of correlation for p and $\bar{p}$, respectively, and let r_G and $r_{\bar{G}}$ denote their sample estimates. The test to be considered is

$$H_0 : \rho_p = \rho_{\bar{p}} \qquad \text{against} \qquad H_a : \rho_p \neq \rho_{\bar{p}}$$

We would like to use the observed significance (p-value) of this test as a quality measure, but the problem is that the sampling distribution of the sample correlation coefficient is not known in general. If x_1 and x_2 follow a bivariate normal distribution, then application of the Fisher z transformation

$$z' = \frac{1}{2} \ln \left(\frac{1+r}{1-r} \right)$$

makes the sampling distribution of z' approximately normal [12]. Its standard error is given by

$$\frac{1}{\sqrt{m-3}}$$

where m is the size of the sample. As a consequence

$$z^* = \frac{z' - \bar{z}'}{\sqrt{\frac{1}{n-3} + \frac{1}{\bar{n}-3}}}$$

approximately follows a standard normal distribution under H_0. Here z' and $\bar{z}'$ are the z-scores obtained through the Fisher z transformation for G and $\bar{G}$, respectively. If both n and $\bar{n}$ are greater than 25, then the normal approximation is quite accurate, and can safely be used to compute the p-values. Because we have to introduce the normality assumption to be able to compute the p-values, they should be viewed as a heuristic measure. Transformation of the original data (for example, taking their logarithm) may make the normality assumption more reasonable. As a quality measure we take 1 minus the computed p-value so that $\varphi_{scd} \in [0, 1]$, and higher values indicate a more interesting subgroup.

3.2 Regression Model

In this section, we discuss some possibilities of EMM with regression models. For ease of exposition, we only consider the linear regression model

$$y_i = a + bx_i + e_i, \tag{1}$$

but this is in no way essential to the methods we discuss.

Significance of Slope Difference (φ_{ssd}). Consider model (1) fitted to a subgroup G and its complement $\bar{G}$. Of course, there is a choice of distance measures between the fitted models. We propose to look at the difference in the slope b between the two models, because this parameter is usually of primary interest when fitting a regression model: it indicates the change in the expected value of y, when x increases with one unit. Another possibility would be to look at the intercept a, if it has a sensible interpretation in the application concerned. Like with the correlation coefficient, we use significance testing to measure the distance between the fitted models. Let b_p be the slope for the regression function of p and $b_{\bar{p}}$ the slope for the regression function of $\bar{p}$. The hypothesis to be tested is

$$H_0 : b_p = b_{\bar{p}} \qquad \text{against} \qquad H_a : b_p \neq b_{\bar{p}}$$

We use the least squares estimate

$$\hat{b} = \frac{\sum(x_i - \bar{x})(y_i - \bar{y})}{\sum(x_i - \bar{x})^2}$$

for the slope b. An unbiased estimator for the variance of $\hat{b}$ is given by

$$s^2 = \frac{\sum \hat{e}_i^2}{(m-2)\sum(x_i - \bar{x})^2}$$

where $\hat{e}_i$ is the regression residual for individual i, and m is the sample size. Finally, we define our test statistic

$$t' = \frac{\hat{b}_G - \hat{b}_{\bar{G}}}{\sqrt{s_G^2 + s_{\bar{G}}^2}}$$

Although t' does not have a t distribution, its distribution can be approximated quite well by one, with degrees of freedom given by (cf. [11]):

$$df = \frac{\left(s_G^2 + s_{\bar{G}}^2\right)^2}{\frac{s_G^4}{n-2} + \frac{s_{\bar{G}}^4}{\bar{n}-2}} \tag{2}$$

Our quality measure $\varphi_{ssd} \in [0, 1]$ is once again defined as one minus the p-value computed on the basis of a t distribution with degrees of freedom given in (2). If $n + \bar{n} \geq 40$ the t-statistic is quite accurate, so we should be confident to use it unless we are analysing a very small dataset.

3.3 Classification Models

In the case of classification, we are dealing with models for which the output attribute y is discrete. In general, the attributes $x_1, ..., x_k$ can be of any type (binary, nominal, numeric, etc). Furthermore, our EMM framework allows for any classification method, as long as some quality measure can be defined in order to judge the models induced. Although we allow arbitrarily complex methods, such as decision trees, support vector machines or even ensembles of classifiers, we only consider two relatively simple classifiers here, for reasons of simplicity and efficiency.

Logistic Regression. Analogous to the linear regression case, we consider the logistic regression model

$$\text{logit}(P(y_i = 1|x_i)) = \ln\left(\frac{P(y_i = 1|x_i)}{P(y_i = 0|x_i)}\right) = a + b \cdot x_i,$$

where $y \in \{0, 1\}$ is a binary class label. The coefficient b tells us something about the effect of x on the probability that y occurs, and hence may be of interest to subject area experts. A positive value for b indicates that an increase in x leads to an increase of $P(y = 1|x)$ and vice versa. The strength of influence can be quantified in terms of the change in the odds of $y = 1$ when x increases with, say, one unit.

To judge whether the effect of x is substantially different in a particular subgroup G_p, we fit the model

$$\text{logit}(P(y_i = 1|x_i)) = a + b \cdot p(i) + c \cdot x_i + d \cdot (p(i) \cdot x_i). \tag{3}$$

Note that

$$\text{logit}(P(y_i = 1|x_i)) = \begin{cases} (a + b) + (c + d) \cdot x_i & \text{if } p(i) = 1 \\ a + c \cdot x_i & \text{if } p(i) = 0 \end{cases}$$

Hence, we allow both the slope and the intercept to be different in the subgroup and its complement. As a quality measure, we propose to use one minus the p-value of a test on $d = 0$ against a two-sided alternative in the model of equation (3). This is a standard test in the literature on logistic regression [12]. We refer to this quality measure as φ_{sed}.

DTM Classifier. The second classifier considered is the *Decision Table Majority* (DTM) classifier [8,7], also known as a *simple decision table*. The idea behind this classifier is to compute the relative frequencies of the y values for each possible combination of values for $x_1, \ldots, x_k$. For combinations that do not appear in the dataset, the relative frequency estimates are based on that of the whole dataset. The predicted y value for a new individual is simply the one with the highest probability estimate for the given combination of input values.

Example 2. As an example of a DTM classifier, consider a hypothetical dataset of 100 people applying for a mortgage. The dataset contains two attributes describing the age (divided into three suitable categories) and marital status of the applicant. A third attribute indicates whether the application was successful, and is used as the output. Out of the 100 applications, 61 were successful. The following decision table lists the estimated probabilities of success for each combination of *age* and *married?*. The support for each combination is indicated between brackets.

	married? = 'no'	*married?* = 'yes'
age = 'low'	0.25 (20)	0.61 (0)
age = 'medium'	0.4 (15)	0.686 (35)
age = 'high'	0.733 (15)	1.0 (15)

As this table shows, the combination *married?* = 'yes'$\wedge$*age* = 'low' does not appear in this particular dataset, and hence the probability estimate is based on the complete dataset (0.61). This classifier predicts a positive outcome in all cases except when *married?* = 'no' and *age* is either 'low' or 'medium'.

For this instance of the classification model we discuss two different quality measures. The *BDeu* (Bayesian Dirichlet equivalent uniform) score, which is a measure for the performance of the DTM classifier on G, and the *Hellinger distance*, which assigns a value to the distance between the conditional probabilities estimated on G and $\bar{G}$.

BDeu Score (φ_{BDeu}). The BDeu score φ_{BDeu} is a measure from Bayesian theory [2] and is used to estimate the performance of a classifier on a subgroup, with a penalty for small contingencies that may lead to overfitting. Note that this measure ignores how the classifier performs on the complement. It merely captures how 'predictable' a particular subgroup is.

The BDeu score is defined as

$$\prod_{x_1,\ldots,x_k} \frac{\Gamma(\alpha/q)}{\Gamma(\alpha/q + n(x_1,...,x_k))} \prod_{y} \frac{\Gamma(\alpha/qr + n(x_1,..,x_k,y))}{\Gamma(\alpha/qr)}$$

where Γ denotes the gamma function, q denotes the number of value combinations of the input variables, r the number of values of the output variable, and $n(x_1,...,x_k,y)$ denotes the number of cases with that value combination. The parameter α denotes the *equivalent sample size*. Its value can be chosen by the user.

Hellinger (φ_{Hel}). Another possibility is to use the Hellinger distance [13]. It defines the distance between two probability distributions $P(z)$ and $Q(z)$ as follows:

$$H(P,Q) = \sum_{z} \left(\sqrt{P(z)} - \sqrt{Q(z)}\right)^2$$

where the sum is taken over all possible values z. In our case, the distributions of interest are

$$P(y \mid x_1,...,x_k)$$

for each possible value combination $x_1,...,x_k$. The overall distance measure becomes

$$\varphi_{Hel}(p) = D(\hat{P}_G, \hat{P}_{\bar{G}}) = \sum_{x_1,\ldots,x_k} \sum_{y} \left(\sqrt{\hat{P}_G(y|x_1,...,x_k)} - \sqrt{\hat{P}_{\bar{G}}(y|x_1,...,x_k)}\right)^2$$

where $\hat{P}_G$ denotes the probability estimates on G. Intuitively, we measure the distance between the conditional distribution of y in G and $\bar{G}$ for each possible combination of input values, and add these distances to obtain an overall distance. Clearly, this measure is aimed at producing subgroups for which the conditional distribution of y is substantially different from its conditional distribution in the overall database.

4 Experiments

This section illustrates exceptional model mining on two real-life datasets, using different quality measures. Although our implementation in Safarii essentially is multi-relational [6], the two dataset we present are propositional. For each test, Safarii returns a configurable number of subgroups ranked according to the quality measure of choice. The following experiments only present the best ranking subgroup and take a closer look at the interpretation of the results.

4.1 Analysis of Housing Data

First, we analyse the Windsor housing data[1] [9]. This dataset contains information on 546 houses that were sold in Windsor, Canada in the summer of 1987. The information for each house includes the two attributes of interest, *lot_size* and *sales_price*, as plotted in Fig. 1. An additional 10 attributes are available to define candidate subgroups, including the number of bedrooms and bathrooms and whether the house is located at a desirable location. The correlation between lot size and sale price is 0.536, which implies that a larger size of the lot coincides with a higher sales price. The fitted regression function is:

$$\hat{y} = 34136 + 6.60 \cdot x$$

As this function shows, on average one extra square meter corresponds to a 6.6 dollar higher sales price. Given this function, one might wonder whether it is possible to find specific subgroups in the data where the price of an additional square meter is significantly less, perhaps even zero. In the next paragraphs, we show how EMM may be used to answer this question.

Significance of Correlation Difference. Looking at the restrictions defined in Section 3.1 we see that the support has to be over 25 in order to be confident about the test results for this measure. This number was used as minimum support threshold for a run of Safarii using φ_{scd}. The following subgroup (and its complement) was found to show the most significant difference in correlation: $\varphi_{scd}(p_1) = 0.9993$.

$$p_1 : drive = 1 \wedge rec\_room = 1 \wedge nbath \geq 2.0$$

This is the group of 35 houses that have a driveway, a recreation room and at least two bathrooms. The scatter plots for the subgroup and its complement are given in Fig. 2. The subgroup shows a correlation of $r_G = -0.090$ compared to $r_{\bar{G}} = 0.549$ for the remaining 511 houses. A tentative interpretation could be that G describes a collection of houses in the higher segments of the markets where the price of a house is mostly determined by its location and facilities. The desirable location may provide a natural limit on the lot size, such that this is not a factor in the pricing. Figure 2 supports this hypothesis: houses in G tend to have a higher price.

[1] Available from the Journal of Applied Econometrics Data Archive at http://econ.queensu.ca/jae/

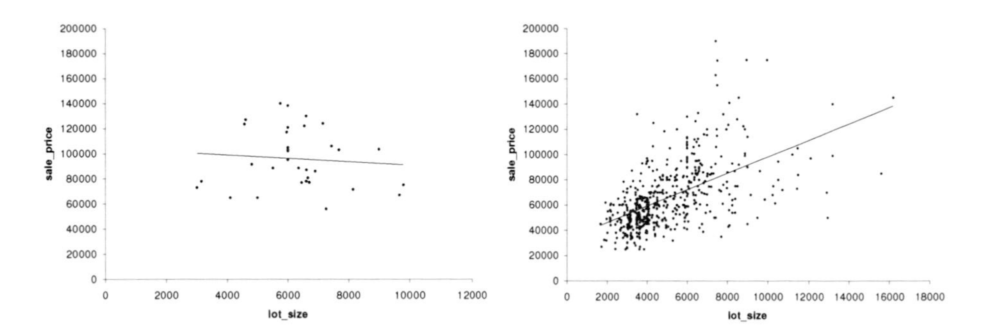

Fig. 2. Housing - φ_{scd}: Scatter plot of *lot_size* and *sales_price* for $drive = 1 \wedge rec\_room = 1 \wedge nbath \geq 2$ (left) and its complement (right)

In general *sales_price* and *lot_size* are positively correlated, but EMM discovers a subgroup with a slightly negative correlation. However, the value in the subgroup is not significantly different from zero: a test of

$$H_0 : b_{p_1} = 0 \qquad \text{against} \qquad H_a : b_{p_1} \neq 0,$$

yields a p-value of 0.61. The scatter plot confirms our impression that *sales_price* and *lot_size* are uncorrelated within the subgroup. For purposes of interpretation, it is interesting to perform some post-processing. In Table 1 we give an overview of the correlations within different subgroups whose intersection produces the final result, as given in the last row. It is interesting to see that the condition $nbath \geq 2$ in itself actually leads to a slight increase in correlation compared to the whole database, but the combination with the presence of a recreation room leads to a substantial drop to $r = 0.129$. When we add the condition that the house should also have a driveway we arrive at the final result with $r = -0.090$. Note that adding this condition only eliminates 3 records (the size of the subgroup goes from 38 to 35) and that the correlation between sales price and lot size in these three records (defined by the condition $nbath \geq 2 \wedge \neg drive = 1 \wedge rec\_room = 1$) is -0.894. We witness a phenomenon similar to Simpson's paradox: splitting up a subgroup with positive correlation (0.129) produces two subgroups both with a negative correlation (-0.090 and -0.894, respectively).

Significance of Slope Difference. In this section, we perform EMM on the housing data using the Significance of Slope Difference (φ_{ssd}) as the quality measure. The highest ranking subgroup consists of the 226 houses that have a driveway, no basement and at most one bathroom:

$$p_2 : drive = 1 \wedge basement = 0 \wedge nbath \leq 1$$

Table 1. Different subgroups of the housing data, and their sample correlation coefficients and supports

Subgroup	r	n
Whole dataset	0.536	546
$nbath \geq 2$	0.564	144
$drive = 1$	0.502	469
$rec\_room = 1$	0.375	97
$nbath \geq 2 \wedge drive = 1$	0.509	128
$nbath \geq 2 \wedge rec\_room = 1$	0.129	38
$drive = 1 \wedge rec\_room = 1$	0.304	90
$nbath \geq 2 \wedge rec\_room = 1 \wedge \neg drive = 1$	−0.894	3
$nbath \geq 2 \wedge rec\_room = 1 \wedge drive = 1$	−0.090	35

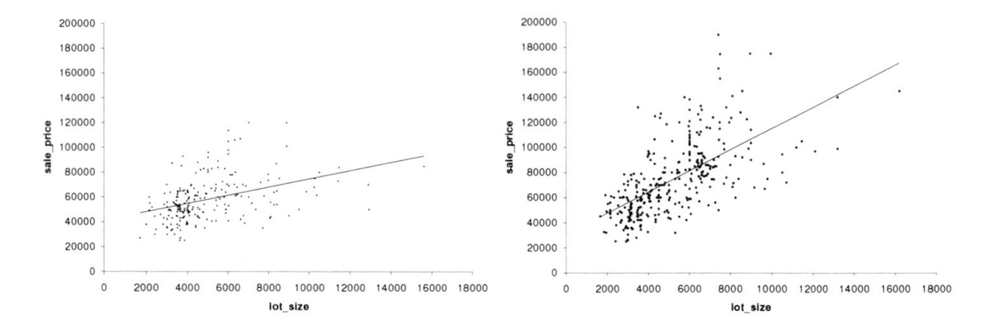

Fig. 3. Housing - φ_{ssd}: Scatter plot of $drive = 1 \wedge basement = 0 \wedge nbath \leq 1$ (left), and its complement (right)

The subgroup G and its complement $\bar{G}$ (320 houses) lead to the following two fitted regression functions, respectively:

$$\hat{y} = 41568 + 3.31 \cdot x$$
$$\hat{y} = 30723 + 8.45 \cdot x$$

The subgroup quality is $\varphi_{ssd} > 0.9999$, meaning that the p-value of the test

$$H_0 : b_{p_2} = b_{\bar{p}_2} \qquad \text{against} \qquad H_a : b_{p_2} \neq b_{\bar{p}_2}$$

is virtually zero. There are subgroups with a larger difference in slope, but the reported subgroup scores higher because it is quite big. Figure 3 shows the scatter plots of *lot_size* and *sales_price* for the subgroup and its complement.

4.2 Analysis of Gene Expression Data

The following experiments demonstrate the usefulness of exceptional model mining in the domain of bioinformatics. In genetics, genes are organised in so-called *gene regulatory networks*. This means that the expression (its effective activity)

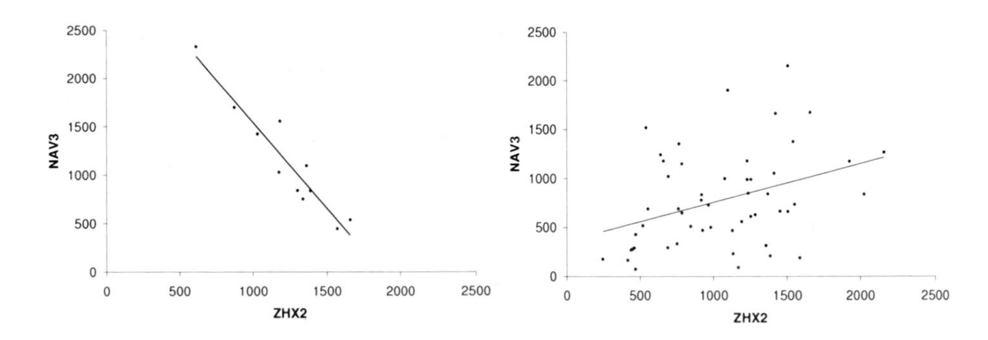

Fig. 4. Gene Expression - φ_{abs}: Scatter plot of 11_band = 'no deletion' $\wedge$ $survivaltime \leq 1919 \wedge XP\_498569.1 \leq 57$ (left; $r = -0.950$) and its complement (right; $r = 0.363$)

of a gene may be influenced by the expression of other genes. Hence, if one gene is regulated by another, one can expect a linear correlation between the associated expression-levels. In many diseases, specifically cancer, this interaction between genes may be disturbed. The Gene Expression dataset shows the expression-levels of 313 genes as measured by an Affymetrix microarray, for 63 patients that suffer from a cancer known as neuroblastoma [10]. Additionally, the dataset contains clinical information about the patients, including age, sex, stage of the disease, etc.

Correlation Model Experiment. As a demonstration of a correlation model, we analyse the correlation between ZHX3 ('Zinc fingers and homeoboxes 2') and NAV3 ('Neuron navigator 3'), in terms of the absolute difference of correlations φ_{abs}. These genes show a very slight correlation ($r = 0.218$) in the whole dataset. The remaining attributes (both gene expression and clinical information) are available for building subgroups. As the φ_{abs} measure does not have any provisions for promoting larger subgroups, we use a minimum support threshold of 10 (15% of the patients). The largest distance ($\varphi_{abs}(p_3) = 1.313$) was found with the following condition:

$$p_3 : 11\_band = \text{'no deletion'} \wedge survivaltime \leq 1919 \wedge XP\_498569.1 \leq 57$$

Figure 4 shows the plot for this subgroup and its complement with the regression lines drawn in. The correlation in the subgroup is $r_G = -0.95$ and the correlation in the remaining data is $r_{\bar{G}} = 0.363$. Note that the subgroup is very "predictable": all points are quite close to the regression line, with $R^2 \approx 0.9$.

DTM Experiment. For the DTM classification experiments on the Gene Expression dataset, we have selected three binary attributes. The first two attributes, which serve as input variables of the decision table, are related to genomic alterations that may be observed within the tumor tissues. The attribute $1p\_band$ (x_1)

describes whether the small arm ('p') of the first chromosome has been deleted. The second attribute, MYCN (x_2), describes whether one specific gene is amplified or not (multiple copies introduced in the genome). Both attributes are known to potentially influence the genesis and prognosis of neuroblastoma. The output attibute for the classification model is $NBstatus$ (y), which can be either 'no event' or 'relapse or deceased'. The following decision table describes the conditional distribution of *NBstatus* given *1p_band* and MYCN on the whole data set:

	MYCN ='amplified'	MYCN = 'not amplified'
$1p\_band$ = 'deletion'	0.333 (3)	0.667 (3)
$1p\_band$ = 'no change'	0.625 (8)	0.204 (49)

In order to find subgroups for which the distribution is significantly different, we run EMM with the Hellinger distance φ_{Hel} as quality measure. As our quality measures for classification do not specifically promote larger subgroups, we have selected a slightly higher minimum support constraint: $minsup = 16$, which corresponds to 25% of the data. The following subgroup of 17 patients was the best found ($\varphi_{Hel} = 3.803$):

$$p_4 : prognosis = \text{'unknown'}$$

	MYCN ='amplified'	MYCN = 'not amplified'
$1p\_band$ = 'deletion'	1.0 (1)	0.833 (6)
$1p\_band$ = 'no change'	1.0 (1)	0.333 (9)

Note that for each combination of input values, the probability of 'relapse or deceased' is increased, which makes sense when the prognosis is uncertain. Note furthermore that the overall dataset does not yield a pure classifier: for every combination of input values, there is still some confusion in the predictions. In our second classification experiment, we are interested in "predictable" subgroups. Therefore, we run EMM with the φ_{BDeu} measure. All other settings are kept the same. The following subgroup ($n = 16$, $\varphi_{BDeu} = -1.075$) is based on the expression of the gene RIF1 ('RAP1 interacting factor homolog (yeast)')

$$p_5 : \text{RIF1} >= 160.45$$

	MYCN ='amplified'	MYCN = 'not amplified'
$1p\_band$ = 'deletion'	0.0 (0)	0.0 (0)
$1p\_band$ = 'no change'	0.0 (0)	0.0 (16)

In this subgroup, the predictiveness is optimal, as all patients turn out to be tumor-free. In fact, the decision table ends up being rather trivial, as all cells indicate the same decision.

Logistic Regression Experiment. In the logistic regression experiment, we take *NBstatus* as the output y, and *age* (age at diagnosis in days) as the predictor x. The subgroups are created using the gene expression level variables. Hence, the model specification is

$$\text{logit}\{P(\mathit{NBstatus} = \text{`relapse or deceased'})\} = a + b \cdot p + c \cdot age + d \cdot (p \cdot age).$$

We find the subgroup

$$p_6 : \text{SMPD1} \geq 840 \wedge \text{HOXB6} \leq 370.75$$

with a coverage of 33, and quality $\varphi_{sed} = 0.994$. We find a positive coefficient of x for the subgroup, and a slightly negative coefficient for its complement. Within the subgroup, the odds of *NBstatus* = 'relapse or deceased' increase with 44% when the age at diagnosis increases with 100 days, whereas in the complement the odds decrease with 8%. More loosely, within the subgroup an increase in age at diagnosis decreases the probability of survival, whereas in the complement an increase in age slightly increases the probability of survival. Such reversals of the direction of influence may be of particular interest to the domain expert.

5 Conclusions and Future Research

We have introduced exceptional model mining (EMM) as an extension of the well-known subgroup discovery framework. By focusing on models instead of single target variables, many new interesting analysis possibilities are created. We have proposed a number of model classes that can be used in EMM, and defined several quality measures for them. We illustrated the use of EMM by its application to two real datasets. Like subgroup discovery, EMM is an exploratory method that requires interaction with a user that is knowledgable in the application domain. It can provide useful insights into the subject area, but does not result in ready-to-use predictive models.

We believe there are many possibilities to extend the work presented in this paper. One could look at different models, for example naive Bayes for classification problems or graphical models for modelling the probability distribution of a number of (discrete) variables. Whatever the selected class of models, the user should specify a quality measure that relates to the more fundamental questions a user may have about the data at hand. In the case of our housing example, the choice for the difference in slope is appropriate, as it captures a relevant aspect of the data, namely a significant change in price per square meter. For similar reasons, we used the difference between the coefficients of the explanatory variable (age at diagnosis) in the subgroup and its complement as a quality measure for logistic regression models.

Specifying an appropriate quality measure that is inspired by a relevant question of the user becomes less straightforward when more complex models are considered, although of course one can always focus on some particular aspect (e.g. coefficients) of the models. However, even for sophisticated models such as support vector machines or Bayesian networks, one can think of measures that make sense, such as the linear separability or the edit distance between two networks [15], respectively.

From a computational viewpoint, it is advisable to keep the models to be fitted simple, since many subgroups have to be evaluated in the search process. For example, fitting a naive Bayes model to a large collection of subgroups can be done quite efficiently, but fitting a support vector machine could prove to be too time consuming.

References

1. Affymetrix (1992), http://www.affymetrix.com/index.affx
2. Heckerman, D., Geiger, D., Chickering, D.: Learning Bayesian Networks: The combination of knowledge and statistical data. Machine Learning 20, 179–243 (1995)
3. Klösgen, W.: Handbook of Data Mining and Knowledge Discovery. Subgroup Discovery, ch. 16.3. Oxford University Press, New York (2002)
4. Friedman, J., Fisher, N.: Bump-Hunting in High-Dimensional Data. Statistics and Computing 9(2), 123–143 (1999)
5. Leman, D., Feelders, A., Knobbe, A.J.: Exceptional Model Mining. In: Daelemans, W., Goethals, B., Morik, K. (eds.) ECML PKDD 2008, Part II. LNCS (LNAI), vol. 5212, pp. 1–16. Springer, Heidelberg (2008)
6. Knobbe, A.: Safarii multi-relational data mining environment (2006), http://www.kiminkii.com/safarii.html
7. Knobbe, A.J., Ho, E.K.Y.: Pattern teams. In: Fürnkranz, J., Scheffer, T., Spiliopoulou, M. (eds.) PKDD 2006. LNCS (LNAI), vol. 4213, pp. 577–584. Springer, Heidelberg (2006)
8. Kohavi, R.: The Power of Decision Tables. In: Proceedings ECML1995, London (1995)
9. Anglin, P.M., Gençay, R.: Semiparametric Estimation of a Hedonic Price Function. Journal of Applied Econometrics 11(6), 633–648 (1996)
10. van de Koppel, E., et al.: Knowledge Discovery in Neuroblastoma-related Biological Data. In: Data Mining in Functional Genomics and Proteomics workshop at PKDD 2007, Warsaw, Poland (2007)
11. Moore, D., McCabe, G.: Introduction to the Practice of Statistics, New York (1993)
12. Neter, J., Kutner, M., Nachtsheim, C.J., Wasserman, W.: Applied Linear Statistical Models. WCB McGraw-Hill, New York (1996)
13. Yang, G., Le Cam, L.: Asymptotics in Statistics: Some Basic Concepts. Springer, Heidelberg (2000)
14. Xu, Y., Fern, A.: Learning Linear Ranking Functions for Beam Search. In: Proceedings ICML 2007 (2007)
15. Niculescu-Mizil, A., Caruana, R.: Inductive Transfer for Bayesian Network Structure Learning. In: Proceedings of the 11th International Conference on AI and Statitics, AISTATS 2007 (2007)

Chapter 10
Online ChiMerge Algorithm

Petri Lehtinen, Matti Saarela, and Tapio Elomaa

Department of Software Systems, Tampere University of Technology
P.O. Box 553 (Korkeakoulunkatu 1), FI-33101 Tampere, Finland
firstname.lastname@tut.fi

Abstract. We show that a commonly-used sampling theoretical attribute discretization algorithm ChiMerge can be implemented efficiently in the online setting. Its benefits include that it is efficient, statistically justified, robust to noise, can be made to produce low-arity partitions, and has empirically been observed to work well in practice.

The worst-case time requirement of the batch version of ChiMerge bottom-up interval merging is $O(n \lg n)$ per attribute. We show that ChiMerge can be implemented in the online setting so that only logarithmic time is required to update the relevant data structures in connection of an insertion. Hence, the same $O(n \lg n)$ total time as in batch setting is spent on discretization of a data stream in which the examples fall into n bins. However, maintaining just one binary search tree is not enough, we also need other data structures. Moreover, in order to guarantee equal discretization results, an up-to-date discretization cannot always be kept available, but we need to delay the updates to happen at periodic intervals. We also provide a comparative evaluation of the proposed algorithm.

1 Introduction

Data streams have become reality in modern computing environments [1,2,3]. They have required to develop new algorithms that can cope efficiently and effectively with the continuous data feed. Naturally, we do not want to reinvent all (the algorithms) of the field from scratch. Rather, there are established and successful machine learning and data mining algorithms that carry over to the new setting without compromise. One must, though, bear in mind that the requirements in online data stream processing may significantly deviate from those of the batch setting: The time limits are tighter because of the high-speed nature of data streams and the algorithms have to be able to tolerate situations changing over time.

No unique model for a data stream exists. For example Aggarwal et al. [4] have debated about the suitability of incremental decision tree learning [5,6] for practical domains. Instead they proposed learning a continuously updating model. In this scenario it is important that the training model adapts quickly to the changing data stream. Also Gao et al. [7,8] have stressed the quick-changing

D.E. Holmes, L.C. Jain (Eds.): Data Mining: Found. & Intell. Paradigms, ISRL 24, pp. 199–216.
springerlink.com

nature of data streams. We will, nevertheless, stick with the one-pass classification model [5,6] and aim for execution time matching that of the batch setting.

Decision tree learning in face of data streams has been tackled to large extent [5,6,9,10,11]. The general methodology of learning decision trees from data streams is known and also drifting concepts, intrinsic to the setting, can be handled. However, some aspects of decision tree learning — like numerical attribute discretization — have been resolved only partly so far [10,12,13,14]. Continuous-valued (numerical) attributes need to be discretized somehow in standard decision tree learning. The number of techniques proposed for discretization is overwhelming and many of the available algorithms work well in practice [15,16,17]. Probably the best-known discretization approaches are unsupervised *equal-width* and *equal-frequency binning*, which overlook the class labels of examples (if provided). The former divides the observed value range into a number of intervals each of which has the same width and the latter into a number of intervals of approximately as many training examples. The user needs to provide the number of desired intervals.

A well-known robust supervised discretization algorithm — taking class labels into account — is Kerber's [18] ChiMerge. It is a *univariate* approach in which only one attribute is examined at a time without regard to the values of the other attributes. Like in standard decision tree learning, the examples are sorted by their value for the numerical attribute in question. In principle each example could make up an individual interval. As examples with the same value for the attribute cannot, anyhow, be distinguished from each other in the univariate setting, we can as well combine all equal-valued examples into one initial interval.

After obtaining the initial intervals, ChiMerge repeatedly merges those two adjacent intervals that appear, in light of a statistical test (χ^2 in the original algorithm), to have the most similar *relative class distribution* (RCD) for the instances. Equal RCD indicates that the numerical attribute at hand does not affect the class label of instances (at this point). Therefore, we have no reason to divide the value range in the cut point candidate being examined. The process continues until a stopping criterion is met. Several subsequent improvements to ChiMerge have been proposed [19,20,21].

ChiMerge is local in its nature since only two adjacent intervals are examined at a time. On the other hand, there is an inherent global component to ChiMerge — the interval combinations need to be examined in the order of their goodness as indicated by the χ^2 statistics. Hence, it is not immediate whether the algorithm can be implemented efficiently online. We will show that it can, though, be done at the price of maintaining some additional data structures. We also need to resort to periodic updates — not always having a discretization that reflects all the examples that have been received.

The basic setting that we examine differs from some other data stream models examined in the literature in the sense that we will not require the learned model to converge at any point. Rather, we follow the normal online learning setting and let the model be updated as long as new training instances are observed.

We will also discuss how Online CHIMERGE can be modified for concept drift and different stream models.

The next section reviews approaches proposed for handling numeric attributes in the algorithms that learn decision trees from data streams. In Section 3 we recapitulate CHIMERGE more thoroughly. After that we show how the algorithm can be implemented efficiently in the online setting. Section 5 presents a comparative evaluation of the proposed approach. Finally, we put forward our concluding remarks and sketch out possible future work.

2 Numeric Attributes, Decision Trees, and Data Streams

Let the streaming data received contain successive training examples each of which consists of instantiations for a pair of random variables $\langle \boldsymbol{X}, Y \rangle$. The k elements of the instance vector $\boldsymbol{X}$ are called *attributes*; $\boldsymbol{X} = \langle A_1, \ldots, A_k \rangle$. An attribute may be nominal-valued or continuous-valued (numerical). In the classification setting the class labels Y usually come from a small nominal set. The aim is to maintain an adaptive anytime model of determining the value of Y based on the attribute values $\boldsymbol{X}$. One is allowed to process the data only in the order that it arrives without storing (all of) it. As the intention is to operate in real time, only (close to) constant processing time per example may be used to update the statistics sufficient to determine which attribute is the appropriate one to be placed in a node of the evolving decision tree.

We abstract the data stream as `DataSource` from which a fresh instance can be requested at all times. If it is a new (labeled) training example, we incorporate it to our data structures and use it (eventually) to update the discretization. If, on the other hand, a test instance (without a class label) is received, we use our anytime hypothesis to classify it.

2.1 VFDT and Numeric Attributes

Research on learning decision trees from data streams was initiated by Domingos and Hulten [5] in introducing the VFDT system. Naturally, machine learning and data mining literature contains earlier attempts to make decision tree learning cope with massive data sets. They include, e.g., subsampling (in main memory) [22,23], incremental algorithms [24,25], and optimizing disk access [26,27]. Let us first consider VFDT and, then, review subsequent proposals for numeric attribute handling.

VFDT learns so-called Hoeffding trees — decision trees with a similarity guarantee to those learned by conventional batch algorithms such as CART [28] and C4.5 [29]. The standard Hoeffding inequality is used to show that the attribute chosen to a node in a Hoeffding tree is, with a high probability, the same as the one that would have been chosen by the batch learner with access to all of the data. VFDT chooses an attribute to the root node based on n first examples, after which the process continues recursively in the leaves down to which the succeeding examples are passed. Hoeffding bounds allow to solve the required n for reaching the user-requested confidence level.

Contrary to our setting, there is a training period in Hoeffding trees during which the tree stabilizes to its final form. VFDT preprunes the tree by expecting at each leaf to be expanded that enough training examples have been seen for statistically secure decision to be made before committing to testing a certain attribute's value. It also computes the attribute evaluation function only after seeing a sequence of new training examples in order to reduce time spent on expensive calculations.

Originally Domingos and Hulten [5] did not elaborate on how to handle numerical attributes in Hoeffding trees. They just proposed that the commonly-used thresholded binary splitting of the numerical value range be applied; i.e., only tests of the form $A_i < t_j$ are used. The value range of a numerical attribute may get multi-way splitted through subsequent binary splits of the induced subintervals. However, their later implementation of VFDT in the VFML package [30] also details numeric attribute handling.

The chosen implementation was based on binning the data into at most one thousand fixed-range intervals. If the limit of a thousand bins is ever reached, subsequent values from the stream are associated with the closest bin. In other words, this method can be seen as a fixed-width histogram technique. After the first thousand unique values observed, static bins are incrementally updated. The bin borders are the potential thresholds on which binary splits can be placed on. Quinlan's [29] *Information Gain* criterion (*IG*) is used as the attribute evaluation function. According to the empirical evaluation of Pfahringer et al. [13] this straightforward approach — with orders of magnitude tighter limit for the maximum number of bins — fares the best out of all the discretization methods they tested.

2.2 Further Approaches

Also Gama et al. [9] put forward an instantiation of VFDT in which *IG* was used to evaluate attributes. Instead of simple binning of VFML, for each numerical attribute A_i a (balanced) binary search tree (BST) is maintained. It records for every potential threshold t_j the class distribution of the binary partition induced by the test $A_i < t_j$. Values existing in the data are used as threshold candidates. Exhaustive evaluation over them is used to choose the test to be placed to the evolving decision tree. However, all threshold candidates for one attribute can be evaluated during a single traversal of the BST.

Obviously, updating the BST takes $O(\lg V)$ time, where V is the number of different values that the attribute in question takes. This price needs to be paid in order to be able to choose the best binary split. One has to sort the values and — as the value range is unknown from the outset — a time proportional to the number of potential cut points needs to be paid per example as long as one does not want to jeopardize finding the best cut point as determined by the attribute evaluation function.

Jin and Agrawal [10] proposed an approach for pruning intervals from the range of a numerical attribute in order to make processing more efficient. They first discretize a numerical value range into equal-width intervals after which a statistical test decides which intervals appear unlikely to include a split point and can, thus, be pruned. In addition they showed that Hoeffding bounds can be reached for *IG* and *Gini* function [28] with a lesser number of samples than in the original VFDT.

Gama et al. [9] also used *functional leaves* in the tree instead of the simple majority class strategy. Before the algorithm has decided which attribute test to assign to a leaf in the evolving tree, Naïve Bayes can be used to give predictions for instances that arrive needing to be classified. For numerical attributes the common approach of discretization into ten equal-width bins (when possible) is used in the naïve Bayes classifiers.

CVFDT [6] adapts the VFDT system to concept drift — concept changing over time. With a changing concept it is necessary to incrementally update the model built for the examples. The real-time operation requirement does not allow to rebuild the model for examples in a sliding window from scratch. Instead, Hulten et al. [6] proposed to build an alternative subtree for those nodes that do not pass the Hoeffding test in light of the sufficient statistics maintained for a sliding window of examples. When the alternate subtree's performance on new examples overtakes that of the old one, it is inserted to the tree. To grow the shadow tree one uses the standard techniques of VFDT, thus ensuring the real-time operation requirement.

In the UFFT system [11] concept drift is detected through the reducing accuracy of the naïve Bayes classifier installed into an internal node. Whenever, a change in the target concept is identified, the subtree rooted at the corresponding node and its associated statistics is pruned into a (functional) leaf, and building of a new subtree may begin anew. In UFFT a binary decision tree is built for each pair of classes and the actual model is a forest of trees. Numerical attributes are handled using the normality assumption as common in naïve Bayesian techniques. The sufficient statistics for each numerical attribute in this case are simply the mean and variance per class.

Gama and Pinto [12] use histograms for data stream discretization. Histograms induce either an equal-width or an equal-frequency discretization of the value range of a numerical attribute. The approach uses two layers of intervals. The first one maintains statistics for an excessive number of intervals and the second one composes the final discretization based on these statistics. The first layer is maintained online by updating the counters in the appropriate interval whenever a new example is received. If a user-defined condition is met, an interval may be split in two; e.g., to keep the intervals of approximately equal width. The second layer produces the final histograms by merging intervals of the first layer. This merging process is not online, but triggers on need basis. Building of the second level discretization is confined on the cut points of the first layer, and may thus be inexact.

Pfahringer et al. [13] have carried out an extensive empirical comparison of different approaches of discretizing numeric value ranges in the data stream setting. They tested Hoeffding trees in three realistic data stream settings: sensor node environment with 100KB of memory, a hand-held device environment in which 32MB of memory is available, and a server setting with 400MB of memory. Four different discretization approaches were compared: The simple VFML binning based on the first examples received [30], the approach of maintaining an exhaustive binary search tree from Gama et al.'s [9] instantiation of VFDT, per-class quantile summaries [31], and Gaussian approximation used, e.g., in UFFT [11]. Over all settings, the approach of VFML with 10 bins was consistently the best approach followed by Gaussian approximation using 10 split points. The exhaustive BST approach suffered from lack of space in these settings of limited memory. The best variant of quantile summaries had a similar performance as the BST approach, but with less space usage.

3 ChiMerge Algorithm

Kerber's [18] ChiMerge algorithm for discretization is a batch algorithm operating bottom-up. It is intended as a preprocessing step to precede execution of a learning algorithm. ChiMerge is based on the following intuitive notions. We look at the given training data in a univariate manner — the values of one attribute and the class labels of the examples at a time — ordered into initial intervals consisting of examples with the same value for the attribute under scrutiny. If the RCDs in two adjacent intervals do not differ significantly, the attribute at hand does not affect the class value. Of course, interval realizations need not have exactly the same RCD, but may differ slightly from each other and still come from the same underlying distribution. To test whether the distributions behind the two intervals are the same, a statistical test is used.

In our current problem a natural *null hypothesis* $\mathcal{H}_0$ is "The RCDs in two adjacent intervals are realizations of the same underlying distribution". We contrast it with the alternative hypothesis $\mathcal{H}_1$: "The RCDs in two adjacent intervals are realizations of different underlying distributions". By a statistical test we seek to either accept or reject the null hypothesis based on how unexpected the data were to $\mathcal{H}_0$. For the statistical test we need to determine a significance level of the test (e.g. 5%), which determines a critical value above which the null hypothesis will be rejected.

Let us now recapitulate the basic (Pearson's) χ^2 statistical test with d degrees of freedom. Let N_{ij} denote the number of instances of class $j \in \{1, \ldots, m\}$ in interval $i \in \{1, \ldots, k\}$. Let $N_i = \sum_{j=1}^{m} N_{ij}$ be the total number of examples in interval i. We consider combining intervals i and $i + 1$. In the two intervals together there are $N = N_i + N_{i+1}$ examples. By $C_j = C_{ij} + C_{(i+1)j}$ we denote the combined number of instances of class j in the two intervals. On the basis of the evidence given by the training sample we would, under the null hypothesis, expect interval i to contain $E_{ij} = N_i C_j / N$ instances of class j.

With these notations, we can write out the formula for the deviation of observed instance counts from the expected ones in comparing two adjacent intervals. Let us denote the candidate intervals with indices $i = 1, 2$.

$$D_{1,2} = \sum_{i=1}^{2} \sum_{j=1}^{m} \frac{(N_{ij} - E_{ij})^2}{E_{ij}}.$$

In other words, we sum together the relative squared differences of observed and expected class occurrences in the two intervals combined. This deviation is approximately distributed as χ^2 statistic with $d = m - 1$ degrees of freedom. Now, D is a real number that can be compared to the critical value of χ^2, which is obtained from a χ^2 table. In using the χ^2 independence test it is statistically justified to set the number of degrees of freedom to be 1 less than the number of classes m. For instance, using the 5% significance level, the critical value of χ^2 with one degree of freedom (two classes) is $\chi^2_{0.05} = 3.84$.

Finally, we compare the obtained deviation value D with the critical value of χ^2 at the chosen significance level. If D exceeds the critical value, we reject the null hypothesis $\mathcal{H}_0$ and choose the alternative hypothesis $\mathcal{H}_1$ instead. In our case, accepting the null hypothesis leads to combining the two intervals under scrutiny and rejecting it means that the cut point is effective and should be left as is.

ChiMerge combines the initial intervals in the order of their probability. In other words, it always searches for the best candidate interval pair, the one with the lowest deviation value. The best pair is merged unless a stopping condition is met. The time complexity of this repeated process is $O(V \lg V)$. Obviously such a time cannot be spent in connection of each new example received from the data stream. Moreover, the need to know the global best candidate means that the approach lacks locality properties and cannot directly be computed efficiently in online processing.

4 Online Version of ChiMerge

The main requirement for the online version of ChiMerge is a processing time that is, per each received training example, logarithmic in the number of intervals. Thus, we would altogether match the $O(n \lg n)$ time requirement of the batch version of ChiMerge. The algorithm OCM attaining the required time is given in Table 1.

OCM uses a balanced binary search tree T into which each example drawn from `DataSource` is (eventually) submitted. Examples with equal value for the numerical attribute under consideration all get directed down to the same node and compose a bin of examples. The BST also updates and maintains the required RCD counts. The first set of initial intervals is obtained by reading M examples from `DataSource` to T before starting the discretization.

In the actual discretization process, one iteration is performed each time a new example is received. Let V denote the number of intervals in T. During the

Table 1. OCM: Online ChiMerge Algorithm

Procedure OCM(M, D_{th})
Input: An integer M giving the number of examples on which initial discretization is based on and real D_{th} which is the χ^2 threshold for interval merging.
Data structures: A binary search tree T, a queue Q, two doubly linked lists L_I and L_D, and a priority queue P.

```
Initialize T, Q, L_I, and L_D as empty;
Read M training examples into tree T;
phase ← 1; b ← TREE-MINIMUM(T);
Make P an empty priority queue of size |T| − 1;
while E ← DataSource() ≠ nil do
  if phase = 1 then ENQUEUE(Q, E)
    else TREE-INSERT(T, E) fi;

  if phase = 1 then - - - - - - - - - - - - - - - - - - - - -
    Insert a copy of b as the last item in L_I;
    if |L_I| > 1 then
      Compute the D-value of the two last intervals in L_I;
      Using the obtained value as a key, add a pointer
        to the two intervals in L_I into P;
    fi
    b ← TREE-SUCCESSOR(T, b);
    if b = nil then phase ← 2 fi

  else if phase = 2 then - - - - - - - - - - - - - - - - - -
    d ← DEQUEUE(Q); TREE-INSERT(T, d);
    (D_{I,J}, ⟨I, J⟩) ← EXTRACT-MIN(P);
    if ⟨I, J⟩ ≠ nil and D_{I,J} < D_th then
      Remove from P the D-values of I and J;
      LIST-DELETE(L_I, I); LIST-DELETE(L_I, J);
      K ← MERGE(I, J);
      Compute the D-values of K with its neighbors in L_I;
      Update the D-values obtained into priority queue P;
    else
      phase ← 3;
    fi

  else - - - - - - - - - - - - - Phase = 3 - - - - - - - - - - - -
    d ← DEQUEUE(Q); TREE-INSERT(T, d);
    e ← LIST-DELETE(L_I, HEAD(L_I));
    LIST-INSERT(L_D, e);
    if EMPTY(Q) then
      phase ← 1; b ← TREE-MINIMUM(T);
      Make P an empty priority queue of size |T| − 1;
    fi
  fi
od
```

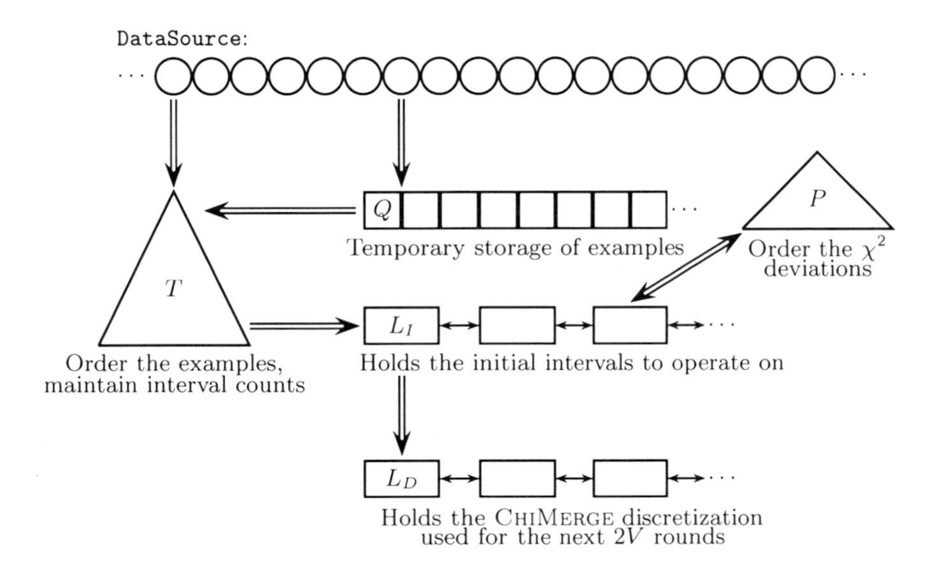

Fig. 1. The data structures of OCM

execution of the algorithm value V monotonically increases as more and more examples are received (unless old values are forgotten in preparation for concept drift; see below).

If each new example drawn from `DataSource` would update the current discretization immediately, this would yield a slowing down of OCM by a factor n as compared to the batch version of the algorithm. Therefore, we update the active discretization only periodically, freezing it for the intermediate period. Examples received during this time can be handled at a logarithmic time and at a constant time per example we are able to prepare the sufficient statistics for the next update of the discretization. The price that needs to be paid is maintaining some other data structures in addition to the BST.

The algorithm continuously takes in new examples from `DataSource`, but instead of just storing them to T, it updates the required data structures simultaneously. We do not want to halt the flow of the data stream because of extra processing of the data structures, but amortize the required work to normal example handling. In addition to the BST, a queue, two doubly linked lists, and a priority queue (heap) are maintained. Figure 1 illustrates these data structures and the flow of data between them. Only standard operations of the data structures [32] are executed in OCM. Recall that function TREE-MINIMUM(T) returns the minimum value stored in T and TREE-SUCCESSOR(T, b) the next smallest value in T after b, if one exists, and `nil` otherwise.

The discretization process works in three phases. In Phase 1 (of length V time steps), the examples from `DataSource` are cached for temporary storage to the queue Q. Meanwhile the initial intervals are collected one at a time from T to a list L_I that holds the intervals in their numerical order. For each pair of two adjacent intervals, the D-value is computed and inserted into the priority queue P. The queue Q is needed to freeze T for the duration of the Phase 1. After seeing V examples, all the initial intervals in T have been inserted to L_I and all the D-values have been computed and added to P. At this point Q holds V (unprocessed) examples.

At the end of Phase 1 all required preparations for interval merging have been done — initial intervals from T await merging in L_I and the pairwise D-values of adjacent intervals have been stored to the priority queue P. Phase 2 implements the merging as in batch ChiMerge, but without stopping the processing of `DataSource`. As a result of each merging, the intervals in L_I as well as the related D-values in P are updated.

In Phase 2 the example received from `DataSource` is submitted directly to T along with another, previously received example that is cached in Q. The order in which the examples from Q are submitted to T is not essential, because they all are inserted to T before the intervals in T are used in discretization again.

The lowest D-value, $D_{I,J}$, corresponding to some adjacent pair of intervals I and J, is drawn from P. If it exceeds the χ^2 merging threshold D_{th}, Phase 2 is complete. Otherwise, the intervals I and J are merged to obtain a new interval K, and the D-values on both sides of K are updated into P.

Consider the case where k iterations of Phase 2 are performed. Obviously $k < V$ because at most $V - 1$ interval mergings can be performed. After k iterations (mergings) there are $V - k$ intervals left in L_I and an equal number of examples in Q. Phase 3 submits the examples still left in Q to T, and copies L_I to another list L_D that saves the result of the discretization.

It is clear that the discretization produced by OCM is equivalent to the one of the batch version: It operates on the same initial intervals using the same merging criterion. Moreover, the statistical significance order in which the initial intervals are examined is the same in both algorithms.

4.1 Time Complexity of Online ChiMerge

Let us now turn to the time consumption of one iteration of Phase 1. The insertion of the received example E to Q clearly takes constant time, as well as the insertion of an interval from T to L_I. Also computing the D-value can be considered a constant-time operation; it takes linear time with respect to the number of classes, which is usually low and fixed in any case. Inserting the obtained value to P is logarithmic in the number of values already in P, and thus requires time $O(\lg V)$. Finding a successor in T also takes time $O(\lg V)$. Thus, the total time consumption of one iteration of Phase 1 is $O(\lg V)$.

Next, consider the time consumption of one iteration of Phase 2. The insertion of the new example E and an example from the queue Q to the BST T both take time $O(\lg V)$. Extracting the lowest D-value from the priority queue P is also an $O(\lg V)$ time operation. As P contains pointers to the items holding intervals I and J in L_I, removing them can be implemented in constant time. The merging of I and J to obtain K can be considered a constant-time operation as well as computing the new D-values for K and its neighbors in L_I. Both depend linearly on the fixed number of classes. Updating each of the new D-values into P takes $O(\lg V)$ time. Thus, the total time consumption of one iteration of Phase 2 is also $O(\lg V)$.

The time consumption of Phase 3 is obviously $O(\lg V)$, since it only inserts examples to T and copies L_I to L_D. Incidentally, observe that within this logarithmic time bound we could build a binary search tree representation of the final discretization, instead of the linked list. It would be quicker to search, when in use, than the list L_D.

As Phase 1 needs V iterations, Phase 2 $(V - k)$ iterations, and Phase 3 k iterations to complete, the result of the discretization is achieved in $2V$ iterations. After the discretization is done, the BST already contains different bins, since $2V$ new examples have been received. At this point, the discretization can be restarted, and a possibly different result is obtained after another $2V$ iterations.

In Phase 1, the examples are accumulated to the queue Q for later processing. In Phase 2, Q is unwound and the examples are inserted to the BST along with the new incoming examples. Exactly V examples are saved in the queue, so its size comparable to the size of the BST. Hence, the $O(\lg V)$ time bound is not compromised.

The requirement of $2V$ iterations to complete the discretization can be reduced by an integral factor, with the cost of more required work per iteration. The cut points can be obtained in $2V/k$ steps if k iterations are performed each time a new example is received. Setting $k = 2V$ makes the algorithm work as if the batch version of ChiMerge was run each time a new example is received.

4.2 Alternative Approaches

First, let us point out that we can easily change OCM to produce (at most) a predefined number N of intervals. We just augment the check concerning the χ^2 threshold D_{th} with one concerning the length of list L_I. The list length can be easily implemented as a constant-time operation using an extra counter. Naturally, if there are less than N bins in the tree T, we also end up having less than N intervals. We will test this version of OCM in the following.

To guarantee results identical to Kerber's [18] original algorithm, above we took a snapshot of the BST T at some point of time. An equivalent discretization was then constructed efficiently on this frozen situation. One could, of course, consider working as proposed above, but without ever freezing T — instead of caching instances to Q, direct them always to T. Then, those bins that are processed later may receive new instances from `DataSource`, while some bins have already been fetched for processing. However, also new bins can be created during the processing of Phase 1. In the worst case this would lead to never reaching Phase 2. Hence, this approach is not really viable.

Another alternative for the algorithm put forward above would be to perform chi-merging in the spirit of VFDT [5]. That is, one would choose some number of initial bins based on the first example received from `DataSource` and only update the bin counts for subsequent examples. Chi-merging would then operate on these bins in the vein as described above.

Table 2. Characteristics of four UCI data sets

Data set	Numerical	Nominal	Classes	Training set	Test set
ADULT	6	8	2	32,561	16,281
CENSUS	7	32	2	199,523	99,762
COVER	10	44	7	387,341	193,671
SHUTTLE	9	–	7	43,500	14,500

When there is no single concept to track from the data stream, but rather the target changes over time [6], it does not suffice to keep stacking incremental changes to the decision tree. At some point one needs to forget old examples that are not instances of the current concept. The simplest approach is to have a sliding window of length W of the most recent examples and maintain a decision tree consistent with them. The overhead for using such a window is constant. Let us consider this scenario without paying attention to details of window length selection and updating.

The straightforward approach is to delete from the BST the oldest example in the window before (or after) inserting a new example to the BST. Deletion of an example causes similar changes to bins as insertion of an example. Hence, the deletion can be handled with local changes in constant time. Of course, we now traverse the BST twice doubling the time requirement of an update. Asymptotically, though, updates are as efficient as in single concept decision trees. Finally, let us point out that in a window of length W there can be at most W different values for a numerical attribute. Thus, in this scenario the maximum overhead for using the BST is a constant of the order $O(\lg W)$.

Another natural heuristic for dealing with concept drift would be to discard the BST once a new discretization has been prepared. Collecting examples from `DataSource` to a new BST would then start anew and after a suitable period a new discretization could be composed (for the changed situation). The success of such a heuristic largely depends on the accuracy of change detection being used.

5 A Comparative Evaluation

We now compare OCM with VFML binning into at most 10 bins [30] (VFML10), which was the superior discretization method in Pfahringer et al.'s [13] test, and with the original BST approach of Gama et al. [9] (BINTREE). Our test environment is Hoeffding trees as implemented by MOA [13,33,34] and we also use its implementation of the comparison discretization methods.

Let us begin by examining some of the larger data sets from the UCI repositories. Three out of the four come divided into separate training and test set. We also divided the remaining one (COVERTYPE) randomly so that 2/3 of the examples are used for training and the remaining 1/3 for testing. Table 2 summarizes the main characteristics of the data sets.

Table 3. Results on four UCI data sets

Algorithm	Size	Nodes	Depth	Accuracy	Size	Nodes	Depth	Accuracy
	ADULT				COVERTYPE			
VFML10	343	114	3	82.78	1,599	245	15	42.53
BINTREE	2,511	167	4	82.58	25,041	344	14	**60.30**
$OCM^{3}_{0.01}$	2,242	108	4	82.56	43,500	610	13	50.59
$OCM^{5}_{0.1}$	2,746	146	5	78.55	61,413	878	9	54.70
$OCM^{5}_{0.01}$	2,367	112	5	**82.80**	59,337	856	11	56.25
$OCM^{5}_{0.001}$	2,651	106	3	82.78	51,995	683	9	58.99
$OCM^{5}_{0.0001}$	2,642	103	3	82.84	59,517	789	11	53.35
$OCM^{5}_{0.00001}$	2,470	131	4	82.71	55,818	777	13	58.99
$OCM^{10}_{0.01}$	2,645	174	6	82.68	65,689	1,083	11	59.22
	CENSUS-INCOME				SHUTTLE			
VFML10	199	884	5	**94.27**	59	17	3	**97.93**
BINTREE	19,328	977	5	**94.27**	163	11	2	94.02
$OCM^{3}_{0.01}$	21,396	517	8	94.24	682	40	8	92.35
$OCM^{5}_{0.1}$	27,135	1,080	8	93.99	688	30	5	94.57
$OCM^{5}_{0.01}$	26,412	877	6	94.03	825	66	6	94.67
$OCM^{5}_{0.001}$	26,498	819	6	94.04	622	25	5	94.53
$OCM^{5}_{0.0001}$	26,611	728	6	94.04	609	22	4	94.53
$OCM^{5}_{0.00001}$	25,582	714	7	94.09	670	35	7	94.64
$OCM^{10}_{0.01}$	25,865	1,405	5	93.90	705	36	7	94.66

Table 3 lists the results obtained for the four test domains. OCM^{x}_{y} stands for the OCM method restricted to produce at most x intervals using χ^2 threshold value y. The columns of Table 3 are the total size (in kilobytes) of the produced Hoeffding tree including all the additional data structures, its total node count, its depth, and finally its classification accuracy on the test data.

We did not include any time measurements to Table 3, because MOA is implemented in Java and, thus, makes reliable time consumption tracking difficult. However, the time consumption of OCM and BINTREE is approximately the same and VFML10 is about 40% more efficient on CENSUS-INCOME and uses circa 60% less time on COVERTYPE. On the smaller sets, ADULT and SHUTTLE, all discretization methods are extremely efficient.

From Table 3 we see that VFML10 typically seems to use an order of magnitude less space than the approaches requiring a BST, even though the difference in node counts is not that large. In fact, VFML10 does not even consistently produce Hoeffding trees with the least number of nodes. BINTREE and OCM need to maintain a BST for every numerical attribute at each leaf of the evolving Hoeffding tree. Hence, it is not surprising that their space consumption is huge in comparison with VFML10, which only needs the ten bins per numerical attribute. The space consumption of OCM tends to be somewhat larger than that of BINTREE. This difference seems to go pretty much hand in hand with the number of nodes in the final tree. The additional data structures required for OCM are mainly responsible for this fact.

Table 4. Results on synthetic integer data

Attrs	3								5			
Values	20		40		80		160		20		40	
	nodes	Acc.	nodes	Acc.	nodes	Acc.	nodes	Acc.	nodes	Acc.	nodes	Acc.
VFML10	1607	64.2	1115	57.4	1076	**53.5**	1070	**51.4**	1079	**56.3**	1082	**54.0**
BinTr	1952	63.8	1217	56.9	1060	52.7	1109	51.1	1076	54.3	1064	53.4
OCM^3	5575	64.1	6331	57.2	5498	52.4	5650	50.8	4732	53.1	6135	52.0
OCM^5	6139	65.5	7908	58.6	6391	52.9	6546	51.0	5527	53.3	6849	52.4
OCM^{10}	6205	65.7	8132	**58.7**	6739	53.1	6672	51.1	5615	53.4	7179	52.5
OCM^{50}	6210	**65.8**	8131	**58.7**	6743	53.1	6672	51.1	5615	53.4	7179	52.5

Observe that, even though OCM uses multi-way splitting of the value range, we have not ruled out recursive partitioning of an attribute's value range that has already been divided. Hence, the OCM trees can be either larger or smaller than Hoeffding trees produced using BinTree. As concerns the parameter settings of OCM, the trend seems to be that tightening the threshold yields smaller trees and allowing more intervals leads to larger trees.

In any case, it is clear that if storage space is a limiting factor, the methods that aim to use exact knowledge of the data stream by maintaining BSTs are not viable alternatives to space-saving heuristics like VFML10. However, an experiment of Elomaa and Lehtinen [14] has demonstrated that the growth rate of the number of bins in data produced using the well known Waveform data generator [28] is only logarithmic in the number of bins.

No clear trend can be read from the depths of the produced trees. Multi-way trees, of course, can be larger than binary trees of equal depth. As concerns the prediction accuracy, VFML10 clearly suffers in the Covertype domain, but has some advantage on Shuttle. The wrong parameter setting hurts OCM, but otherwise (e.g., using $\text{OCM}^5_{0.01}$ or $\text{OCM}^5_{0.001}$) it appears competitive with the other techniques on these real-world domains. Covertype with its 44 binary attributes is the only domain in which clear performance differences are observed.

In our second set of tests we control the characteristics of the examples in order to recognize the important factors for the success of the discretization algorithms. We use synthetic data generated using RandomTreeGenerator of MOA. One million training and test examples are generated online in all test. The other characteristics of the data — like the type of attributes, their number, values per integer domain, and the number of classes — are varied.

We expect OCM to be at its best when the numerical attributes in the data are not really continuous-valued (real), but rather discrete-valued (integer). In such a case there will not be too many initial intervals to operate on, and there is real statistical significance in interval merging. Let us start by testing a setting in which there are only integer-valued attributes. There are two classes in these tests and the χ^2 threshold for OCM is always 0.01, so we leave it unmarked.

Table 4 shows the results in case of 3 and 5 integer-valued attributes with growing numbers of different values for the attributes. The first observation to

Table 5. Results on synthetic real data

Classes	2						5		10		20	
Atts	3		5		10		3		3		3	
	nodes	Acc.	nodes	Acc.	nodes	Acc.	nodes	Acc.	nodes	Acc.	nodes	Acc.
VFML10	371	99.8	281	99.8	443	**99.5**	374	98.2	275	98.0	179	95.5
BINTR	203	**99.9**	182	**99.9**	N/A	N/A	215	**99.2**	134	**99.0**	125	**99.2**
OCM^5	3716	97.3	4240	95.2	4607	92.9	2490	95.8	1563	96.6	1046	96.6
OCM^{10}	3815	98.2	2722	97.7	4171	95.7	2069	95.7	2045	95.9	1163	96.7
OCM^{50}	4525	97.8	3753	97.5	6427	94.7	3427	95.7	2485	96.7	1169	96.4

be made is that the prediction accuracies are quite low. This is an artifact caused by the fact that we needed to trick the RandomTreeGenerator to produce integer-valued attributes. Hoeffding trees of OCM have 5–7 times more nodes than those of VFML10 and BINTREE. Hence, the cost of using multi-way discretization turns out to be quite high. In prediction accuracy OCM has an advantage as long as the number of possible integer values is low, but loses it to VFML10 when the number grows, and also as the number of attributes is increased.

Table 5 lists the results when all generated attributes are real-valued. We expect this setting to be unfavorable to OCM, since interval mergings are presumably very rare. At the same time we also test whether increasing the number of classes has a significant impact on the results. This time OCM trees are already an order of magnitude larger than those of VFML10 and BINTREE. The prediction accuracies of all discretization methods are clearly higher than in case of pure integer attributes. Using BINTREE leads consistently to the most accurate Hoeffding trees. However, its space consumption is so high that already when there are only ten real-valued attributes the MOA implementation runs out of space. As expected, OCM produces somewhat less accurate trees than the comparison methods. VFML10 seems to be hit worst by increasing number of classes, while the results of OCM even keep improving.

Also in other tests conducted under different settings we found BINTREE to produce quite consistently slightly more accurate Hoeffding trees than VFML10. Hence, without an explicit limit for the available memory, exact cut point evaluation appears to be worth the effort.

In light of this brief evaluation, it is quite clear that the possible advantages of OCM are overshadowed by its drawbacks, mainly the large space consumption. However, using a different evaluation function (because of the known downsides of *IG*) and a more heuristic approach could lead to better results.

6 Conclusion

Decision tree learning from a data stream has been, on the high level, solved. However, numeric attribute learning — to some extent an open problem even in the batch setting — still needs some attention. Using the trivial ten-fold binning based on the first examples received is intellectually disappointing, even if it might work well in practice [13]. We have considered how to implement Kerber's [18] ChiMerge algorithm efficiently in the online setting. It is intuitively quite an appealing approach. The downside in the proposed algorithm is the fact that it is based on maintaining a balanced binary search tree recording the observed values of attributes (plus some other data structures). Thus, the space requirement can turn out to be prohibitive in some data stream scenarios [13].

It would be interesting to explore whether, e.g., a combination of a simple heuristic like VFML10 and OCM would lead to better accuracies space efficiently. Another obvious open problem is to examine which other successful batch learning algorithms can be implemented efficiently in the online model of computation. A more subtle question is whether they then suit the data stream model with strict requirements. As a more specific question, it would be interesting to examine whether the proposed approach can accommodate the improvements that have been proposed to ChiMerge.

Acknowledgments. This work has been supported by Academy of Finland. We thank Bernhard Pfahringer for divulging MOA to our use.

References

1. Muthukrishnan, S.: Data Streams: Algorithms and Applications. Foundations and Trends in Theoretical Computer Science, vol. 1(2). Now Publishers, Hanover (2005)
2. Aggarwal, C.C. (ed.): Data Streams: Models and Algorithms. Advances in Database Systems, vol. 31. Springer, Heidelberg (2007)
3. Gama, J., Gaber, M.M. (eds.): Learning from Data Streams: Processing Techniques in Sensor Networks. Springer, Heidelberg (2007)
4. Aggarwal, C.C., Han, J., Wang, J., Yu, P.S.: On demand classification of data streams. In: Proc. Tenth ACM SIGKDD International Conference on Knowledge Discovery and Data Mining, pp. 503–508. ACM Press, New York (2004)
5. Domingos, P., Hulten, G.: Mining high-speed data streams. In: Proc. Sixth ACM SIGKDD Conference on Data Mining and Knowledge Discovery, pp. 71–80. ACM Press, New York (2000)
6. Hulten, G., Spencer, L., Domingos, P.: Mining time-changing data streams. In: Proc. Seventh ACM SIGKDD Conference on Data Mining and Knowledge Discovery, pp. 97–106. ACM Press, New York (2001)
7. Gao, J., Fan, W., Han, J.: On appropriate assumptions to mine data streams: Analysis and practice. In: Proc. 7th IEEE International Conference on Data Mining, pp. 143–152. IEEE Computer Society Press, Los Alamitos (2007)
8. Gao, J., Fan, W., Han, J., Yu, P.S.: A general framework for mining concept-drifting data streams with skewed distributions. In: Proc. Seventh SIAM International Conference on Data Mining. SIAM, Philadelphia (2007)
9. Gama, J., Rocha, R., Medas, P.: Accurate decision trees for mining high-speed data streams. In: Proc. Ninth ACM SIGKDD Conference on Data Mining and Knowledge Discovery, pp. 523–528. ACM Press, New York (2003)
10. Jin, R., Agrawal, G.: Efficient decision tree construction for streaming data. In: Proc. Ninth ACM SIGKDD Conference on Data Mining and Knowledge Discovery, pp. 571–576. ACM Press, New York (2003)

11. Gama, J., Medas, P., Rodrigues, P.: Learning decision trees from dynamic data streams. In: Proc. 2005 ACM Symposium on Applied Computing, pp. 573–577. ACM Press, New York (2005)
12. Gama, J., Pinto, C.: Dizcretization from data streams: Applications to histograms and data mining. In: Proc. 2006 ACM Symposium on Applied Computing, pp. 662–667. ACM Press, New York (2006)
13. Pfahringer, B., Holmes, G., Kirkby, R.: Handling numeric attributes in hoeffding trees. In: Washio, T., Suzuki, E., Ting, K.M., Inokuchi, A. (eds.) PAKDD 2008. LNCS (LNAI), vol. 5012, pp. 296–307. Springer, Heidelberg (2008)
14. Elomaa, T., Lehtinen, P.: Maintaining optimal multi-way splits for numerical attributes in data streams. In: Washio, T., Suzuki, E., Ting, K.M., Inokuchi, A. (eds.) PAKDD 2008. LNCS (LNAI), vol. 5012, pp. 544–553. Springer, Heidelberg (2008)
15. Dougherty, J., Kohavi, R., Sahami, M.: Supervised and unsupervised discretization of continuous features. In: Proc. Twelfth International Conference on Machine Learning, pp. 194–202. Morgan Kaufmann, San Francisco (1995)
16. Liu, H., Hussain, F., Tan, C.L., Dash, M.: Discretization: An enabling technique. Data Mining and Knowledge Discovery 6(4), 393–423 (2002)
17. Yang, Y., Webb, G.I.: Discretization methods. In: The Data Mining and Knowledge Discovery Handbook. Springer, Heidelberg (2005)
18. Kerber, R.: ChiMerge: Discretization of numeric attributes. In: Proc. Tenth National Conference on Artificial Intelligence, pp. 123–128. AAAI Press, Menlo Park (1992)
19. Richeldi, M., Rossotto, M.: Class-driven statistical discretization of continuous attributes. In: ECML 1995. LNCS, vol. 912, pp. 335–338. Springer, Heidelberg (1995)
20. Liu, H., Setiono, R.: Feature selection via discretization. IEEE Transactions on Knowledge and Data Engineering 9, 642–645 (1997)
21. Tay, F.E.H., Shen, L.: A modified Chi2 algorithm for discretization. IEEE Transactions on Knowledge and Data Engineering 14(3), 666–670 (2002)
22. Catlett, J.: Megainduction: A test flight. In: Proc. Eighth International Workshop on Machine Learning, pp. 596–599. Morgan Kaufmann, San Mateo (1991)
23. Provost, F., Jensen, D., Oates, T.: Efficient progressive sampling. In: Proc. Fifth ACM SIGKDD International Conference on Knowledge Discovery and Data Mining, pp. 23–32. ACM Press, New York (1999)
24. Utgoff, P.: Incremental induction of decision trees. Machine Learning 4, 161–186 (1989)
25. Utgoff, P., Berkman, N.C., Clouse, J.A.: Decision tree induction based on efficient tree restructuring. Machine Learning 29(1), 5–44 (1997)
26. Mehta, M., Agrawal, R., Rissanen, J.: SLIQ: A fast scalable classifier for data mining. In: EDBT 1996. LNCS, vol. 1057, pp. 18–32. Springer, Heidelberg (1996)
27. Shafer, J.C., Agrawal, R., Mehta, M.: SPRINT: A scalable parallel classifier for data mining. In: Proc. Twenty-Second International Conference on Very Large Databases, pp. 544–555. Morgan Kaufmann, San Francisco (1996)
28. Breiman, L., Friedman, J.H., Olshen, R.A., Stone, C.J.: Classification and Regression Trees. Wadsworth, Pacific Grove (1984)
29. Quinlan, J.R.: C4.5: Programs for Machine Learning. Morgan Kaufmann, San Francisco (1993)
30. Hulten, G., Domingos, P.: VFML — a toolkit for mining high-speed time-changing data streams (2003)

31. Greenwald, M., Khanna, S.: Space-efficient online computation of quantile summaries. In: SIGMOD 2001 Electronic Proceedings, pp. 58–66 (2001)
32. Cormen, T.H., Leiserson, C.E., Rivest, R.L., Stein, C.: Introduction to Algorithms, 2nd edn. MIT Press, Cambridge (2001)
33. Kirkby, R.: Improving Hoeffding Trees. PhD thesis, University of Waikato, Department of Computer Science, New Zealand (2008), `http://adt.waikato.ac.nz/public/adt-uow20080415.103751/index.html`
34. Univ. of Waikato New Zealand: MOA: Massive On-line Analysis (2008), `http://www.cs.waikato.ac.nz/~abifet/MOA/`

Chapter 11
Mining Chains of Relations*

Foto Aftrati[1], Gautam Das[2], Aristides Gionis[3], Heikki Mannila[4], Taneli Mielikäinen[5], and Panayiotis Tsaparas[6]

[1] National Technical University of Athens
afrati@softlab.ece.ntua.gr
[2] University of Texas at Arlington
gdas@cse.uta.edu
[3] Yahoo! Research, Barcelona
gionis@yahoo-inc.com
[4] University of Helsinki
mannila@cs.helsinki.fi
[5] Nokia Research Center, Palo Alto
taneli.mielikainen@nokia.com
[6] Microsoft Research, Mountain View
panats@microsoft.com

Abstract. Traditional data mining methods consider the problem of mining a single relation that relates two different attributes. For example, in a scientific bibliography database, authors are related to papers, and we may be interested in discovering association rules between authors based on the papers that they have co-authored. However, in real life it is often the case that we have multiple attributes related through *chains* of relations. For example, authors write papers, and papers belong to one or more topics, defining a three-level chain of relations.

In this paper we consider the problem of mining such relational chains. We formulate a generic problem of finding selector sets (subsets of objects from one of the attributes) such that the projected dataset—the part of the dataset determined by the selector set—satisfies a specific property. The motivation for our approach is that a given property might not hold on the whole dataset, but holds when projecting the data on a subset of objects. We show that many existing and new data mining problems can be formulated in the framework. We discuss various algorithms and identify the conditions when apriori technique can be used. We experimentally demonstrate the effectiveness and efficiency of our methods.

1 Introduction

Analysis of transactional datasets has been the focus of many data mining algorithms. Even though the model of transactional data is simple, it is powerful enough to express many datasets of interest: customers buying products, documents containing words, students registering for courses, authors writing papers,

* A preliminary version of the paper appeared in ICDM'05.

D.E. Holmes, L.C. Jain (Eds.): Data Mining: Found. & Intell. Paradigms, ISRL 24, pp. 217–246.
springerlink.com

genes expressed in tissues, and many more. A large amount of work has been done on trying to analyze such two-attribute datasets and to extract useful information such as similarities, dependencies, clusters, frequent sets, association rules, etc [2, 5]. At the same time, there have been many attempts to generalize existing data mining problems on datasets with more complex schemas. For instance, multi-relational data mining [15, 17, 18, 19, 21] has been considered an extension to the simple transactional data model. However, addressing the problem in the full generality has been proved to be a daunting task.

In this paper, we focus on the specific problem of finding selector sets from one of the attributes of a multi-relational dataset, such that the projections they define on the dataset satisfy a specific property. As an example, consider a dataset with attributes A (authors), P (papers), and T (topics), and relations $R_1(A, P)$ on authors writing papers, and $R_2(P, T)$ on papers concerning topics. An interesting pattern, e.g., "authors x and y frequently write papers together" might not be true for the whole dataset, but it might hold for a specific topic t. Therefore, it is meaningful to consider projections of the bibliographic data on particular topics and search for interesting patterns (e.g., frequent author sets) that occur on the papers of those topics. Additionally, the schema resulting from combining the two relations $R_1(A, P)$ and $R_2(P, T)$ is rich enough so that one can express patterns that go beyond frequent sets and associations. For example, one of the problems we introduce in a later section asks for finding subsets of topics and corresponding authors who have written more papers than anyone else one those topics. Arguably such prolific authors are candidates of being the most *authoritative* researchers on the corresponding topics. Searching for combinations of {topics, authoritative authors} is a new and interesting data mining problem.

In our approach we model datasets as graphs, and patterns to be mined as graph properties. We formulate a generic problem, which in our graph terminology is as follows: *find subsets of nodes so that the subgraph resulting from projecting the data graph on those nodes satisfies a given property.* Our motivation is that the above formulation is a generalization of existing data mining problems, in the sense that commonly studied problems are instances of our generic problem for certain graph properties. Furthermore, in this paper we introduce a number of additional properties—instantiations to our generic problem—that lead to new and challenging problems.

Our contributions can be summarized as follows:

- We introduce a novel approach to mining multi-relational data. Our formulation is quite powerful and it can express many existing problems in data mining and machine learning. For example, finding frequent itemsets, association rules, as well as classification problems can be cast as special cases of our framework.
- In addition to expressing already existing problems, the proposed framework allows us to define many new interesting problems. We express such mining problems in terms of graph properties. We discuss many examples of specific

problems that can be used to obtain useful results in real applications and datasets.
- We give conditions under which monotonicity properties hold, and thus, a level-wise method like apriori (see, e.g., [47]) can be used to speed-up the computations. Many of the problems we consider are NP-hard — many of them are hard instances of node removal problems [60]. For such problems we propose an Integer Programming (IP) formulation that can be used to solve medium-size instances by using existing IP solvers.
- To demonstrate the utility of our model we perform experiments on two datasets: a bibliographic dataset, and the IMDB dataset. Our experiments indicate that our algorithms can handle realistic datasets, and they produce interesting results.

The general problem we consider can be defined for complex database schemas. However, for concreteness we restrict our exposition in cases of three attributes connected by a chain of two relations—as in the example of the bibliographic dataset. Such an extension is one of the simplest that one can make to the traditional transactional model. However, even this restricted setting can be useful in modeling many interesting datasets, and the resulting problems are computationally hard. Thus, we believe that exploring the simple model of two-relation chains can provide valuable insights before proceeding to address the problem for more complex multi-relational schemas. In this paper, we only discuss briefly extensions to more complex schemas in Section 3.4.

The rest of the paper is organized as follows. We start our discussion by presenting the related work in Section 2. In Section 3 we formally define our data mining framework and we give examples of interesting problems. In Section 4.1 we demonstrate a characterization of monotonicity that allows us to identify when a problem can be solved efficiently using a level-wise pruning algorithm. In Section 4.2 we describe Integer Programming formulations that allows us to solve small- and medium-size instances for many of our problems. Section 4.3 contains more details about the algorithms we implement and in Section 5 we discuss the results of our experiments. Finally Section 6 is a short conclusion.

2 Related Work

Mining of frequent itemsets and association rules on single binary tables such as market basket databases has been a very popular area of study for over a decade [2,5]. There has also been some effort on investigating data mining problems at the other end of the spectrum, i.e., *multi-relational mining* [15,17,18,19, 21,11,24,32,10,34,8]. The approach taken by researchers has been to generalize apriori-like data mining algorithms to the multi-relational case using inductive logic programming concepts. Our work also has connections with work in mining from multidimensional data such as OLAP databases [53] and with the more recent multi-structural databases [22]. In the latter, algorithms are presented for very general analytical operations that attempt to select and segment the data in interesting ways along certain dimensions. While such approaches have been extremely interesting in concept, our goal is more focused—we proceed from a single table case to the special case of multiple tables defined by chains of relations which often occur in real-world problems.

The work closest to our work is [35] where the authors introduce *compositional data mining* where they cascade data mining primitive operations over chains of relations. The primitive operations they consider is a bi-clustering operation and a re-description operation. Informally they look for patterns (bi-clusters) that emerge in one relation, after applying operations up in the chain of relations. The re-description operator is similar to to the selection predicates we consider, making their work closely related to ours. However, their work does not aim to optimize the selection process as in our case, but rather enumerate all possible mined patterns.

Our work on mining layered graphs also has connections with the widely studied general area of *graph mining*. Various types of graph mining problems have been investigated, such as mining frequent subgraphs [16, 29, 28, 30, 31, 33, 41, 56, 57, 59, 58, 61, 36, 63], link analysis of web graphs [50, 39, 62, 51, 6, 49, 20], extraction of communities [25, 4, 55, 40, 44], identification of influencers [37, 38, 1, 42, 13, 46, 43, 12, 54, 26], and so on. The work in [45] tries to summarize k-partite graphs, by defining clusters per level. As with multi-relational mining, our approach is more focused than these general efforts—we specifically investigate layered graphs, making the case that many interesting real-world problems can be modeled using such graphs, and develop interesting algorithmic techniques that can leverage the structure of such graphs. We also approach the problem from a different perspective, since we focus on the problem of finding selectors that make patterns emerge in the projected datasets, rather than looking for patterns in the whole dataset.

3 The General Framework

In the most general case of a database schema we assume attributes $A_1, A_2, \ldots, A_n$ and relations $R_1, R_2, \ldots, R_m$ on the attributes. Transactional data, the object of study of most data mining algorithms, can be viewed as an elementary schema having two attributes A (items) and B (transactions) and a single binary relation $R(A, B)$ (transactions contain items). There are at least three different, but equivalent, ways to view the relation R: (i) a usual database table T on A and B, (ii) a binary co-occurrence matrix M, with rows on A and columns on B, such that $M[a, b]$ is 1 if $(a, b) \in R$ and 0 otherwise, and (iii) a bipartite graph $G = (A, B; E)$ with edges $(a, b) \in E$ if and only if $(a, b) \in R$. In this paper, we find it convenient to work with the graph representation of schemas.[1]

As we noted in the introduction, we focus on a simple extension of the model to three attributes A, B and C and a chain of two relations $R_1(A, B)$ and $R_2(B, C)$. Thus, we assume a graph $G = (A, B, C; E_1, E_2)$ with three sets of nodes A, B and C corresponding to the three attributes and having one node

[1] Graph representation works well as long as all relations have two attributes. For relations with more than two attributes, one would need to talk about hypergraphs.

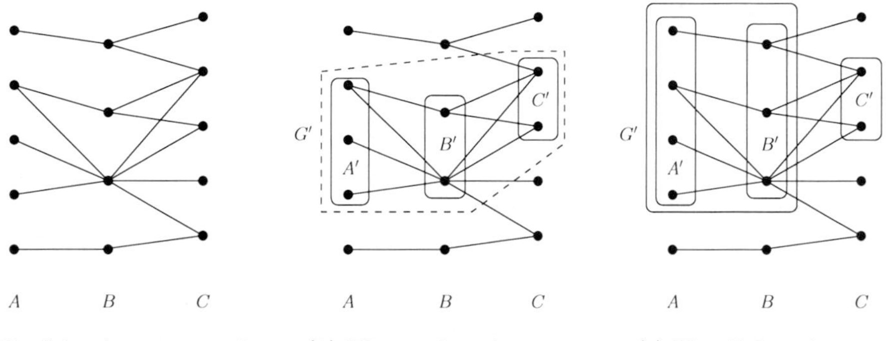

(a) The 3-level representation (b) The conjunctive case (c) The disjunctive case

Fig. 1. A graphical representation of the general framework: selecting a subset of nodes in the third level induces a bipartite subgraph between the first two levels. In this example, the *conjunctive interpretation* has been used to define the induced subgraph.

for each value in the domain of the attribute. The graph also has two sets of edges, E_1 connecting nodes in A and B, and E_2 connecting nodes in B and C. We call such a graph a *three-level graph.*

Examples of datasets that can be modeled with a three-level graph structure include: AUTHORS writing PAPERS about TOPICS; Web USERS answering online QUESTIONS associated with TAGS; ACTORS playing in MOVIES belonging to GENRES; TRANSCRIPTION-FACTOR-BINDING-SITES occurring at the promoter sequences of GENES that are expressed in TISSUES; and DOCUMENTS containing PARAGRAPHS containing WORDS.

The general data mining framework we consider is graphically depicted in Figure 1, and it is informally defined as follows. Consider the three-level graph $G = (A, B, C; E_1, E_2)$ shown in Figure 1(a). Given a subset $C' \subseteq C$ of nodes from level C, one can induce a subgraph G' from G by taking $B' \subseteq B$ and $A' \subseteq A$, such that every node in A' and B' is reachable from a node in C'. There are (at least) two different ways to define the sets A' and B' depending on whether we require that every node in A' and B' is reachable by *every* node in C' (the conjunctive case – Figure 1(b)), or that every node in A' and B' is reachable by *some* node in C' (the disjunctive case – Figure 1(c)). In each case, we obtain a different subgraph G', with different semantics. Now we are interested on whether the induced subgraph G' satisfies a given property, for example, "G' contains a clique $K_{s,t}$", or "all nodes in A' have degree at least k". The intuition is that the induced subgraph corresponds to a projection of the data, while the graph property corresponds to an interesting pattern. Thus, the generic data mining problem is the following: given a specific property Ψ, to find the selector set C' so that the induced subgraph G' satisfies Ψ.

3.1 Motivation

In this section we discuss the motivation behind our definition and we provide evidence that common data mining and machine learning problems can be cast in our framework.

First consider the traditional transactional data model, e.g., market-basket data. In the graph representation, the data form a bipartite graph $G = (I, T; E)$ with items in the set I, transactions in the set T, and an edge $(i, t) \in E$ if transaction $t \in T$ contains the item $i \in I$. Consider now the problem of finding a frequent itemset of s items with support threshold f. Such an itemset should appear in at least $f|T|$ transactions, giving rise to a $K_{s,f|T|}$ bipartite clique in the graph G. Thus, the problem of finding frequent itemsets corresponds to finding cliques in the bipartite data graph. Furthermore, answering the question whether the dataset contains a frequent itemset of size s with support f, corresponds to answering whether the input graph G contains a $K_{s,f|T|}$ clique. In other words, it corresponds to testing a *property* of the graph G.

Another well-studied problem in data mining is the problem of finding association-rules. An association rule $A \Rightarrow B$ with confidence c holds in the data if the itemset B appears in at least a c-fraction of the transactions in which the itemset A appears. Assume now that we want to find association rules with $|A| = k$ and $|B| = s$. We will show how this problem can be formulated as a selection problem in the three-level framework. Consider the graph representation $G = (I, T; E)$ of the transaction data, as defined before. Now, consider a set of items $A \subseteq I$. The set A induces a subgraph $G_A = (I_A, T_A; E_A)$, with $T_A = \{t : (i, t) \in E \text{ for all } i \in A\}$, $I_A = \{j : j \notin A, \text{ and } (j, t) \in E \text{ for some } t \in T_A\}$, and $E_A = \{(i, t) \in E : i \in I_A \text{ and } t \in T_A\}$. In other words, the subgraph G_A induced by A contains all transactions (T_A) that contain all items in A and all other items (I_A) in those transaction except those in A. The task is to find itemsets A (of size k) such that the induced subgraph G_A contains a $K_{s,c|T_A|}$ clique. The itemset B on the item side of the clique, together with the itemset A define an association rule $A \Rightarrow B$, with confidence c. So, the problem of finding association rules can be formulated as selecting a set of nodes so that the induced subgraph satisfies a given property.

In our next example, we show how a canonical machine-learning problem can also be formulated in our framework, and this time as a three-level graph problem. Consider a dataset of n "examples" $\mathcal{E} = \{\langle \mathbf{d}_i : c_i \rangle, i = 1, \ldots, n\}$, where each example is defined by a datapoint $\mathbf{d}_i$ over a set of attributes and c_i is a class label from a small set C of labels. Think of $\mathbf{d}_i$ as a person's entries to a credit card application questionnaire and the label c_i recording if the credit card was granted or not. The learning problem is to find a set of rules that correctly predict the credit card granting decision for a new applicant $\mathbf{x}$. For instance, such a rule combination could be "**if** `x.income > 50K` **and** `x.age` $\geq$ `18` **then** `yes`".

We now map the above learning problem to a three-level graph mining problem. The graph $G = (C, D, R; E_1, E_2)$ is constructed as follows. The examples in $\mathcal{E}$ induce the subgraph $(C, D; E_1)$. The set C consists of all possible class labels.

Alternatively the class labels can be considered as the possible properties of the data points. D is the set of datapoints, i.e., D has one vertex for each datapoint $\mathbf{d}_i$. There is an edge $(c, d) \in E_1$ iff the datapoint $d \in D$ has property $c \in C$.

The vertex set R captures the set of potential rules (or features). A rule r is a mapping $r : D \to \{0, 1\}$. For example if r is the rule "$\texttt{x.age} \geq \texttt{18}$", then $r(d) = 1$ for all datapoints that correspond to applicants older than 18, and $r(d) = 0$ for all applicants under 18. If the rules are restricted to be in a specific class, say, conjunctions of conditionals on single attributes of size at most three, then one can enumerate all potential rules. There is an edge $(d, r) \in E_2$ iff $r(d) = 1$. Hence, in the disjunctive interpretation, a subset of R induces a disjunction of rules, while in the conjunctive interpretation a conjunction of rules.

There are many classifier learning tasks that can be formulated for such three-level graph by posing additional constraints on the vertex and edge sets. Let us consider the credit card example mentioned above. For simplicity, we assume that there are only two classes, $C = \{\texttt{yes}, \texttt{no}\}$ corresponding on whether the credit card was granted. A person $d \in D$ is connected to the class `yes` if the person's credit card was approved and `no` if the card was declined. Hence, a person can be connected to one, two or none of the classes. There are a few natural formulations of the learning task. For example, the goal in the learning can be to find the set of rules that captures all persons connected to the class `yes` and no persons connected the class `no`, i.e., to find the *consistent classifier* characterizing the people who have been granted the credit card. Note that necessary condition of such set to exist is that each person is connected exactly to one of the classes. In practice there are often misclassifications and multiple class labels for the same data point. Hence, a more practical variant of the learning task would be to construct a rule set that captures people who should (should not) be granted the credit card, i.e., the people who are connected only to the class `yes` (`no`).

The classification problem example is only meant to convey intuition and motivation by casting a well known problem in our general framework. Many important issues such as selecting the collection of rules, avoiding overfitting the data, etc., are not discussed here. However a further discussion of this problem and precise definitions can be found in subsequent sections (Section 3.3 and Section 4.3).

3.2 Problem Definition

Before proceeding to formally define our problem, we make a comment on the notation: as a working example in the rest of the paper we use the bibliography dataset (AUTHORS – PAPERS – TOPICS). Therefore, we appropriately denote the three attributes appearing in the formulation by A, P, and T. The names of the problems and the graph properties are also inspired by the bibliography dataset, but this is only for improving the readability—most of problems are meaningful to many other datasets.

We start with attributes A, P and T, relations $E_1(A, P) \subseteq A \times P$ and $E_2(P, T) \subseteq P \times T$, and the corresponding three-level graph $G = (A, P, T; E_1, E_2)$.

Let $S \subseteq T$ be a subset of T. The set S acts as a selector over the sets P and A. First, for a single node $t \in T$, we define

$$P_t = \{p \in P : (p,t) \in E_2\}, \text{ and}$$
$$A_t = \bigcup_{p \in P_t} A_p = \bigcup_{p \in P_t} \{a \in A : (a,p) \in E_1\}.$$

That is, the sets P_t and A_t are the subsets of nodes in P and A, respectively, that are reachable from the node $t \in T$. (The set A_p is the subset of nodes in A that are reachable from the node $p \in P$.) We can extend the definition to the subsets P_S and A_S that is reachable from the set $S \subseteq T$. Extending the definition to sets requires to define the *interpretation* of the selector S. We consider the following two simple cases.

Disjunctive Interpretation. In the disjunctive interpretation ($\mathcal{D}$), the subsets P_S and A_S are the set of nodes that are reachable from *at least* one node in S. Therefore, we have

$$P_S^{\mathcal{D}} = \bigcup_{t \in S} P_t \quad \text{and} \quad A_S^{\mathcal{D}} = \bigcup_{p \in P_S^{\mathcal{D}}} A_p.$$

Conjunctive Interpretation. In the conjunctive interpretation ($\mathcal{C}$), the subsets P_S and A_S are the set of nodes that are reachable from *every* node in S. Therefore, we have

$$P_S^{\mathcal{C}} = \bigcap_{t \in S} P_t \quad \text{and} \quad A_S^{\mathcal{C}} = \bigcup_{p \in P_S^{\mathcal{C}}} A_p.$$

Now, let $\mathcal{I}$ denote the interpretation, which can be either conjunctive ($\mathcal{C}$), or disjunctive ($\mathcal{D}$), or any other possible interpretation. Given the selector set $S \subseteq T$ and the subsets $A_S^{\mathcal{I}}$ and $P_S^{\mathcal{I}}$, we can define the *induced* three-level graph $G_S^{\mathcal{I}} = (A_S^{\mathcal{I}}, P_S^{\mathcal{I}}, S; E_{1,S}^{\mathcal{I}}, E_{2,S}^{\mathcal{I}})$, where

$$E_{1,S}^{\mathcal{I}} = \{(a,p) \in E_1 : a \in A_S^{\mathcal{I}} \text{ and } p \in P_S^{\mathcal{I}}\}, \text{ and}$$
$$E_{2,S}^{\mathcal{I}} = \{(p,t) \in E_2 : p \in P_S^{\mathcal{I}} \text{ and } t \in S\}.$$

We also define the *induced* bipartite subgraph $B_S^{\mathcal{I}} = (A_S^{\mathcal{I}}, P_S^{\mathcal{I}}; E_{1,S}^{\mathcal{I}})$, which consists of the first two levels of G_S.

Hence, the selector set S selects a subset $P_S^{\mathcal{I}}$ of P and the set $P_S^{\mathcal{I}}$ induces the bipartite graph $B_S^{\mathcal{I}}$ by selecting all edges in E_1 and nodes in A that are adjacent to some node in $P_S^{\mathcal{I}}$, regardless of the interpretation. (There is no need for any additional interpretations for $A_S^{\mathcal{I}}$ or $B_S^{\mathcal{I}}$ as any further restrictions for $B_S^{\mathcal{I}}$ can be implemented as additional requirements to the property Ψ that $B_S^{\mathcal{I}}$ is required to satisfy.)

We are interested in finding selector sets S for which the induced subgraph $G_S^{\mathcal{I}}$ satisfies certain properties. Let $\mathcal{L}_G^{\mathcal{I}} = \{G_S^{\mathcal{I}} : S \subseteq T\}$ denote the set of all possible induced three-level graphs under interpretation $\mathcal{I}$. We define a property

Ψ as any subset of the set $\mathcal{L}_G^{\mathcal{I}}$. We say that the graph G_S satisfies Ψ if $G_S \in \Psi$. For the following, to ease the notation, we will often omit the superscript $\mathcal{I}$, when it is immaterial to the discussion.

For some specific property Ψ we can define the following data mining problem.

Definition 1 (Ψ Problem). *Given a three-level graph $G = (A, P, T; E_1, E_2)$, and the interpretation $\mathcal{I}$ find a selector set $S \subseteq T$ such that the induced subgraph $G_S^{\mathcal{I}}$ satisfies the property Ψ.*

The definition of the Ψ problem, requires finding any *feasible* solution $S \subseteq T$, such that the graph $G_S^{\mathcal{I}}$ satisfies the property Ψ. It is often the case that there are multiple feasible solutions to the Ψ problem, and we are interested in finding a feasible solution that satisfies an additional requirement, e.g., find the minimal, or maximal selector set $S \subseteq T$ that is a feasible solution to the Ψ problem. Formally, let $g : \mathcal{L}_G \to \mathbb{R}$, be a real-valued function on the set of graphs $\mathcal{L}_G$. We are then interested in finding a feasible solution S, such that the function $g(G_S)$ is optimized. Therefore, we define the following problem.

Definition 2 (g-Ψ Problem). *Given a three-level graph $G = (A, P, T; E_1, E_2)$, and the interpretation $\mathcal{I}$ find a selector set S such that the induced subgraph $G_S^{\mathcal{I}}$ satisfies the property Ψ, and the function g is optimized.*

This problem definition is general enough to capture different optimization problems. For example finding the maximum (or minimum) selector set such that G_S satisfies the property Ψ, corresponds to the case where $g(G_S) = |S|$, and we want to maximize (or minimize $g(G_S)$).

3.3 Examples of Properties

In this section we provide examples of interesting properties, some of which we will consider in the remainder of the paper. For the following definitions, we assume that the graph $G = (A, P, T; E_1, E_2)$ is considered as input. Additionally most of the properties require additional input parameters, i.e., they are defined with respect to threshold parameters, prespecified nodes of the graph, etc. Such parameters are mentioned explicitly in the definition of each property.

Given a selector set $S \subseteq T$ we have already defined the three-level induced subgraph $G_S = (A_S, P_S, S; E_{1,S}, E_{2,S})$, and the induced bipartite counterpart $B_S = (A_S, P_S; E_{1,S})$ (for some interpretation, whose index we omit here). Several of the properties we define, are actually properties of the bipartite graph B_S.

- AUTHORITY(c): Given a node $c \in A$, the graph $G_S = (A_S, P_S, S; E_{1,S}, E_{2,S}) \in \mathcal{L}_G$ satisfies AUTHORITY(c) if $c \in A_S$, and c has the maximum degree among all nodes in A_S. That is, given a specific author $c \in A$ we want to find a set of topics S for which the author c has written more papers than any other author, and thus, author c qualifies to be an authority for the combination of topics S. In a Questions'n Answers (QNA) system, where users answer questions online, we are interested in finding the set of TAGS for which a certain user c has answered the most questions.

- BESTRANK(c): Given a node $c \in A$, the graph $G_S = (A_S, P_S, S; E_{1,S}, E_{2,S}) \in \mathcal{L}_G$ satisfies BESTRANK(c) if $c \in A_S$, and for every other graph $G_R \in \mathcal{L}_G$, c is *ranked* at least as highly in G_S as in G_R. The rank of a node c in a graph G_S is the number of nodes in A_S with degree strictly higher than the degree of c, plus 1. This property is meant to be a relaxation of the AUTHORITY(c) property: since for a specific author c there might be no combination of topics on which c is an authority, we are interested in finding the combination T_c of topics for which author c is the "most authoritative". There might be other authors more authoritative than c on T_c but this is the best that c can do.
- CLIQUE: The graph $G_S \in \mathcal{L}_G$ satisfies CLIQUE if the corresponding bipartite graph B_S is a bipartite clique. Here we are interested in topics in which all papers have been written by the same set of authors. This property is more intuitive for the case of a biological dataset consisting of attributes TISSUES-GENES-TFBSs, where we look for TBFS's which regulate genes that are all expressed over the same tissues. It also makes sense in the QNA setting, where we are looking for a set of tags that define communities of users that answer the same questions.
- FREQUENCY(f, s): Given threshold value $f \in [0, 1]$, and an integer value s the graph $G_S = (A_S, P_S, S; E_{1,S}, E_{2,S}) \in \mathcal{L}_G$ satisfies the property FREQUENCY(f, s) if the corresponding bipartite graph B_S contains a bipartite clique $K_{s,f|P_S|}$. The intuition here is that a bipartite clique $K_{s,f|P_S|}$ implies a frequent itemset of size s with frequency threshold f on the induced subgraph. For this property, it is also interesting to consider the g-Ψ problem, where we define the objective function g to be the number of $K_{s,f|P_S|}$ cliques, and then look for the selector set that maximizes the value of the function g, that is, it maximizes the number of frequent itemsets.
- MAJORITY: The graph $G_S = (A_S, P_S, S; E_{1,S}, E_{2,S}) \in \mathcal{L}_G$ satisfies MAJORITY if for every $a \in A_S$ we have $|E^a_{1,S}| \geq |E^a_1 \setminus E^a_{1,S}|$, that is, for every node a in A_S, the majority of edges in G incident on a are included in the graph G_S. In the author-paper-topic context this means that in the induced subgraph for each selected author, the majority of its papers are selected by the selector topic set.
- POPULARITY(b): Given a positive integer b, the graph $G_S = (A_S, P_S, S; E_{1,S}, E_{2,S}) \in \mathcal{L}_G$ satisfies POPULARITY(b) if $|A_S| \geq b$. That is, we want to find topics for which more than b authors have written papers about.
- IMPACT(b): Given a positive integer b, the graph $G_S = (A_S, P_S, S; E_{1,S}, E_{2,S}) \in \mathcal{L}_G$ satisfies IMPACT(b) if for all nodes $a \in A_S$, the degree of a in the induced subgraph G_S is at least b. Here, the intention is to search for topics on which all authors have written at least b papers—and thus, hopefully, also have impact.
- ABSOLUTEIMPACT(b): Given a positive integer b, a graph $G_S = (A_S, P_S, S; E_{1,S}, E_{2,S}) \in \mathcal{L}_G$ satisfies ABSOLUTEIMPACT(b) if for all nodes $a \in A_S$, the degree of a in G is at least b. Note that the difference with the previous

definition is that we now consider the degree of node a in the graph G, rather than the induced subgraph G_S.

- CollaborationClique: A graph $G_S = (A_S, P_S, S; E_{1,S}, E_{2,S}) \in \mathcal{L}_G$ satisfies the property CollaborationClique if for every pair of nodes $a, b \in A_S$, there exists at least one node $p \in P_S$, such that $(a,p) \in E_{1,S}$ and $(b,p) \in E_{1,S}$. In other words, each pair of authors have co-authored at least one paper on the topics of S.
- Classification(c): In this setting we assume that the first level A is the set of class labels, the second level P is the set of examples, and the third level T is the set of features. Given a node $c \in A$, a graph $G_S = (A_S, P_S, S; E_{1,S}, E_{2,S}) \in \mathcal{L}_G$ satisfies Classification(c) if $P_S = \{p \in P : (c,p) \in E_1\}$ and $A_S = \{c\}$. That is, the selector set, must be such that an example $p \in P$ is selected if and only if it belongs to class c. Note that this implicitly assumes that each example is associated with a single class label, otherwise there is no feasible solution. Weaker properties can also be defined, if we allow some of the examples of other classes to be selected, or if we do not require all of the examples of class c to be selected. Those weaker versions can be defined using constraints on the number of false positives and false negatives. Also, one can look for feature sets characterizing multiple classes or combinations of classes, hence being related to multi-task learning [9].
- ProgramCommittee(Z, l, m): For this property, we break the convention that the selector operates on the set of topics, and we will assume that we select from the set of authors. This does not change anything in our definitions, since we can just swap the roles of the sets A and T. We are given a set $Z \subseteq T$ (topics of a conference), and values l and m. We say that the induced subgraph $G_S = (S, P_S, T_S; E_{1,S}, E_{2,S}) \in \mathcal{L}_G^{\mathcal{D}}$ satisfies the property ProgramCommittee(Z, l, m) if $T_S = Z$ (exactly the given topic set is selected), $|S| = m$, (m members in the program committee), and every node $t \in Z$ is connected to at least l nodes in S (for each topic there are at least l experts in the committee). Notice that this is the only example where we make use of the selector set S to define the property. Also, this is the only example in which we need to specify the interpretation $\mathcal{I}$, since the problem makes little sense in the case of the conjunctive interpretation.

3.4 Extensions of the Model

There are several ways in which our model can be extended to include more complex cases. Here we outline some of the possible extensions.

Boolean interpretations in between of disjunctive and conjunctive interpretations. Disjunctive and conjunctive interpretations are two extreme ways of selecting the nodes in P. Let S be the selector set. A node $p \in P$ belongs in $P_S^{\mathcal{D}}$ if and only if there is at least one edge from p to a node in S, and $p \in P$ belongs in $P_S^{\mathcal{D}}$ if and only if $(p,t) \in E$ for each $t \in S$. Hence, $P_S^{\mathcal{D}}$ contains all nodes in P covered by S and $P_S^{\mathcal{C}}$ contains all nodes in P that form a bi-clique with S.

There is a natural interpretation in between of these two extreme interpretations that unifies both the disjunctive and conjunctive interpretations. In the unifying interpretation the set $P_S^\delta \subseteq P$ of elements selected by S consists of all elements in P that are connected to at least δ-fraction of the nodes in S, i.e.,

$$P_S^\delta = \{p \in P : |\{t \in S : (p,t) \in E\}| \geq \delta |S|\}.$$

The conjunctive interpretation is obtained by setting δ to be 1, and the disjunctive interpretation by setting $\delta = 1/|S|$.

Weighted Graphs. In our definitions so far we have assumed that the graphs (or relations) are not weighted. A natural extension is to consider the case that the edges between the nodes of the various levels have weights, that is, the tuples in the corresponding relations E_1 and E_2 are associated with a weight. These weights carry some semantics, and we should modify our definitions to take them into account.

If there is a weight $w(p,t) \in (0,1]$ for each edge $(p,t) \in E_2$, the selection of node $p \in P$ can be done similarly as in Section 3.4: p is selected iff

$$\sum_{(p,t)\in E_2, t \in S} w(p,t) \geq \delta |S|.$$

Consider the case that each edge $(p,t) \in E_2$ is associated with a probability $Pr(p,t)$, and an element $t \in T$ selects a node p with probability $Pr(p,t)$. In that case we can express probabilistic versions of the interpretations. In the conjunctive interpretation, given a selector set S, we have that $p \in P_S$ with probability

$$\prod_{t:(p,t)\in E_2} Pr(p,t),$$

while in the disjunctive interpretation we have that $p \in P_S$ with probability

$$1 - \prod_{t:(p,t)\in E_2} (1 - Pr(p,t)).$$

We can also assume that relation E_1 is weighted. For example, in a dataset of tissues-genes-TBFS's, we may also have information about the expression levels of each gene on each tissue. There are several problems that generalize nicely in this setting, such as, Authority, BestRank, Majority, Impact, AbsoluteImpact. These problems involve looking at the degree of a node $a \in A$, which can naturally be replaced by the weighted degree, and the rest of the definition carries through. Furthermore, we can associate weights to the nodes of the graph, to model, e.g., the costs or the importance of the nodes.

It is also interesting to consider the Classification problem in the weighted case, where we assume that weight of an edge $(c,d) \in E_1$ is the probability that the example d belongs to class c. We can redefine the selection problem, to look for a set S of features such that the probability of the examples to belong to the chosen class c in the subgraph induced by S is maximized.

More Complex Schemas. The focus of this paper has been on mining three-level chains of relations. However, our definitions can be naturally extended into more complex schemas, involving more attributes and relations. In this general setting we have m attributes $A_1, \ldots, A_m$, and k binary relations $E_1, \ldots, E_k$. Thus we obtain a graph $G = (A_1, \ldots, A_m; E_1, \ldots, E_k)$. We assume that the relations are such that the resulting graph is connected. If A_s is the selector attribute, a node $s \in A_s$ selects a node in another attribute A_i, if there is a path between them in the graph G. Given a selector set $S \subseteq A_s$, and an interpretation, we can naturally extend the definitions in Section 3.2 to define the induced subgraph G_S, and then look for properties of this graph.

Schemas that would be interesting to explore in future work include the following.

- Longer chains of relations.
- Schemas in the form of k-partite graphs.
- Star schemas, where the selector attribute is one of the spikes of the star.
- Wheel graphs, where the selector attribute is the center of the wheel.

Implicit Topics. Sometimes the set of topics can be very large but still it can be decided efficiently whether a given paper p is connected to a given topic t, e.g., in polynomial time in the size of the graph $(A, P; E_1)$.

This is the case, for example, in learning boolean formulas in disjunctive (or conjunctive) normal form. Namely, for each topic $i \in T$ there is a monomial m_i over ℓ variables and there is a binary vector $b_j \in \{0,1\}^\ell$ associated to each paper $j \in P$. A topic $i \in T$ is connected to a paper $j \in P$ if and only if b_j satisfies the m_i. Hence, the problem corresponds the CLASSIFICATION problem (see Section 4.3) where the topics and their links to the papers are not given explicitly but by a polynomial-time algorithm determining for any topic $t \in T$ and paper $p \in P$ whether or not $(p, t) \in E_2$.

4 Algorithmic Tools

In this section we study characteristics of the various properties, and we show how they can help us in performing data mining tasks efficiently. We identify cases where level-wise methods (like the apriori algorithm) can be used and we propose an integer programming formulation that can be used in many problems. Finally we focus in four specific problems and discuss methods for their solution in more detail.

4.1 A Characterization of Monotonicity

The objective in this subsection is to identify cases where one can use standard level-wise methods, like the apriori algorithm and its variants. Given a three-level graph $G = (A, P, T; E_1, E_2)$, and an interpretation $\mathcal{I} \in \{\mathcal{C}, \mathcal{D}\}$, recall that $\mathcal{L}^{\mathcal{I}}$ is the set of all possible induced graphs under interpretation $\mathcal{I}$, for all possible selector sets $S \subseteq T$. We first give the following definitions for *monotonicity* and *anti-monotonicity*.

Definition 3. *A property Ψ is* monotone *on the set $\mathcal{L}_G^{\mathcal{I}}$ if the following is true: if for some selector set $S \subseteq T$ we have $G_S^{\mathcal{I}} \in \Psi$, then for all $R \subseteq S$ we have $G_R^{\mathcal{I}} \in \Psi$.*

A property Ψ is anti-monotone *on the set $\mathcal{L}_G^{\mathcal{I}}$ if the following is true: if for some selector set $S \subseteq T$ we have $G_S^{\mathcal{I}} \in \Psi$, then for all $R \supseteq S$ we have $G_R^{\mathcal{I}} \in \Psi$.*

The concept of monotonicity can be used to gain considerable efficiency in the computations by enumerating all possible sets of selectors in an incremental fashion (generate a set after having generated all of its subsets). Once it is found that the property Ψ is not satisfied for some selector set S, then the search space can be pruned by discarding from consideration all supersets of S. Many different implementations of this idea can be found in the literature [5]. Here we relate monotonicity and anti-monotonicity with the concept of *hereditary* properties on graphs.

Definition 4. *A property Ψ is* hereditary *on a class $\mathcal{G}$ of graphs with respect to node deletions, if the following is true: if $G = (V, E)$ is a graph that satisfies Ψ, then any subgraph $G' = (V', E')$ of G, induced by a subset $V' \in V$ also satisfies the property.*

A property Ψ is anti-hereditary *on a class $\mathcal{G}$ of graphs with respect to node deletions, if the following is true: if $G = (V, E)$ is a graph that does not satisfy Ψ, then any subgraph $G' = (V', E')$ of G, induced by a subset $V' \in V$ also does not satisfy the property.*

We can show that if a graph property Ψ is hereditary, it implies that the property is also monotone with respect to the disjunctive interpretation and anti-monotone with respect to the conjunctive interpretation.

Theorem 1. *Any hereditary property is monotone on the set $\mathcal{L}_G^{\mathcal{D}}$, and anti-monotone on the set $\mathcal{L}_G^{\mathcal{C}}$.*

Any anti-hereditary property is anti-monotone on the set $\mathcal{L}_G^{\mathcal{D}}$, and monotone on the set $\mathcal{L}_G^{\mathcal{C}}$.

Proof. Consider a hereditary property Ψ, and also consider any selector sets S and R such that $S \subseteq R \subseteq T$. We have $G_S^{\mathcal{D}} \subseteq G_R^{\mathcal{D}}$ and $G_R^{\mathcal{C}} \subseteq G_S^{\mathcal{C}}$. Since Ψ is hereditary it follows that if $G_R^{\mathcal{D}} \in \Psi$ then $G_S^{\mathcal{D}} \in \Psi$. Similarly, if $G_S^{\mathcal{C}} \in \Psi$ then $G_R^{\mathcal{C}} \in \Psi$. Thus, Ψ is monotone on $\mathcal{L}_G^{\mathcal{D}}$, and anti-monotone on $\mathcal{L}_G^{\mathcal{C}}$.

The rest of the theorem follows from the fact that an anti-hereditary property is a complement of a hereditary property.

The implication of the theorem is that, usually, given a property Ψ, one can check easily if Ψ is (anti-)hereditary or not. If it is (anti-)hereditary, then we know that a level-wise algorithm can be devised for solving the graph mining problem for this property [47]. For example, CLIQUE is hereditary, since removing any nodes from a clique graph we are still left with a clique. Additionally, the following results are immediate.

Proposition 1. *The properties* CLIQUE *and* ABSOLUTEIMPACT *are monotone on* $\mathcal{L}_G^{\mathcal{D}}$ *and anti-monotone on* $\mathcal{L}_G^{\mathcal{C}}$*. The property* POPULARITY *is anti-monotone on* $\mathcal{L}_G^{\mathcal{D}}$ *and monotone on* $\mathcal{L}_G^{\mathcal{C}}$*.*

On the other hand, by constructing simple counterexamples, one can show that the properties AUTHORITY, BESTRANK, FREQUENCY, MAJORITY, IMPACT, CLASSIFICATION and COLLABORATIONCLIQUE are neither monotone nor anti-monotone on $\mathcal{L}_G^{\mathcal{D}}$ or $\mathcal{L}_G^{\mathcal{C}}$. Thus, level-wise methods do not suffice to solve the corresponding problems.

4.2 Integer Programming Formulations

Computing the *maximal*, *minimal*, or *any* selector set is an NP-hard problem for most of the examples given in Section 3.3. In Section 4.1 we showed that if the property under consideration is hereditary, then the task of enumerating all solution sets (therefore also the maximal and the minimal sets) can be done efficiently by a level-wise approach.

In this section we give IP formulations for some of the examples given in Section 3.3. Solvers for IP and LP have been in the core of extensive research in operations research and applied algorithms, and highly optimized methods are available [48]. We found that small- and medium-size instances of the problems we consider can be solved quite efficiently using an off-the-shelf IP solver.[2] Notice also that in the IP formulation we typically ask for one solution (often by imposing an objective function to optimize), as opposed to enumerating all solutions like in the previous section.

Let $G = (A, P, T; E_1, E_2)$ denote the three-level graph that represents the relational chain. For each element $i \in T$, we define a variable $t_i \in \{0, 1\}$, where $t_i = 1$ if the element i is selected and zero otherwise. Furthermore for each element $j \in P$ we define a variable $p_j \in \{0, 1\}$. We need also to add constraints on these variables.

First, we implement the selection of elements in P. In the disjunctive interpretation we require that if an element $i \in T$ is chosen, then the set $P_i^T = \{j \in P : (j, i) \in E_2\}$, consisting of all the papers in P that belong to topic i, is also chosen. This condition is enforced by requiring that

$$p_j \geq t_i \text{ for all } j \in P_i^T.$$

[2] In practice, we solve IPs using the Mixed Integer Programming (MIP) solver `lp_solve` obtained from `http://groups.yahoo.com/group/lp_solve/`.

Furthermore, we require that for each $j \in P$ that is chosen, at least one $i \in T$ is chosen, such that $(j, i) \in E_2$. Let $T_j^P = \{i \in T : (j, i) \in E_2\}$ be the set of topics to which paper j belongs. Hence, we have that

$$\sum_{i \in T_j^P} t_i \geq p_j \text{ for all } j \in P.$$

The constraints guarantee that if the variables $t_i \in [0, 1]$ take values in $\{0, 1\}$ then the variables $p_j \in [0, 1]$ will also take values in $\{0, 1\}$. Thus, in the disjunctive interpretation we can relax the constraints $p_j \in \{0, 1\}$ to $p_j \in [0, 1]$ for all $j \in P$.

In conjunctive interpretation we require that a paper in P can be selected if and only if it is connected to all nodes in the selector set S. This can be expressed by the inequalities

$$\sum_{i \in T_j^P} t_i \geq |T_j^P| p_j \qquad \text{and} \qquad |T_j^P| - \sum_{i \in T_j^P} t_i \geq 1 - p_j.$$

The constraints guarantee that if the variables $p_j \in [0, 1]$ take values in $\{0, 1\}$ then the variables $t_i \in [0, 1]$ will also take values in $\{0, 1\}$. Thus, in the conjunctive interpretation we can relax the constraints $t_i \in \{0, 1\}$ to $t_i \in [0, 1]$ for all $i \in T$.

Finally, for each element $k \in A$, we similarly define a variable $a_k \in \{0, 1\}$ and impose the same constraints as for the p_j variables in the disjunctive interpretation. Let $A_j^P = \{k : (k, j) \in E_1\}$ be the set of authors of paper j, and $P_k^A = \{j : (k, j) \in E_1\}$ be the set of papers authored by author k. Then we have

$$a_k \geq p_j \qquad \text{and} \qquad \sum_{j \in P_k^A} p_j \geq a_k$$

for all $k \in A_j^P$, and again the constraints $a_k \in \{0, 1\}$ can be relaxed to $a_k \in [0, 1]$ for all $k \in A$.[3] We also define variable x_k, that captures the degree of the node $k \in A$ in the subgraph induced by the selected nodes in T, i.e., $x_k = \sum_{j \in P_k^A} p_j$.

We now show how to express some of the properties we discussed in Section 3.3 by imposing restrictions on the different variables.

- Authority(c): We impose the constraints $x_c \geq x_k$ for all $k \in A - \{c\}$. Note that the potential topics are the topics that author c has at least one paper. That is, we can restrict the search for a good topic set to the subgraph induced by the topics of author c.
- Clique: We impose the constraint that $a_k = \sum_{j \in P} p_j$ for all $k \in A$.
- Frequency(f, s): We define variables z_k for selecting a subset of selected authors and y_j for selecting a subset of selected papers. These variables are used to define the clique. First, we express that only selected authors and

[3] In fact, by allowing some of the variables to be real-valued, we can used Mixed Integer Programming (MIP) instead of IP and improve the performance considerably.

papers can be selected. That is, $z_k \in \{0, a_k\}$ for all $k \in A$, and $y_j \in \{0, p_j\}$ for all $j \in P$. Second, we add constraints requiring that the number of authored in the clique is s and that the number of papers in the clique is at least $f|P_S|$, i.e., $\sum_{k \in A} z_k = s$ and $\sum_{j \in P} y_j \geq f \sum_{j \in P} p_j$. Finally, we require that the variables z_k and y_j define a clique: $\sum_{k \in A, (k,j) \in E_1} z_k = s y_j$ for all $j \in P$.
- MAJORITY: We impose the constraint that $(1 - a_k)|P_k^A| + x_k \geq |P_k^A|/2$ for all $k \in A$.
- POPULARITY(b): We impose the constraint that $\sum_{k \in A} a_k \geq b$.
- IMPACT(b): We impose the constraint that $x_k \geq b$ for all $k \in A$.
- ABSOLUTEIMPACT(b): We impose the constraint that $|P_k^A| \geq b a_k$ for all $k \in A$.
- COLLABORATIONCLIQUE: Let us denote the set of co-authors of author $k \in A$ by $C_k = \{k' \in A : \exists j \in P_k^A \text{ s.t. } (k,j), (k',j) \in E_1\}$. Then we impose the constraints $a_k|A| + c - \sum_{k' \in C_k} a_{k'} \leq |A|$ for all $k \in A$, and $c = \sum_{k \in A} a_k$ where c is a real-valued variable.
- PROGRAMCOMMITTEE(Z, l, m): Let $A_i^T = \{k \in A : \exists j \in P_k^A \text{ s.t. } (j,i) \in E_2\}$. We add the constraints $\sum_{k \in A} a_k \leq m$, and $\sum_{k \in A_i^T} a_k \geq l$ for all $i \in Z$. For this problem, we need also the constraints $a_k \in \{0,1\}$ for all $k \in A$ since there are no topic set selection involved in the program. Note also that we can neglect the authors outside the set $\bigcup_{i \in Z} A_i^T$.

4.3 Case Studies

In this subsection, we focus on four specific problems among those listed in Section 3.3 and we look into detailed aspects of their solution. Two of them are selected to perform experiments with on real datasets. These experiments are reported in the next section.

The FREQUENCY **Problem.** Recall that the FREQUENCY problem is as follows. Given the graph $G = (A, P, T, E_1, E_2)$ a value s, and a threshold value f, we want to find a subset of nodes $S \subseteq T$ so that in the induced subgraph $G_S = (A_S, P_S, S; E_{1,S}, E_{2,S})$ there exist frequently occurring "itemsets" $V \subseteq A_S$ of size s. In other words, for itemset V to be frequent according our definition, it needs to be the case that V is frequent on the restriction of the graph imposed by a selector set S. Thus, finding frequent itemsets V with frequency threshold f in the three-level graphs is equivalent to fining *association rules* $S \Rightarrow V$ with confidence threshold f.

One only needs to add the restriction that the premise set S is selected from node set T and the conclusion set V is selected from node set A, but this only prunes the possible search space. There are many algorithms for association-rule mining in the literature [5] and any of them would be applicable in our setting with the above-mentioned modification.

The AUTHORITY **Problem.** For a single author c, we solve the authority problem using MIP. As the optimization objective function g, we consider maximizing the number of authors related to the topic set $S \subseteq T$, that is, $g(G_S) = |A_S|$, for $G_S = (A_S, P_S, S; E_{1,S}, E_{2,S})$.

The requirement that the author has the largest number of papers in the induced subgraph can sometimes be too restrictive. One could also, for example, minimize the absolute distance between the highest degree $\max_{k \in A_S} x_k$ of the authors and the degree x_c of the author c, or minimize $\sum_{k \in A_S}(x_k - x_c)$.

The rank alone, however, does not tell everything about the authority of an author. For example, the number of authors and papers in the induced subgraph matter. Thus, it makes sense to search for ranks for all different topic sets.

A set of papers fully determines the set of authors and a set of topics fully determines the set of papers. It is often the case that different sets of topics induce the same set of papers. Thus, we do not have to compute the rankings of the authors for all sets of topics to obtain all different rankings; it suffices to compute the rankings only once for each distinct set of papers that results by a combination of topics. The actual details of how to do this depend on which interpretation we use.

Conjunctive interpretation. In the conjunctive interpretation, the subgraph induced by a topic set S contains a paper $j \in P$ if and only if $S \subseteq T_j^P$, that is, S is a subset of the set of topics to which paper j belongs. Thus, we can consider each paper $j \in P$ as a topic set T_j^P. Finding all topic sets that induce a non-empty paper set in the conjunctive interpretation can be easily done using a bottom-up apriori approach. The problem can be cast as a frequent-set mining task in a database consisting the topic sets T_j^P of the papers $j \in P$ with frequency threshold $f = 1/|P|$ (so that a chosen topic set is related to at least one paper). Any frequent set mining algorithms can be used, e.g., see [5]. Furthermore, we can easily impose a minimum frequency constraint for the topic sets, i.e., we can require that a topic set should be contained in at least $f|P|$ sets $T_j^P, j \in P$ for a given frequency threshold $f \in [0, 1]$. In addition to being a natural constraint for the problem, this often decreases considerably the number of topic sets to be ranked.

However, it is sufficient to compute the rankings only once for each distinct set of papers. It can be shown that the smallest such collection of topic sets consists of the topic sets $S \subseteq T$ such that $S = \bigcap_{i \in S, j \in P_i^T} T_j^P$. Intuitively, this means that the set S is closed under the following operation: take the set of papers that are connected to all topics in S. Then for each paper j compute T_j^P, the set of topics to which paper j belongs, and then take the intersection of T_j^P's. This operation essentially computes the nodes in T that are reachable from S when you follow an edge from S to P, and then back to T. The intersection of T_j^P's should give the set S. In frequent set mining such sets are known as the closed sets, and there are many efficient algorithms discovering (frequent) closed sets [5]. The number of closed frequent itemsets can be exponentially smaller than the number of all frequent itemsets, and actually in practice the closed frequent itemsets are often only a fraction of all frequent itemsets.

Disjunctive interpretation. In the disjunctive interpretation, the subgraph induced by the topic set S contains a paper $j \in P$ if and only if S hits the paper, i.e., $S \cap T_j^P \neq \emptyset$. Hence, it is sufficient to compute the rankings only for those topic sets S that hit strictly more papers than any of their subsets. By definition, such sets of topics correspond to minimal hypergraph transversals and their subsets in the hypergraph $\left(T, \{T_j^P\}_{j \in P}\right)$, i.e., the partial minimal hypergraph transversals.

Definition 5. *A hypergraph is a pair $H = (X, \mathcal{F})$ where X is a finite set and $\mathcal{F}$ is a collection of subsets of X. A set $Y \subseteq X$ is a hypergraph transversal in H if and only if $Y \cap Z \neq \emptyset$ for all $Z \in \mathcal{F}$. A hypergraph transversal Y is minimal if and only if no proper subset of it is a hypergraph transversal.*

All partial minimal hypergraph transversals can be generated by a level-wise search because each subset of a partial minimal hypergraph transversal is a partial minimal hypergraph transversal. Furthermore, each partial minimal transversal in the hypergraph $\left(T, \{T_j^P\}_{j \in P}\right)$ selects a different set of papers than any of its sub- or superset.

Theorem 2. *Let $Z' \subsetneq Z \subsetneq Y$ where Y is a minimal hypergraph transversal. Then $P_Z^{\mathcal{D}} \neq P_{Z'}^{\mathcal{D}}$.*

Proof. Let Y be a minimal hypergraph transversal and assume that $Z' \cap Z$ hits all same sets in the hypergraph as Z for some $Z' \subsetneq Z \subsetneq Y$. Then $Y \setminus (Z \setminus Z')$ hits the same set in the hypergraph as Y, which is in contradiction with the assumption that Y is a minimal hypergraph transversal.

The all minimal hypergraph transversals could be enumerate also by discovering all *free* itemsets in the transaction database representing the complement of the bipartite graph $(P, T; E_2)$ where topics are items and papers transactions. (Free itemsets are itemsets that have strictly higher frequency in the data than any of their strict subsets. Free frequent itemsets can be discovered using the level-wise search [7].) More specifically, the complements of the free itemsets in such data correspond to the minimal transversals in a hypergraph $H = (X, \mathcal{F})$:

$$\bigcup \{Z \in \mathcal{F} : Z \cap Y \neq \emptyset\} = X \setminus \bigcap \{X \setminus Z \in \mathcal{F} : Z \cap Y \neq \emptyset\},$$

i.e., that the union of sets $Z \in \mathcal{F}$ intersecting with the set Y is the complement of the intersection of the sets $X \setminus Z \in \mathcal{F}$ such that Z intersects with Y.

In the disjunctive interpretation of the AUTHORITY problem we impose an additional constraint for the topic sets to make the obtained topic sets more meaningful. Namely, we require that for a topic set to be relevant, there must be at least one author that has written papers about all of the topics. This further prunes the search space and eases the candidate generation in the level-wise solution.

The ProgramCommittee Problem. For the exact solution to the ProgramCommittee problem we use the MIP formulation sketched in Section 4.2. That is, we look for a set of m authors such that for each topic in a given set of topics Z there are at least l selected authors with a paper on this topic. Among such sets of authors, we aim to maximize the number of papers of the authors on the topics in Z. To simplify considerations, we assume, without loss of generality, that the topic set T of the given three-level graph $G = (A, P, T; E_1, E_2)$ is equal to Z and that all authors and papers are connected to the topics.

Although the ProgramCommittee problem can be solved exactly using mixed integer programming techniques, one can also obtain approximate solutions in polynomial time in the size of G. The ProgramCommittee problem can be decomposed into the following subproblems.

First, for any solution to the ProgramCommittee problem we require that for each topic in Z there are at least l selected authors with papers about the topic. This problem is known as the minimum set multicover problem [52]:

Problem 1 (Minimum set multicover). Given a collection $\mathcal{C}$ of subsets of S and a positive integer l, find the collection $\mathcal{C}' \subseteq \mathcal{C}$ of the smallest cardinality such that every element in S is contained in at least l sets in $\mathcal{C}'$.

The problem is NP-hard and polynomial-time inapproximable within a factor $(1 - \epsilon) \log |S|$ for all $\epsilon > 0$, unless NP $\subseteq$ $\textsc{Dtime}(n^{\log \log n})$ [23]. However, it can be approximated in polynomial time within a factor $H_{|S|}$ where $H_{|S|} = 1 + 1/2 + \ldots + 1/|S| \leq 1 + \ln |S|$ [52]. Hence, if there is a program committee of size at most m covering each topic in Z at least l times, we can find such a program committee of size at most $mH_{|Z|}$.

Second, we want to maximize the number of papers (on the given set Z of topics) by the selected committee. This problem is known as the maximum coverage problem [23]:

Problem 2 (Maximum coverage). Given a collection $\mathcal{C}$ of subsets of a finite set S and a positive integer k, find the collection $\mathcal{C}' \subseteq \mathcal{C}$ covering as many elements in S as possible.

The problem NP-hard and polynomial-time inapproximable within the factor $(1 - 1/e) - \epsilon$ for any $\epsilon > 0$, unless NP = P. However, the fraction of covered elements in S by at most k sets in $\mathcal{C}$ can be approximated in polynomial time within a factor $1 - 1/e$ by a greedy algorithm [23]. Hence, we can find a program committee that has at least $1 - 1/e$ times the number of papers as the program committee of the same size with the largest number of papers.

Neither of these solutions is sufficient for our purposes. The minimum set multicover solution ensures that each topic has sufficient number of experts in the program committee, but does not provide any guarantees on the number of papers of the program committee. The maximum coverage solution maximizes the number of papers of the program committee, but does not ensure that each topic has any program committee members.

By combining the approximation algorithms for the minimum set multicover and maximum coverage problems, we can obtain an $(1 + H_{|Z|}, 1 - 1/e)$-approximation algorithm for the PROGRAMCOMMITTEE problem, i.e., we can derive an algorithm such that the size of the program committee is at most $(1 + H_{|Z|}m)$ and the number of the papers of the program committee is within a factor $1 - 1/e$ of the program committee of size m with the largest number of papers. The algorithm is as follows:

1. Select a set $A' \subseteq A$ of at most $mH_{|Z|}$ authors in such a way that each topic in Z is covered by at least l authors (using the approximation algorithm for the minimum set multicover problem). Stop if such a set does not exist.
2. Select a set $A'' \subseteq A$ of m authors that maximizes the coverage of the papers (using the approximation algorithm for the maximum coverage).
3. Output $A' \cup A''$.

In other words, first we select at most $mH_{|Z|}$ member to the program committee in such a way that each topic of the conference is covered by sufficiently many program committee members and then we select authors that cover large fraction of papers on some of the topics of the conference, regardless of which particular topic they have been publishing of.

Clearly, $|A' \cup A''| \leq (1+H_{|Z|})m$ and the number of papers covered by the sets in $A' \cup A''$ is within a factor $1 - 1/e$ from the largest number of papers covered by any subset of A of cardinality m.

The algorithm can be improved in practice in several ways. For example, we might not need all sets in A to achieve the factor $1 - 1/e$ approximation of the covering the papers with m authors. We can compute the number h of papers needed to be covered to achieve the approximation factor $1 - 1/e$ by the approximation algorithm for the maximum coverage problem. Let the number of paper covered by A' be h'. Then we need to cover only $h'' = h - h'$ papers more. This can be done by applying the greedy set cover algorithm to the instance that does not contain the papers covered by the authors in A'. The set of authors obtained by this approach is at most as large as $A' \cup A''$. The solution can be improved also by observing that for each covered paper only one author is needed and each topic has to be covered by only l authors. Hence, we can remove one by one the authors from $A' \cup A''$ as far as these constraints are not violated.

The CLASSIFICATION Problem. The classification problem is equal to learning monomials and clauses of explicit features. These tasks correspond to conjunctive and disjunctive interpretations of the CLASSIFICATION problem, respectively.

Conjunctive interpretation. Finding the largest (or any) set $F_{\max} \subseteq T$ corresponding to examples $E \subseteq P$ of a certain class $c \in A$ can be easily obtained by taking all nodes in T that contain all examples of class c, if such a subset exists. (Essentially the same algorithm is well-known also in PAC-learning [3].)

The problem becomes more interesting if we set $g(G_S) = |S|$ and we require the solution S that minimizes g. The problem of obtaining the smallest set $F_{\min} \subseteq T$ capturing all examples of class c and no other examples is known to be NP-hard [3]. The problem can be recast as a minimum set cover problem as follows. Let $\bar{E}_c \subseteq P$ denote the set of examples of all classes other than c. Also let $F_c \subseteq T$ denote the set of features linking to the examples of the class c. Now consider the bipartite graph $B = (\bar{E}_c, F_c; E)$, where $(p,t) \in E$ if $(p,t) \notin E_2$. For any feasible solution S for the classification problem, the features in S must cover the elements in $\bar{E}_c$ in the bipartite graph B. That is, for each $e \in \bar{E}_c$ there exists $f \in S$, such that $(e,f) \in E$, that is, $(e,f) \notin E_2$. Otherwise, there exists an example $e \in \bar{E}_c$ such that for all for all $f \in S$, $(e,f) \in E_2$, and therefore, e is included in the induced subgraph G_S, thus violating the CLASSIFICATION property. Finding the minimum cover for the elements in $\bar{E}_c$ in the bipartite graph B is an NP-complete problem. However, it can be approximated within a factor $1 + \ln |F_c|$ by the standard greedy procedure that selects each time the feature that covers the most elements [14]. (This algorithm is also well-known in the computational learning theory [27].)

Disjunctive interpretation. First note that it is straightforward to find the largest set of features, which induces a subgraph that contains only examples of the target class c. This task can be performed by simply taking all features that disagree with all examples of other classes. Once we have this largest set, then one can find the smallest set, by selecting the minimum subset of sets that covers all examples of the class c. This is again an instance of the set cover problem, and the greedy algorithm [14] can be used to obtain the best approximation factor (logarithmic).

5 Experiments

We now describe our experiments with real data. We used information available on the Web to construct two real datasets with three-level structure. For the datasets we used we found it more interesting to perform experiments with the AUTHORITY problem and the PROGRAMCOMMITTEE problem. Many other possibilities of real datasets with three-level graph structure exist, and depending on the dataset different problems might be of interest.

5.1 Datasets

Bibliography Datasets. We crawled the ACM digital library website[4] and we extracted information about two publication forums: Journal of ACM (JACM) and ACM Symposium on Theory of Computing (STOC). For each published paper we obtained the list of authors (attribute A), the title (attribute P), and the list of topics (attribute T). For topics we arbitrarily selected to use the *second level* of the "Index Terms" hierarchy of the ACM classification. Examples of topics include "analysis of algorithms and problem complexity", "programming languages", "discrete mathematics", and "numerical analysis". In total, in the JACM dataset we have 2 112 authors, 2 321 papers, and 56 topics. In the STOC dataset we have 1 404 authors, 1 790 papers, and 48 topics.

[4] `http://portal.acm.org/dl`

IMDB Dataset. We extract the IMDB[5] actors-movies-genres dataset as follows. First we prune movies made for TV and video, TV serials, non-English-speaking movies and movies for which there is no genre. This defines a set of "valid" movies. For each actor we find all the valid movies in which he appears, and we enter an entry in the actor-movie relation if the actor appears in one of the top 5 positions of the credits, thus pruning away secondary roles and extras. This defines the actor-movie relation. For each movie in this relation we find the set of genres it is associated with, obtaining the movies-genres relation. In total, there are 45 342 actors, 71 912 movies and 21 genres.

5.2 Problems

The AUTHORITY **Problem.** For the AUTHORITY problem, we run the level-wise algorithms described in Section 4.3 on the two bibliography datasets and the IMDB dataset. For compactness, whatever we say about authors, papers, and topics, applies also to actors, movies, and genres, respectively. For each author a and for each combination of topics S that a has written a paper about (under the disjunctive or the conjunctive interpretation), we compute the rank of author a for S. If an author a has written at least one paper on *each* topic of S, and a is ranked first in S, we say that a is an *authority* on S. Given an author a, we define the collection of topic sets $\mathcal{A}(a) = \{S : a \text{ is authority for } S\}$, and $\mathcal{A}^0(a)$ the collection of minimal sets of $\mathcal{A}(a)$, that is, $\mathcal{A}^0(a) = \{S : S \in \mathcal{A}\}$, and there is no $S' \in \mathcal{A}$ such that $S' \subsetneq S\}$. Notice that for authors who are not authorities, the collections $\mathcal{A}(a)$ and $\mathcal{A}^0(a)$ are empty.

A few statistics computed for the STOC dataset are shown in Figure 2. In the first two plots we show the distribution of the number of papers, and the number of topics, per author. One sees that the distribution of the number of papers is very skewed, while the number of topics has a mode at 3. We also look at the collections $\mathcal{A}(a)$ and $\mathcal{A}^0(a)$. If the size of the collection $\mathcal{A}^0(a)$ is large it means that author a has many interests, while if the size of $\mathcal{A}^0(a)$ is small it means that author a is very focused on few topics. Similarly, the average size of sets inside $\mathcal{A}^0(a)$ indicates to what degree an author prefers to work on combination of topics, or on single-topic core areas. In the last two plots of Figure 2 we show the distribution of the size of the collection $\mathcal{A}(a)$ and the scatter plot of the average set size in $\mathcal{A}(a)$ vs. the average set size in $\mathcal{A}^0(a)$.

The author with the most papers in STOC is Wigderson with 36 papers. The values of the size of $\mathcal{A}^0$ and the average set size in $\mathcal{A}^0$ for Wigderson is 37 and 2.8, respectively, indicating that he tends to work in many different combinations of topics. On the other hand, Tarjan who is 4th in the overall ranking with 25 papers, has corresponding values 2 and 1.5. That is, he is very focused on two combinations of topics: "data structures" and ("discrete mathematics", "artificial intelligence"). These indicative results match our intuitions about the authors.

---

[5] `http://www.imdb.com/`

We observed similar trends when we searched for authorities in the JACM and IMDB datasets, and we omit the results to avoid repetition. As a small example, in the IMDB dataset, we observed that Schwarzenegger is an authority of the combinations ("action", "fantasy") and ("action", "sci-fi") but he is not an authority in any of those single genres.

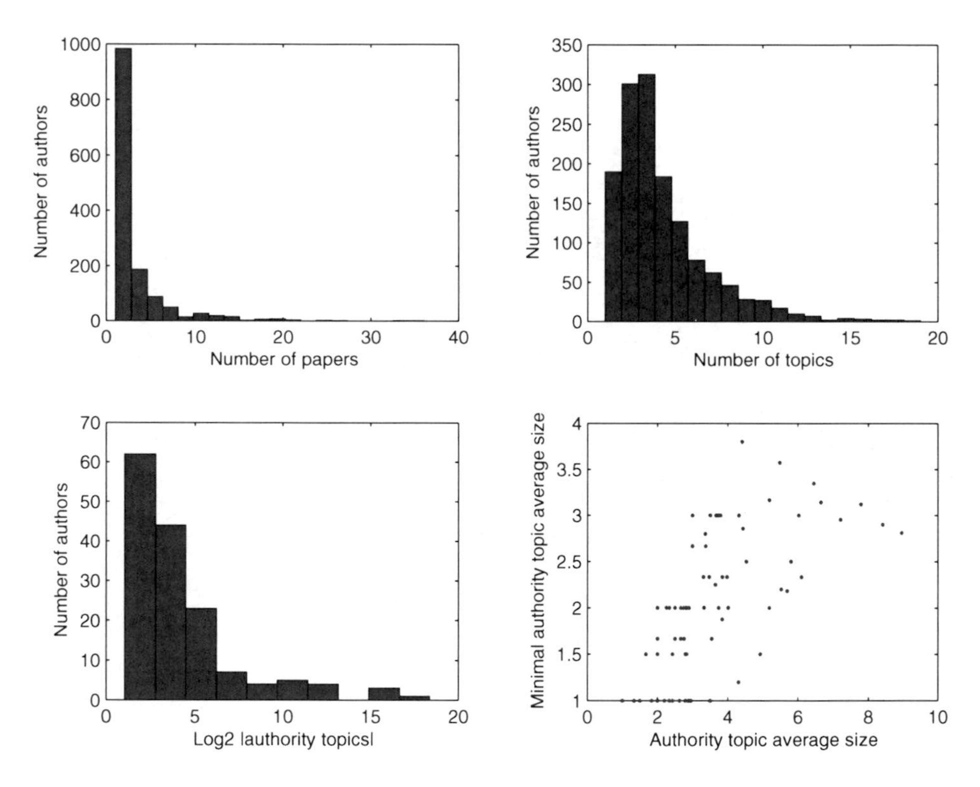

Fig. 2. A few statistics collected on the results from the Authority problem on the STOC dataset

The ProgramCommittee Problem. The task in this experiment is to select program committee members for a subset of topics (potential conference). In our experiment, the only information used is our three-level bibliography dataset; in real life many more considerations are taken into account. Here we give two examples of selecting program committee members for two fictional conferences. For the first conference, which we called Logic-AI, we used as seed the topics "mathematical logic and formal languages", "artificial intelligence", "models and principles", and "logics and meanings of programs". For the second conference, which we called Algorithms-complexity, we used as seed the topics "discrete mathematics", "analysis of algorithms and problem complexity", "computation by abstract devices", and "data structures". In both cases we requested a committee of 12 members requiring topics to be covered by at least 4 of the PC members. The objective was to maximize the total number of papers written by the PC members. The committee members for the LOGIC-AI conference, ordered by their number of papers, were

> Vardi, Raz, Vazirani, Blum, Kearns, Kilian,
> Beame, Goldreich, Kushilevitz, Bellare,
> Warmuth, and Smith.

The committee for the ALGORITHMS-COMPLEXITY conference was

> Wigderson, Naor, Tarjan, Leighton, Nisan,
> Raghavan, Yannakakis, Feige, Awerbuch, Galil,
> Yao, and Kosaraju.

In both cases, all constraints are satisfied and we observe that the committees are composed by well-known authorities in the fields. The running time for solving the IP in both cases is less than 1 second on a 3GHz Pentium 4 with 1GB memory, making the method very attractive to even larger datasets – for example, the corresponding IP for the IMDB dataset (containing hundreds of thousands variables in the constraints) is solved in 4min.

6 Conclusions

In this paper we introduce an approach to multi-relational data mining. The main idea is to find selectors that define projections on the data such that interesting patterns occur. We focus on datasets that consist of two relations that are connected into a chain. Patterns in this setting are expressed as graph properties. We show that many of the existing data mining problems can be cast as special cases of our framework, and we define a number of interesting novel data mining problems. We provide a characterization of properties for which one can apply level-wise methods. Additionally, we give an integer programming formulation of many interesting properties that allow us to solve the corresponding problems efficiently for medium-size instances of datasets in practice. In Table 1, the data mining problems we define in our framework are listed together with the property that defines them and the algorithmic tools we propose for their solution. Finally, we report experiments on two real datasets that demonstrate the benefits of our approach.

The current results are promising, but there are still many interesting questions on mining chains of relations. For example, the algorithmics of answering data mining queries on three-level graphs has many open problems. Level-wise search and other pattern discovery techniques provide efficient means to enumerate all feasible solutions for monotone and anti-monotone properties. However, the pattern discovery techniques are not limited to monotone and anti-monotone properties: it is sufficient that there is a relaxation of the property that is monotone or anti-monotone. Hence, finding monotone and anti-monotone relaxations of the properties that are not monotone nor anti-monotone themselves is a potential direction of further research. Although many data mining queries on three-level graphs can be answered quite efficiently using off-the-shelf MILP solvers

Table 1. Summary of problems and proposed algorithmic tools. Input is $G = (A, P, T; E_1, E_2)$. Given a selector set $S \subseteq T$ we have defined $G_S = (A_S, P_S, S; E_{1,S}, E_{2,S})$, and $B_S = (A_S, P_S; E_{1,S})$. By S we denote the selector set which is a solution and by R any selector set. D_c^S (D_c^R resp.) is the degree of c in G_S (G_R resp.) and D_c is the degree of c in G. The asterisk means that experiments are run on variants of these problems and also that these problems are discussed in more detail in this paper.

Problem	Property of G_S	Algorithmic tools
AUTHORITY(c) *	c has max degree in G_S	non-monotone, IP
BESTRANK(c)	$D_c^S \geq D_c^R$	non-monotone
CLIQUE	B_S bipartite clique	level-wise, IP
FREQUENCY(f, s)	B_S contains bipartite clique $K_{s,f\|P_S\|}$	non-monotone, IP association-rule mining
MAJORITY	every $a \in A_S$ has $\|E_{1,S}^a\| \geq \|E_1^a \setminus E_{1,S}^a\|$	non-monotone, IP
POPULARITY(b)	$\|A_S\| \geq b$	level-wise, IP
IMPACT(b)	for all $a \in A_S$, $D_a^S \geq b$	non-monotone, IP
ABSOLUTEIMPACT(b)	for all $a \in A_S$, $D_c \geq b$	level-wise, IP
COLLABORATIONCLIQUE	for every $a, b \in A_S$, at least one $p \in P_S$, s.t. $(a, p) \in E_{1,S}$ and $(b, p) \in E_{1,S}$	non-monotone, IP
CLASSIFICATION(c)	$P_S = \{p \in P : (c, p) \in E_1\}$ and $A_S = \{c\}$	non-monotone
PROGRAMCOMMITTEE(Z, l, m) *	$A_S = Z$, $\|S\| = m$, and every $t \in Z$ is connected to at least l nodes in S	IP

in practice for instances of moderate size, more sophisticated optimization techniques for particular mining queries, both in theory and in practice. Answering to multiple data mining queries on three-level graphs and updating the query answers when the graphs are interesting questions with practical relevance in data mining systems for chains of relations.

We have demonstrated the use of the framework using two datasets, but further experimental studies with the framework solving large-scale real-world data mining tasks would be of interest. We have done some preliminary studies on some biological datasets using the basic three-level framework. In real-world applications it would often be useful to extend the basic three-level graph framework in order to the actual data better into account. Extending the basic model to weighted edges, various interpretations, and more complex schemas seem a promising and relevant future direction in practice. There is a trade-off between the expressivity of the framework and the computational feasibility of the data mining queries. To cope with complex data, it would be very useful to have semi-automatic techniques to discover simple views to complex database schemas that capture relevant mining queries in our framework, in addition to generalizing our query answering techniques to more complex database schemas.

References

1. Agarwal, N., Liu, H., Tang, L., Yu, P.S.: Identifying the influential bloggers in a community. In: WSDM (2008)
2. Agrawal, R., Imielinski, T., Swami, A.N.: Mining association rules between sets of items in large databases. In: Buneman, P., Jajodia, S. (eds.) Proceedings of the 1993 ACM SIGMOD International Conference on Management of Data, Washington, D.C, May 26-28, pp. 207–216. ACM Press, New York (1993)
3. Anthony, M., Biggs, N.: Computational Learning Theory: An Introduction. Cambridge University Press, Cambridge (1997)
4. Backstrom, L., Huttenlocher, D.P., Kleinberg, J.M., Lan, X.: Group formation in large social networks: membership, growth, and evolution. In: KDD, pp. 44–54 (2006)
5. Bayardo, R.J., Goethals, B., Zaki, M.J. (eds.): FIMI 2004, Proceedings of the IEEE ICDM Workshop on Frequent Itemset Mining Implementations, Brighton, UK, November 1. ser. CEUR Workshop Proceedings, vol. 126 (2004), CEUR-WS.org
6. Borodin, A., Roberts, G.O., Rosenthal, J.S., Tsaparas, P.: Link analysis ranking: Algorithms, theory, and experiments. ACM Transactions on Internet Technologies 5(1) (February 2005)
7. Boulicaut, J.-F., Bykowski, A., Rigotti, C.: Free-sets: A condensed representation of boolean data for the approximation of frequency queries. Data Mining and Knowledge Discovery 7(1), 5–22 (2003)
8. Calders, T., Lakshmanan, L.V.S., Ng, R.T., Paredaens, J.: Expressive power of an algebra for data mining. ACM Trans. Database Syst. 31, 1169–1214 (2006)
9. Caruana, R.: Multitask learning. Machine Learning 28(1), 41–75 (1997)
10. Cerf, L., Besson, J., Robardet, C., Boulicaut, J.-F: Data peeler: Contraint-based closed pattern mining in n-ary relations. In: SIAM International Conference on Data Mining, pp. 37–48 (2008)
11. Cerf, L., Besson, J., Robardet, C., Boulicaut, J.-F.: Closed patterns meet n-ary relations. ACM Trans. Knowl. Discov. Data 3, 3:1–3:36 (2009)
12. Chen, W., Wang, C., Wang, Y.: Scalable influence maximization for prevalent viral marketing in large-scale social networks. In: KDD. ACM, New York (2010)
13. Chen, W., Wang, Y., Yang, S.: Efficient influence maximization in social networks. In: KDD (2009)
14. Chvátal, V.: A greedy heuristic for the set-covering problem. Mathematics of Operations Research 4(3), 233–235 (1979)
15. Clare, A., Williams, H.E., Lester, N.: Scalable multi-relational association mining. In: Proceedings of the 4th IEEE International Conference on Data Mining (ICDM 2004), pp. 355–358. IEEE Computer Society, Los Alamitos (2004)
16. Cook, D.J., Holder, L.B.: Graph-based data mining. IEEE Intelligent Systems 15(2), 32–41 (2000)
17. Costa, V.S., Srinivasan, A., Camacho, R., Blockeel, H., Demoen, B., Janssens, G., Struyf, J., Vandecasteele, H., Laer, W.V.: Query transformations for improving the efficiency of ILP systems. Journal of Machine Learning Research 4, 465–491 (2003)
18. Dehaspe, L., de Raedt, L.: Mining association rules in multiple relations. In: Lavrac, N., Dzeroski, S. (eds.) ILP 1997. Proceedings, ser. Lecture Notes in Computer Science, vol. 1297, pp. 125–132. Springer, Heidelberg (1997)

19. Dehaspe, L., Toivonen, H.: Discovery of frequent DATALOG patterns. Data Mining and Knowledge Discovery 3(1), 7–36 (1999)
20. Deng, H., Lyu, M.R., King, I.: A generalized co-hits algorithm and its application to bipartite graphs. In: Proceedings of the 15th ACM SIGKDD International Conference on Knowledge Discovery and Data Mining, pp. 239–248. ACM, New York (2009)
21. Dzeroski, S., Lavrac, N. (eds.): Relational Data Mining. Springer, Heidelberg (2001)
22. Fagin, R., Guha, R.V., Kumar, R., Novak, J., Sivakumar, D., Tomkins, A.: Multi-structural databases. In: Li, C. (ed.) Proceedings of the Twenty-fourth ACM SIGACT-SIGMOD-SIGART Symposium on Principles of Database Systems, Baltimore, Maryland, USA, June 13-15, pp. 184–195. ACM, New York (2005)
23. Feige, U.: A threshold of ln n for approximating set cover. Journal of the ACM 45(4), 634–652 (1998)
24. Garriga, G.C., Khardon, R., De Raedt, L.: On mining closed sets in multi-relational data. In: Proceedings of the 20th International Joint Conference on Artifical Intelligence, pp. 804–809. Morgan Kaufmann Publishers Inc., San Francisco (2007)
25. Gibson, D., Kleinberg, J.M., Raghavan, P.: Inferring web communities from link topology. In: HYPERTEXT 1998. Proceedings of the Ninth ACM Conference on Hypertext and Hypermedia: Links, Objects, Time and Space - Structure in Hypermedia Systems, Pittsburgh, PA, USA, June 20-24, pp. 225–234. ACM Press, New York (1998)
26. Goyal, A., Lu, W., Lakshmanan, L.V.: Celf++: optimizing the greedy algorithm for influence maximization in social networks. In: WWW, pp. 47–48. ACM Press, New York (2011)
27. Haussler, D.: Quantifying inductive bias: AI learning algorithms and Valiant's learning framework. Artificial Intelligence 36(2), 177–221 (1988)
28. Horváth, T.: Cyclic pattern kernels revisited. In: Ho, T.-B., Cheung, D., Liu, H. (eds.) PAKDD 2005. LNCS (LNAI), vol. 3518, pp. 791–801. Springer, Heidelberg (2005)
29. Horváth, T., Gärtner, T., Wrobel, S.: Cyclic pattern kernels for predictive graph mining. In: Kim, W., Kohavi, R., Gehrke, J., DuMouchel, W. (eds.) Proceedings of the Tenth ACM SIGKDD International Conference on Knowledge Discovery and Data Mining, Seattle, Washington, USA, 2004, August 22-25, pp. 158–167. ACM Press, New York (2004)
30. Huan, J., Wang, W., Prins, J.: Efficient mining of frequent subgraphs in the presence of isomorphism. In: Proceedings of the 3rd IEEE International Conference on Data Mining (ICDM 2003), Melbourne, Florida, USA, December 19-22, pp. 549–552. IEEE Computer Society Press, Los Alamitos (2003)
31. Huan, J., Wang, W., Prins, J., Yang, J.: SPIN: mining maximal frequent subgraphs from graph databases. In: Kim, W., Kohavi, R., Gehrke, J., DuMouchel, W. (eds.) Proceedings of the Tenth ACM SIGKDD International Conference on Knowledge Discovery and Data Mining, Seattle, Washington, USA, 2004, August 22-25, pp. 581–586. ACM Press, New York (2004)
32. Jaschke, R., Hotho, A., Schmitz, C., Ganter, B., Gerd, S.: Trias–an algorithm for mining iceberg tri-lattices. In: Proceedings of the Sixth International Conference on Data Mining, pp. 907–911. IEEE Computer Society, DC, USA (2006)
33. Jeh, G., Widom, J.: Mining the space of graph properties. In: Proceedings of the Tenth ACM SIGKDD International Conference on Knowledge Discovery and Data Mining, Seattle, Washington, USA, 2004, August 22-25, pp. 187–196. ACM Press, New York (2004)

34. Ji, L., Tan, K.-L., Tung, A.K.H.: Mining frequent closed cubes in 3d datasets. In: Proceedings of the 32nd International Conference on Very Large Data Bases, VLDB Endowment, pp. 811–822 (2006)
35. Jin, Y., Murali, T.M., Ramakrishnan, N.: Compositional mining of multirelational biological datasets. ACM Trans. Knowl. Discov. Data 2, 2:1–2:35 (2008)
36. Kang, U., Tsourakakis, C.E., Faloutsos, C.: Pegasus: A peta-scale graph mining system. In: ICDM, pp. 229–238 (2009)
37. Kempe, D., Kleinberg, J.M., Tardos, É.: Maximizing the spread of influence through a social network. In: KDD (2003)
38. Kempe, D., Kleinberg, J.M., Tardos, É.: Influential nodes in a diffusion model for social networks. In: ICALP (2005)
39. Kumar, R., Raghavan, P., Rajagopalan, S., Sivakumar, D., Tomkins, A., Upfal, E.: The web as a graph. In: Proceedings of the Nineteenth ACM SIGMOD-SIGACT-SIGART Symposium on Principles of Database Systems, Dallas, Texas, USA, May 15-17, pp. 1–10. ACM Press, New York (2000)
40. Kumar, R., Raghavan, P., Rajagopalan, S., Tomkins, A.: Trawling the web for emerging cyber-communities. Computer Networks 31(11-16), 1481–1493 (1999)
41. Kuramochi, M., Karypis, G.: Frequent subgraph discovery. In: Cercone, N., Lin, T.Y., Wu, X. (eds.) Proceedings of the 2001 IEEE International Conference on Data Mining, San Jose, California, USA, November 29 - December 2, pp. 313–320. IEEE Computer Society Press, Los Alamitos (2001)
42. Lappas, T., Liu, K., Terzi, E.: Finding a team of experts in social networks. In: KDD (2009)
43. Lappas, T., Terzi, E., Gunopulos, D., Mannila, H.: Finding effectors in social networks. In: KDD (2010)
44. Leskovec, J., Lang, K.J., Mahoney, M.W.: Empirical comparison of algorithms for network community detection. In: WWW (2010)
45. Long, B., Wu, X., Zhang, Z., Yu, P.S.: Unsupervised learning on k-partite graphs. In: Knowledge Discovery and Data Mining, pp. 317–326 (2006)
46. Mannila, H., Terzi, E.: Finding links and initiators: A graph-reconstruction problem. In: SDM (2009)
47. Mannila, H., Toivonen, H.: Levelwise search and borders of theories in knowledge discovery. Data Minining and Knowledge Discovery 1(3), 241–258 (1997)
48. Martin, A.: General mixed integer programming: Computational issues for branch-and-cut algorithms. In: Computational Combinatorial Optimization, pp. 1–25 (2001)
49. Newman, M.E.J., Girvan, M.: Finding and evaluating community structure in networks. Phys. Rev. E 69(2), 026113 (2004)
50. Page, L., Brin, S., Motwani, R., Winograd, T.: The PageRank citation ranking: Bringing order to the web. Stanford University, Tech. Rep. (1998)
51. Pandurangan, G., Raghavan, P., Upfal, E.: Using pageRank to characterize web structure. In: Ibarra, O.H., Zhang, L. (eds.) COCOON 2002. LNCS, vol. 2387, pp. 330–339. Springer, Heidelberg (2002)
52. Rajagopalan, S., Vazirani, V.V.: Primal-dual RNC approximation algorithms for set cover and covering integer programs. SIAM Journal on Computing 28(2), 525–540 (1998)
53. Sarawagi, S., Sathe, G.: i^3: Intelligent, interactive investigation of OLAP data cubes. In: Chen, W., Naughton, J.F., Bernstein, P.A. (eds.) Proceedings of the 2000 ACM SIGMOD International Conference on Management of Data, Dallas, Texas, USA, May 16-18, p. 589. ACM Press, New York (2000)

54. Theodoros, L., Kun, L., Evimaria, T.: A survey of algorithms and systems for expert location in social networks. In: Aggarwal, C.C. (ed.) Social Network Data Analytics, pp. 215–241. Springer, Heidelberg (2011)
55. Tong, H., Papadimitriou, S., Sun, J., Yu, P.S., Faloutsos, C.: Colibri: fast mining of large static and dynamic graphs. In: Proceeding of the 14th ACM SIGKDD International Conference on Knowledge Discovery and Data Mining (2008)
56. Wang, C., Wang, W., Pei, J., Zhu, Y., Shi, B.: Scalable mining of large disk-based graph databases. In: Kim, W., Kohavi, R., Gehrke, J., DuMouchel, W. (eds.) Proceedings of the Tenth ACM SIGKDD International Conference on Knowledge Discovery and Data Mining, Seattle, Washington, USA, August 22-25, pp. 316–325. ACM Press, New York (2004)
57. Washio, T., Motoda, H.: State of the art of graph-based data mining. SIGKDD Explorations 5(1), 59–68 (2003)
58. Yan, X., Han, J.: Closegraph: mining closed frequent graph patterns. In: Getoor, L., Senator, T.E., Domingos, P., Faloutsos, C. (eds.) Proceedings of the Ninth ACM SIGKDD International Conference on Knowledge Discovery and Data Mining, Washington, DC, USA, August 24-27, pp. 286–295. ACM Press, New York (2003)
59. Yan, X., Yu, P.S., Han, J.: Graph indexing: A frequent structure-based approach. In: Weikum, G., König, A.C., Deßloch, S. (eds.) Proceedings of the ACM SIGMOD International Conference on Management of Data, Paris, France, June 13-18, pp. 335–346. ACM Press, New York (2004)
60. Yannakakis, M.: Node-and edge-deletion NP-complete problems. In: Lipton, R.J., Burkhard, W., Savitch, W., Friedman, E.P., Aho, A. (eds.) Proceedings of the tenth annual ACM symposium on Theory of computing, San Diego, California, United States, May 01-03, pp. 253–264. ACM Press, New York (1978)
61. Zaki, M.J.: Efficiently mining frequent trees in a forest. In: Proceedings of the Eighth ACM SIGKDD International Conference on Knowledge Discovery and Data Mining, Edmonton, Alberta, Canada, July 23-26, pp. 71–80. ACM Press, New York (2002)
62. Zheng, A.X., Ng, A.Y., Jordan, M.I.: Stable algorithms for link analysis. In: Croft, W.B., Harper, D.J., Kraft, D.H., Zobel, J. (eds.) SIGIR 2001: Proceedings of the 24th Annual International ACM SIGIR Conference on Research and Development in Information Retrieval, New Orleans, Louisiana, USA, September 9-13, pp. 258–266. ACM Press, New York (2001)
63. Zou, Z., Gao, H., Li, J.: Discovering frequent subgraphs over uncertain graph databases under probabilistic semantics. In: Proceedings of the 16th ACM SIGKDD International Conference on Knowledge Discovery and Data Mining, pp. 633–642. ACM Press, New York (2010)

Author Index

Printed by Publishers' Graphics LLC